COLLABORATIVE BRAIN INJURY INTERVENTION

Positive Everyday Routines

COLLABORATIVE BRAIN INJURY INTERVENTION

Positive Everyday Routines

Mark Ylvisaker, Ph.D.

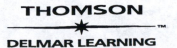

THOMSON
™
DELMAR LEARNING

Australia Canada Mexico Singapore Spain United Kingdom United States

COPYRIGHT © 1998

by Thomson Delmar Learning, a part of the Thomson Corporation. The Thomson Learning logo is a registered trademark used herein under license.

Printed in the United States of America
6 7 8 9 10 XXX

For more information, contact Thomson Delmar Learning, 5 Maxwell Drive, Clifton Park, NY 12065; or find us on the World Wide Web at http://www.delmarlearning.com

Library of Congress Cataloging-in-Publication Data
Ylvisaker, Mark, 1944–
      Collaborative brain injury intervention: positive everyday
routines / by Mark Ylvisaker and Timothy Feeney.
          p.   cm.
      Includes bibliographical references and index.

      1. Brain damage—Patients—Rehabilitation. I. Veeney, Timothy.
II. Title.
RC387.5.Y58   1998
616.8'043—dc21

                                                98-30364
                                                CIP
      ISBN-13: 978-1-5659-3733-8
      ISBN-10: 1-5659-3733-3 (pbk. : alk. paper)

Contents

Foreword

Research culminating in the "Decade of the Brain" has led to an explosion of knowledge about how the healthy brain works and how brain damage and disease disrupt its normal operation. Yet our ability to apply the theories and empirical findings from this basic research to clinical rehabilitation practice is still very limited. Organized attempts to rehabilitate individuals with brain damage, particularly those with traumatic brain injury, are relatively recent. They have relied, of necessity, on trial and error and common sense to develop a variety of treatments, service systems, and environmental supports for individuals with disability as a result of brain injury. We now stand poised, however, to develop more rational approaches to brain injury rehabilitation that draw upon the important advances in neuroscience research.

Early work with individuals with brain injury tended to focus on medical, physical, and motor deficits, since these were often the most obvious problems and also problems that clinicians had some skill in treating. But long-term studies of individuals with brain injury have consistently shown that it is the cognitive, behavioral, and social problems that cause the most long-term disability and place the greatest stress on caregivers. We have known far less about how to approach these problems.

The recent advances in many areas of psychology and neuroscience offer the possibility of theory-based treatment. While successes in a trial-and-error mode help patients, they teach us little, and failures teach us nothing. In contrast, treatments based on sound theories advance our knowledge when they succeed, and even tell us something when they fail—namely, how our theories and concepts need revision. Ylvisaker and Feeney provide a theoretical framework for understanding the cognitive and behavioral problems of brain injury and for rationally designing therapies. I think their theoretical perspective is mostly right. But, even if parts of it are wrong, they have put us on a path which will help us learn systematically from our failures as well as our successes.

The title of Drs. Ylvisaker and Feeney's book, *Collaborative Brain Injury Intervention: Positive Everyday Routines*, is very apt, since the book illustrates collaboration and thereby integration in several important ways. Recent research in cognitive, behavioral, and neuropsychology has much to say about how to conduct rehabilitation for individuals with brain injury, but each discipline sees the problem from a different angle and paints an incomplete picture. The authors succeed admirably in integrating these different perspectives into a coherent view of the nature of the problem and the approach to treatment. Rehabilitation service is often fragmented, with different team members treating different "pieces" of the affected individual, and different service components (hospitals, outpatient programs, vocational programs) adopting different treatment approaches. The authors suggest a collaborative treatment approach that should help to unify the work of different disciplines and services over time in the service of the client's real-world needs. Much rehabilitation work has also focused on treating specific impairments in isolation in the hope that improving each impairment would translate into global functional improvement. The authors make a powerful case that such an approach is fundamentally flawed, and support an integrated treatment approach that sees individuals' impairments, and their strengths, in the context of the environments and tasks in which they perform. Finally, the authors recognize that many of the apparently distinct problems experienced by individuals with brain injury can be traced to difficulties with executive function. By unifying these heterogenous problems under a single conceptual category, the authors provide the possibility of an integrated approach to treating a broad range of problems.

This book will also be of interest to clinicians experiencing the changes in health care brought about by managed care—and that is likely to be all clinicians! While the pressure to move patients out of the hospital and into their homes is experienced as a stress by many of us, it also provides opportunities for innovation. Ylvisaker and Feeney provide a wealth of tools for working with clients outside the walls of the hospital or clinic, in the environments where they need to live and work, and give realistic and vivid case illustrations to accompany their suggestions.

As clinicians with a command of a broad research literature, Ylvisaker and Feeney are ideal guides to a new era of rehabilitation care and a new integrated approach to providing treatment. They have grasped many of the important advances from the Decade of the Brain and have designed innovative ways of applying them to the real-world needs of those with brain injuries. In doing so, they never lose sight of the environment that their clients must return to, and the whole and integrated lives that they wish to lead.

John Whyte, M.D., Ph.D.
Director
Moss Rehabilitation Research Institute
Philadelphia, Pennsylvania

Preface

ROOTS

This book is rooted in the real world of services and supports for children and adults with chronic impairment after brain injury. The intervention principles and practices that we describe have grown out of our combined 35 years of experience with collaborative brain injury rehabilitation in medical and community settings, rehabilitation and psychiatric hospitals, schools (preschool through college), day programs, jails and prisons, substance abuse programs, vocational training and work settings, and community residences, including family homes.

Many of the people with whom we have worked carried a pessimistic prognosis for success in achieving their chosen academic, vocational, and social goals. Furthermore, many of them were considered by staff to be very difficult to work with. Nevertheless, we have consistently approached our work optimistically and have grown increasingly optimistic over the years. We write this book for people who are similarly enthusiastic about serving children and adults with chronic impairment and are seeking person-centered procedures to use in providing that service in a creative, collaborative, and real-worldly manner.

In highlighting the book's practical sources and goals, we do not wish to promote an antitheoretical or antiexperimental bias in brain injury rehabilitation. On the contrary, in Chapter 1 we locate our work within a specific theoretical framework and call attention to an impressive body of research that supports the application of this framework to brain injury rehabilitation. In Chapter 3, we describe careful experimental procedures used to identify effective interventions. However, when all is said and done, the ultimate measure of the value of intervention theories and procedures is their ability to substantially improve the real lives of real people with disability.

POPULATION

Most of the individuals we describe in this book had disability caused by traumatic brain injury. More specifically, damage to the frontal and limbic regions of the brain—the areas most vulnerable in closed head injury—resulted in some degree of impairment in the domain of functions in which cognition, communication, and behavior intersect and become virtually impossible to disentangle. Construed broadly, the term *executive functions* captures much of the disability in this tricky domain.

The difficulties experienced by the people we use to illustrate our approach to rehabilitation appear in some cases to load in the cognitive domain of impairment (Chapters 4 and 5), in other cases in the behavioral domain (Chapter 6), in yet other cases in the communication and social skills domain (Chapter 7). However, most of the case illustrations could have appeared in any of our four intervention chapters. This reality underscores the need to understand disability comprehensively and to avoid the temptation to describe complex and interrelated problems from the perspective of a single profession.

The broad areas of impairment addressed in this book invite the attention of many professions—behavioral psychology, neuropsychology, speech-language pathology, occupational therapy, cognitive rehabilitation, social work and counseling psychology, physiatry and psychiatry, vocational rehabilitation, special education, recreation therapy, and others—as well as family members, funders of services, and case managers. The interrelatedness of the themes invites each of these groups to approach their work in this area in a spirit of collaboration.

Many—but certainly not all—of these individuals had problems that could be classified as "neurobehavioral." However, we wish to avoid such potentially misleading, divisive, and pessimistic labels. This and other commonly used neurodiagnostic terms (e.g., "pseudopsychopathic personality") easily interfere with a careful delineation of the organic and nonorganic contributors to presenting problems, with an experimental approach to identifying the relative contributions of cognitive, behavioral, and communication components of the problem, and with a spirit of optimism in working with individuals as they attack the obstacles they face.

We illustrate our approach to rehabilitation with individuals whose brain injuries would be classified as severe by most standards, but whose neurological recovery was sufficient to support community reintegration, with considerable support in many cases. However, the general approach and many of the specific procedures are also often useful for individuals with persistent mild disability after injuries judged initially to be relatively minor. In contrast, the approach is not directly applicable to people whose disability is exclusively physical—except in the important sense that they may need to be more strategic in the conduct of their affairs than would have been the case with no brain injury. Our discussion of executive system intervention may be useful in working with these individuals despite no specific impairment in this domain.

REHABILITATION THROUGH EVERYDAY ROUTINES

Our primary theme is that rehabilitation for people with chronic cognitive, behavioral, and communication impairment after

brain injury is best provided by collaborating with everyday people in the life of the person with disability to create positive, supported everyday routines of action and interaction in the context of everyday activities. We use the term *everyday people* descriptively (i.e., these are the people who interact with the person with disability on a routine, everyday basis) and honorifically (i.e., these are the people who have the greatest potential to influence the life of that individual). The collaboration that dominates this functional approach to rehabilitation includes collaboration among professionals, between professionals and the person with disability (and family), and between the person with disability and members of his or her network of support. In this approach to intervention, specialists in rehabilitation play the role of consultant to everyday people at least as much as their traditional role as treating therapist. This theme is presented in Chapter 1 and illustrated throughout the book.

EFFECTIVENESS

In Chapter 1, we offer a theoretical rationale for our approach to rehabilitation and cite supportive bodies of experimental literature from several clinical fields. Crosspopulation inferences must be used cautiously; however, wise clinicians pay close attention to the history of intervention studies in fields that bear important resemblance to their own. We also support our approach indirectly by making reference to studies that raise serious questions about alternative approaches. Finally, throughout the book, we offer supportive case material which, we acknowledge, is at best illustrative and suggestive, falling short of experimental validation. Our work with several hundred children and adults with chronic disability after brain injury convinces us of the merits of the procedures we describe in this book. We understand that additional experimental validation is required for these procedures to meet stringent efficacy standards for this population.

THE SPIRIT OF REHABILITATION

In Chapter 8 we highlight the importance of optimism, creativity, flexibility, and enthusiasm for problem solving in brain injury rehabilitation. Rehabilitation for the people about whom this book is written is more than the mechanical application of technical procedures. In our judgment, it involves a commitment to enter the lives of people with disability, to create collaborative relationships with them and the everyday people in their lives, and to support them in part by serving as an ongoing source of optimism, creativity, flexibility, and enthusiasm in the face of obstacles that often seem overwhelming. We hope that this spirit of rehabilitation is evident in the book alongside the procedures that may require greater technical expertise for their implementation.

SOME GUIDELINES FOR READING THIS BOOK

Our four intervention chapters (Chapters 4, 5, 6, and 7) constitute the practical core of the book. In each chapter, we describe prin-

ciples of intervention and present case illustrations. We have attempted to tie the case material as directly as possible to the principles with which they are associated. This attempt explains some differences in the organization of these four chapters. We identify case illustrations in terms of the amount of support the individuals needed at that time (as opposed to the more customary identifying terms mild, moderate, and severe disability), a stylistic convention that is growing in popularity in work with people with chronic disability. In Chapter 4 we offer operational definitions for levels of support.

All of the case illustrations come from our work as clinicians and consultants. In some cases, but not all, we worked together. However, in every case description, we use the plural "we" to refer to one or the other or both of us, a decision motivated in part by stylistic considerations and in part by the need to underscore the extent to which our professions (behavioral psychology and speech-language pathology) and other professions merge in the practical world of providing services and supports to people with complex disability.

With the exception of Jason Lewin, we have changed the names of the individuals we present and, in some cases, we also changed other potentially identifying information to protect confidentiality. In no case did we change clinically relevant information.

Acknowledgments

Our greatest debt of gratitude is to the individuals with brain injury and their families who have taught us how to serve them best. Many of the people whose stories are told in this book reviewed what we wrote about them and helped us to describe them accurately and in a way that is consistent with how they perceived their rehabilitation. In particular, we thank Jason Lewin for telling his important story in the epilogue and for designing the book's cover.

Several individuals have provided valuable suggestions in response to earlier drafts of this book. We thank them for their help while accepting total responsibility for the book's inevitable errors. Ann Glang, Linda Davern, Michele Reilly, John Dziewit, and Susan Fitzpatrick offered particularly helpful insights. We thank John Whyte for taking time from his very busy life to write a Foreword and for providing several constructive suggestions. We thank the New York State Department of Health for their support of the Sage Statewide Neurobehavioral Resource Project, a project that has given us the freedom to pursue the approach to brain injury rehabilitation described in this book. Special thanks to Pat Greene, Bill Reynolds, and Bruce Rosen for their ongoing support for our work and for their commitment to the development of high quality community-based services for people with brain injury. We thank Marie Linvill of Singular Publishing Group for maintaining her good humor in the face of many missed deadlines, lame excuses, and pathetic attempts on our part to take the spotlight off deadlines with silly jokes.

Our families deserve a thank you much louder than we would ever be able to shout it. Jessica Ylvisaker is responsible for much of the artwork. Kathy Ylvisaker is an ongoing source of inspiration, support, and good ideas about how to serve people with disability. Ben Ylvisaker continues to bless us with his technical expertise and willingness to lose at golf, even when losing requires considerable creativity.

Joe and Kathy Feeney have been constant sources of encouragement and have managed to keep their sense of humor in full bloom for the past 30-odd years while trying to answer their often-asked question, "What's he done now?" Sarah and Katie Feeney endure their father's moodiness and have learned to appear happy playing cards and basketball in order to raise his spirits. Chris Feeney suffers through her spouse's crankiness, self-doubt, odd hours, frequent absentmindedness, and wild-eyed enthusiasm for his work with decency, wit, and unconditional love.

We dedicate this book to our families:
Kathy, Jessica, and Ben Ylvisaker;
Chris, Sarah, and Katie Feeney

CHAPTER 1

Introduction to Functional, Everyday Intervention: Theory, Research, and Practice

The purpose of this book is to provide readers with an approach to rehabilitation for individuals, both children and adults, with disability after traumatic brain injury (TBI), an approach that is functional and practical, yet at the same time consistent with current theory in several domains, including neuropsychology, educational psychology, behavioral psychology, cognitive neuroscience, and communication science. This is a tall order and we recognize that such a mission may appear overly ambitious. But this is our goal.

The individuals for whom we recommend this approach are those with mild-to-severe chronic disability in the broad domain of functioning in which cognitive, executive system, behavioral, and communication issues overlap and intermingle in their negative effect on academic, vocational, and social life. From a pathophysiologic perspective, this group primarily includes those with damage to frontal or frontolimbic regions of the brain, the most common sites of damage in closed head injury (see Chapter 2). Individuals with acquired brain injury from other causes, including stroke, tumor, and anoxia, are candidates for the approaches presented in this book, assuming chronic disability in the listed domains of functioning. Although we use the terms

brain injury and TBI to designate this population, the intervention themes are in many cases applicable to children and adults with developmental disability in the same domains of functioning. More specifically, individuals with congenital impairment directly linked to frontal lobe dysfunction (e.g., ADHD) are strong candidates for the approach.

In this introductory chapter, we introduce our topic with a dilemma that demands resolution in the rehabilitation of individuals with frontal lobe injury or developmental impairment. We then propose a resolution to this dilemma, using the concept of positive everyday routines, which dominates the book from beginning to end. This introduction is followed by a discussion of Vygotsky's theory of teaching, learning, and cognitive and self-regulatory development, which we offer as a theoretical support for the rehabilitation practices that we describe in subsequent chapters. We follow this theoretical discussion with a summary of critical differences between a conventional and a functional approach to rehabilitation and the implications of our approach for the most critical test of any approach to rehabilitation, namely generalization to relevant domains of everyday life and maintenance over time.

...apter with a discussion of ...sability, and handicap in the ...ctional, routine-based inter... ...list the premises that underlie ... ...h to intervention that we illustrate in ... remainder of the book. Although we believe that responsible clinicians should be able to place their rehabilitation procedures within a theoretical framework that is current and supported by research, we wish to emphasize that the procedures discussed and illustrated in this book do not stand or fall with the theories evoked to support them. Indeed, we hope that many of these procedures could be honored with the title *common sense*, with roots in thousands of years of human beings developing effective ways of teaching, of managing their behavior, and of helping others to manage their own behavior.

POSITIVE EVERYDAY ROUTINES: ESCAPING THROUGH THE HORNS OF A DILEMMA

The title of this book and of its four intervention chapters (Chapters 4 through 7) contains the phrase *positive everyday routines*. Our goal in this section is to explain our use of the concept of everyday routines and begin to argue for its usefulness in escaping through the horns of a destructive dilemma that threatens TBI rehabilitation. This dilemma (depicted in Figure 1–1), derives from the work of Damasio (1994) and serves as a useful and striking introduction to many of the themes of this book. The concept of everyday routines has a natural home in both cognitive and behavioral theory (see below) and holds the potential to contribute to a practical marriage of these two apparently improbable theoretical bedfellows.

In social, vocational, academic, and personal contexts, successful self-directed behavior would seem to be a consequence of good decisions, effective habits, or some combination of the two. Whether the behavior is a common activity of daily living, like eating lunch, or an apparently more complex social, academic, or vocational activity, success can potentially be achieved with relatively automatic, habitual behaviors or by using deliberate decision making, carefully evaluating possible courses of action and ruling them in or out based on a deliberate weighing of their benefits, costs, and other relevant considerations.

The Dilemma: Horn #1: High Reason

In his insightful book on human rationality and frontal lobe injury, Antonio Damasio (1994) outlined two possible answers to the question. "How do people sort through a vast array of potentially relevant considerations and ultimately make decisions about how to act?" One possibility (existing at one extreme of a continuum of possibilities), with a noble philosophical lineage but little basis in reality, is that people faced with the necessity of making a decision (1) identify a set of possible courses of action; (2) marshal their knowledge of the world to predict consequences of these actions, including costs and benefits for themselves and others; (3) weigh the relative merits of each possible choice; (4) deduce the best alternative; (5) act on that choice; and (6) attend to the consequences so that additional knowledge will be available for future decision making. The less emotionality infects this process, the more rational it is and the better the outcome. This hypothesis emphasizes abstract, knowledge-based expertise, and is perhaps most clearly observed in the real world in institutional and corporate strategic planning.

Damasio's first observation about this *high-reason* hypothesis is that it is rarely descriptive of how typical people in typical situations make decisions about how to act. To be sure, when decisions are important and people have little history to guide their decision making, they may reflect on alternatives, weigh their relative merits, consult with others, and in general apply serious

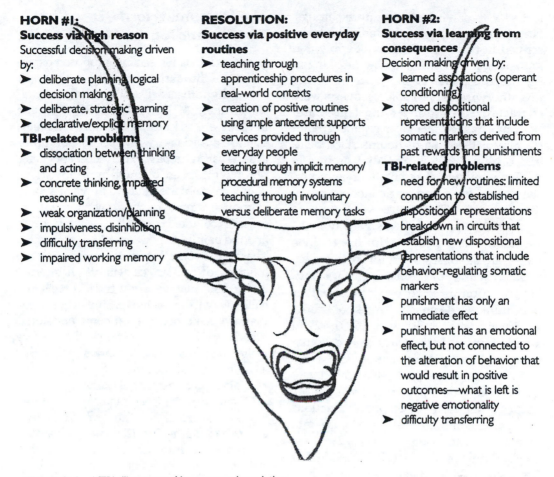

HORN #1:

Success via high reason

Successful decision making driven by:

➤ deliberate planning, logical decision making
➤ deliberate, strategic learning
➤ declarative/explicit memory

TBI-related problems:

➤ dissociation between thinking and acting
➤ concrete thinking, impaired reasoning
➤ weak organization/planning
➤ impulsiveness, disinhibition
➤ difficulty transferring
➤ impaired working memory

RESOLUTION:

Success via positive everyday routines

➤ teaching through apprenticeship procedures in real-world contexts
➤ creation of positive routines using ample antecedent supports
➤ services provided through everyday people
➤ teaching through implicit memory/procedural memory systems
➤ teaching through involuntary versus deliberate memory tasks

HORN #2:

Success via learning from consequences

Decision making driven by:

➤ learned associations (operant conditioning)
➤ stored dispositional representations that include somatic markers derived from past rewards and punishments

TBI-related problems

➤ need for new routines: limited connection to established dispositional representations
➤ breakdown in circuits that establish new dispositional representations that include behavior-regulating somatic markers
➤ punishment has only an immediate effect
➤ punishment has an emotional effect, but not connected to the alteration of behavior that would result in positive outcomes—what is left is negative emotionality
➤ difficulty transferring

Figure 1–1. A TBI dilemma and its proposed resolution.

thought to decisions that affect action. However, even in these cases of deliberate decision making, there must be other forces at work that contribute to the outcome. Theoretically, there are indefinitely many possible alternatives; therefore, effectively calculating consequences in order to make the best decision would require massive amounts of information and powerful statistical analyses. Practical considerations, such as time and resources in human working memory, place fierce limits on deliberate decision making in ordinary circumstances.

Following frontal lobe injury, which is common in TBI, conditions for high-reason decision making are threatened by many neuropsychological factors. First, many people with prefrontal injury are plagued by what Hans Teuber (1964) characterized as the *riddle of the frontal lobes*, namely, the curious dissociation between knowing and doing. That is, all the factual and social knowledge in the world may not lead them to a concrete decision and to action based on their knowledge (Damasio, 1990; Damasio, Tranel, & Damasio, 1991). Damasio (1994) included this striking phenomenon as a component of the "Gage Matrix," named after the famous 19th century frontal lobe patient, Phineas Gage, described by his physician, Harlowe (1868). Gage, and many with injuries like his, including most of the individuals included as case illustrations in this book, retained adequate factual and social knowledge and was able to reason effectively in clinical or laboratory settings. However, like many of the individuals described in this book, he did not apply that knowledge to practical decision making in his life and therefore the years following his otherwise remarkable recovery were characterized by unrelenting failure and personal tragedy. Damasio's patient Elliot (Damasio, 1994), with circumscribed bilateral orbital and ventromedial prefrontal damage following removal of a tumor, stands as a vivid and tragic modern representative of the Gage matrix.

In addition to this knowledge–action dissociation, many people with frontal lobe injury are seriously disinhibited (often associated with orbitofrontal injury), resulting in action directed by impulse rather than thinking (Damasio, Tranel, & Damasio, 1990; Grattan & Eslinger, 1990, 1992). In addition, many have injury-related limitations on their working memory and attentional control (often associated with dorsolateral and dorsomedial prefrontal injury), reducing the number of possible actions and considerations that can figure into their decision making (Damasio, 1989; Eslinger, Biddle, & Grattan, 1997; Eslinger & Damasio, 1985; Eslinger & Grattan, 1993). Those with damage to the dorsal prefrontal initiation/activation centers of the left hemisphere may require external activation in order to apply their knowledge to action. Some, including many with right hemisphere frontal lobe injury, have difficulty perceiving and interpreting social cues, further reducing their ability to make effective decisions about how to act in a social context (Brazzeli, Colombo, DellaSala, & Spinnler, 1994). Finally, many with widespread injury after TBI have depleted knowledge stores (posterior injury), or inefficient access to that knowledge, adding yet another reason to be pessimistic about High Reason as their road to effective decision making and successful action (Hunkin, Parkin, Bradley, Burrows, Aldrich, Jansari, & Burdon-Cooper, 1995).

The Dilemma: Horn #2: The *Somatic Marker* Hypothesis

Damasio labels his second proposed explanation of human rationality the *somatic marker* hypothesis (Damasio, 1994; Damasio, Tranel, & Damasio, 1991). Somatic markers are visceral and emotional states that are associated with specific stimuli or actions based on past experience. For example, having been burned by a hot stove, young children are likely to move in a more cautious manner in that environment because of the stored connection between stoves and the painful experience of being burned. That is, the somatic marker stored with the memory of hot stoves sets off an internal alarm bell that automatically directs the child away from the stove. Similarly, actions that achieve a positive outcome are stored in memory with a connection to the positive feeling states or somatic markers that serve as a "beacon of incentive" (Damasio, 1994, p. 174) to guide future decisions.

Of course there is a large universe of theory and research in the area of experienced-based learning that can and should be integrated into the somatic marker hypothesis. Damasio's contribution has been to begin to describe the neurological basis for learning from consequences and to shed light on those whose experience-based learning is impaired as a result of brain damage. The stimulus-response laws and learned associations described by behavioral psychologists become neurologically based *dispositional representations* in Damasio's neuropsychological framework. The dispositional representations responsible for guiding social behavior seem to require for their formation and storage the ventromedial prefrontal cortex, precisely the area most directly damaged in Gage, Elliot, and many people with closed head injury.

For years, clinicians working directly with individuals with frontal lobe injury or immaturity, including those with closed head injury (Feeney & Ylvisaker, 1997) and attention deficit, hyperactivity disorder (ADHD) (Hallowell & Ratey, 1994), have questioned the efficiency in these populations of learning from consequences. Some have attributed this weakness to cognitive impairment. For example, Cohen and colleagues (1985) associated ineffective contingency-based behavior management with the student's weak understanding of cause-effect relationships, an unlikely explanation in light of the minimal cognitive requirements in animals for learning from consequences and because people like Gage and Elliot retained strong intellects despite minimal ability to profit from experience, including severely punishing experiences.

Using experimental procedures, Alderman (1996) concluded that weakness in the central executive component of working memory may explain the failure of many individuals with frontal lobe injury to respond to traditional operant training techniques, including reinforcement, extinction, and time-out interventions. Although working memory impairments may be a component of the explanation, the fact that Damasio's Elliot and others who do not benefit efficiently from feedback nevertheless perform well on all measures of working memory suggests that there must be more to the explanation than that offered by Alderman.

Ineffective formation, storage, and retrieval of dispositional representations that connect the intellectual components of knowledge with behavior-guiding somatic markers may explain the frustrating reality of people failing to profit from the consequences of their actions. Damasio's laboratory experiments with adults with ventromedial prefrontal injury showed them to respond only immediately to punishment, and not in a way that served to guide intelligent decision making over the long term (Bechara, Damasio, Damasio, & Anderson, 1994; Damasio et al., 1990). Our experience is consistent with this finding. Many of the people with whom we have worked have failed to respond—or in some cases have responded negatively (see Ylvisaker, Feeney, & Szekeres, 1998)—to traditional contingency-based behavior management. In many cases, when their behavior is punished, they may retain a diffuse negative emotionality associated with the deliverer of the punishment, but *not* encode and retain the intended disposition to refrain from the action that resulted in the punishment. Furthermore, even in cases in which intensive application of consequences successfully modifies behavior in contrived training contexts (e.g., within a neurobehavioral treatment program), transfer to real-life settings and interactions is unlikely.

We do not wish to suggest that Damasio's neuropsychological account is the only possible neurological theory that would support our positive, proactive, everyday routine-based approach to cognitive and psychosocial rehabilitation after TBI. For example, Grafman's theory of prefrontal storage of managerial knowledge units, including scripts, plans, themes, and other event complexes, could serve as an alternative neuropsychological foundation (Grafman, 1995). Whatever the ultimate theoretical explanation, the critical reality is that many people with TBI have difficulty acting in a successful way in everyday life when they rely on decision making that is dependent on high reason, on their reinforcement history, or on a mix of these options. In cases of severe prefrontal injury, this difficulty is often profound and debilitating; in cases of less severe prefrontal injury, the associated weakness in self-management may be less obvious than that of Gage and Elliot, but may nevertheless have a profound impact on academic, vocational, and social life. If high reason, effective, automatic triggering of somatic markers, or a combination of the two exhausted available options, the dilemma posed in Figure 1–1 would be destructive indeed for many people with frontal lobe injury.

Escaping Through the Horns of the Dilemma

In Damasio's account of human practical reason, somatic markers and deliber soning form a partnership: Somatic markers stored as dispositional representations dramatically reduce the domain of potential actions and considerations that could support potential actions, making it possible for one to choose among the few remaining alternatives by means of a calculation within a limited set of costs, benefits, societal rules, and other considerations. Unfortunately, many people with frontal lobe injury are so compromised in the components of high reason and so inefficient in learning from consequences of their actions (i.e., laying down new somatic markers to guide future decisions and actions) and in accessing existing dispositional representations that the partnership between high reason and somatic markers fails as a guide to successful action. To be sure, this dilemma does not describe the situation of everybody with TBI. However, some degree of impairment in the domains of functioning gored by the two horns of this dilemma is sufficiently common among those with chronic disability after TBI that escaping through the horns of the dilemma is a matter of considerable urgency.

We perceive two possible escape routes: (a) others exerting control over the individual or (b) creating positive everyday routines using antecedent-focused procedures.

Others Exerting Control Over the Individual with TBI

One possible escape is to take decision making and internal control away from people with this complex of disabilities and surround them with systems of near total external control. Barkley (1997) makes essentially this recommendation to parents of children with ADHD in his call for the parents to serve as their child's prosthetic executive system. Many clinicians make a similar recommendation in working with people with TBI during the confused stages of their recovery, urging professionals to refrain from contributing to patients' confusion by expecting that they make decisions or plan any components of their day. Meichenbaum observed that the same external

control management decision is frequently made by staff who work with adults with chronic disability after TBI, although the decision is not always conscious and deliberate (Meichenbaum, 1993). That is, many staff and family members fall into the role of prosthetic frontal lobes without a clear understanding of the potentially negative consequences of the role that they come to play.

To be sure, external control is an appropriate response in cases of severely restricted self-control, for example, in young infants. However, the ever-present dangers associated with high levels of external control are learned helplessness and oppositionality. It is a long-standing principle that the more opportunities for decision making are removed from people, the more they become dependent on the decision making of others, or the more oppositional and defiant they become, or both. Furthermore, potential for internal control and effective decision making exists on a continuum from none to total, with thousands of distinct points in between. An important goal for clinicians, family members, and others is to identify where individuals should be on this continuum of external-to-internal control and then implement procedures designed to move them as quickly as possible in the direction of internal control. Many of the intervention procedures described in this book are motivated by this goal.

Supporting Successful Decision Making Through Positive Everyday Routines

The second possible escape through the horns of the angry bull dilemma in Figure 1–1 is the approach to rehabilitation presented in this book. Everyday people in the lives of individuals with TBI help them to establish successful routines in the context of a life that is generally satisfying. To achieve success in their daily routines, antecedent supports of the sort described in Chapters 4 through 7 are typically required. Those supports may relate mainly to executive functions (see the discussion of executive system routines in Chapter 4), to cognitive functions (see the discussion of advance organizers and cognitive prostheses in Chapter 5), to behavior (see the antecedent management approaches described in Chapter 6), or to communication (see the discussion of social supports and communication alternatives to challenging behavior in Chapter 7).

Within the context of meaningful everyday activities, relevant everyday people in the person's life (e.g., family members, direct care staff, employment supervisors, teaching staff, peers) facilitate the individual's acquisition and internalization of skills, strategies, and other behaviors that are patiently practiced to the point of habituation. In behavioral terms, the individual acquires *behavior chains* in which each link serves as a discriminative stimulus for the next. However, because the teaching relies on antecedent supports within an otherwise satisfying life, there is reduced focus on learning from consequences. In cognitive terms, the individual internalizes knowledge structures in the form of *behavior-guiding scripts*. The goal is for positive and successful behavior—including so-called higher level cognitive and executive system behavior as well as everyday social behavior—to be routine in the sense that turning off the alarm, getting out of bed, and proceeding through a morning bathroom sequence is routine for most people.

Teaching and supporting positive behavior through everyday routines requires that everyday people in the person's life (e.g., family members, direct care staff, teachers, friends) are well trained and well supported so that they can in turn provide needed supports successfully. Their role is not to teach or train in a traditional sense, but rather to facilitate incremental improvement through procedures similar to those used by a master craftsperson coaching and mentoring an apprentice (see below). Because the teaching is through routines and not explicit instruction, learning is through the typically more intact procedural memory and implicit memory systems

as opposed to the more vulnerable explicit and declarative memory systems. A consistent finding in studies of individuals with TBI is that one of the most vulnerable structures in the brain is the hippocampus (Bigler, 1990; Pang, 1985), often as a result of secondary hypoxic injury (see Chapter 2). The hippocampus plays the most critical role in consolidating new memory traces and directing them elsewhere in the brain for ultimate storage. Declarative memory (i.e., *knowing that*, or memory for facts) and explicit memory (i.e., memories stored along with a recollection of the acquisition of the information) appear to rely on the intactness of the hippocampus (Bechara, Tranel, Damasio, Adolphs, Rockland, & Damasio, 1995; Gluck & Meyers, 1995). In contrast, implicit memory (i.e., memories stored without conscious recollection of having been exposed to the information) and procedural learning (i.e., *knowing how to* versus knowing that) do not appear to rely on intactness of the hippocampus and therefore are often better preserved after TBI (Cummings, 1993).

Because supports are available for successful task completion, effective teaching can occur without the need for failure or for limited success in only a percentage of the learning trials. Traditional training paradigms (see section on apprenticeship below) are based on differential reinforcement of task performance: rewards for success as opposed to no response, reteaching, or punishment for failure. As Wilson and colleagues (1994, 1996) have found, most people with severe explicit and declarative memory problems learn most effectively under conditions of errorless learning. Indeed, errors have a particularly pernicious influence on people who do not remember the learning experience in that the incorrect information or inappropriate action may be retained as a memory trace without an associated memory for the experience that resulted in the learning, thereby making it harder to extinguish the memory for the incorrect information. Errorless learning may also be useful for people who do not have severe memory impairment, although there are certainly cases in which errors present occasions for robust learning.

In the absence of attention to the creation of positive everyday routines, people with chronic disability after TBI and the everyday people in their lives often develop *negative* routines that hold the potential to spiral out of control, interfering with learning and positive behavior. For example, unsupported performance of difficult tasks easily results in failure and the perceived need to escape the punishing failure situation; this perception in turn may lead to the acquisition of challenging behaviors that serve the purpose of signaling escape. Or people with disability may experience insufficient sense of control over events in their life, leading them to exert control, in turn leading caregivers and supervisors to impose greater control, resulting in stronger resistance and challenging behavior. Or service providers may step in and help the person with disability with such frequency that he or she progressively grows more dependent and helpless. The general point is that everyday routines have a powerful effect on life, on development, on internalization of behavior-guiding cognitive representations, and ultimately on recovery after brain injury. Positive everyday routines support success in the present and improved functioning in the future; negative everyday routines contribute to failure in the present and regression in the future. Therefore, rehabilitation specialists have a high calling to work with people with disability and the everyday people in their lives to make everyday routines as positive as possible.

Routines and Behavioral Theory

From a behavioral perspective, a routine is a behavior chain in which each link—each discrete behavior—is a discriminitive stimulus for the next link and a conditioned reinforcer for the previous link (Halle & Spradlin, 1993). For example, assembling needed items to prepare lunch, preparing the lunch, and eating it may involve a large number of discrete behaviors, each of which triggers the next, with the ultimate product being a rewarding experience, namely eating lunch. In everyday life, many routines are so thoroughly habituated that they require no thought or planning whatsoever. For example, the sequence of events initiated by the morning alarm and ending several minutes later with the individual dressed and ready for the day often happens automatically. Once established, routines successfully guide behavior in the absence of any need for explicit reinforcement of any specific behavior in the chain, provided the routine is generally positive, relatively easy to accomplish, and generally associated with satisfying experiences.

An important goal of training in the field of developmental disabilities is the creation of routines with sufficient flexibility that environmental stimuli can vary within reasonable limits without disrupting successful completion of the routine. Increasingly, behavioral specialists recommend identifying an appropriate instructional universe (i.e., a range of stimulus and response variation that is realistic in relation to the individual's everyday environment) and teaching behavior chains (routines) in that variable universe rather than in a laboratory or other artificial setting in which stimulus and response classes are unrealistically narrow and within which concrete associations may be formed that actually interfere with transfer to natural contexts (Horner & Budd, 1985; Horner, Dunlap, & Koegel, 1988; O'Neill & Reichle, 1993). We refer to this method of teaching (i.e., general case instruction) simply as teaching behaviors or facilitating the acquisition of skills in everyday contexts, capitalizing on the variation that is normal within those contexts and guaranteeing a functional outcome of the training (see section on generalization below). These observations have led many authorities in the field of mental retardation (e.g., Wetzel & Hoschouer, 1984) and autism (e.g., Brown, 1991) to create service delivery systems in which services are delivered mainly in the context of everyday routines, using direct care staff as the primary deliverers of the services and supports.

The downward behavioral spiral observed in many children and adults after TBI can often be understood as a result of a dynamic initially created by disability-induced disruption of the individual's well rehearsed pretrauma positive routines. The disrupted routines may be as simple as getting dressed or as complex as carrying out the responsibilities of a job. The individual's negative behavior in reaction to these disruptions, failures, and frustrations may elicit punishment from others, or possibly a reward in the form of positive attention or escape from an aversive situation. In either case, the new posttrauma routines are thereby additionally disrupted, with a growing sense of failure and alienation over time.

Many people with TBI—as well as many with developmental disabilities—are rigidly dependent on routines to the point that minor variations or deviations create anxiety, agitation and serious behavioral reactions (Lhermitte, 1983; Lhermitte, Pillon, & Serdaru, 1986). In such cases, family members and professionals alike may try to avoid establishing routines on the grounds that they will inevitably become rigid rituals and, in the long run, cause more problems than they resolve. Our answer to this challenge is not to avoid routines, but rather to recognize the individual's need for routine and help to create "metaroutines" or routines for dealing with changes in routines. This concept is illustrated with child and adult case material in Chapter 4. Von Cramon and von Cramon (1994) described a creative application of this concept in their successful intervention for a physician (pathologist) with frontal lobe injury and associated executive system impairment.

Routines and Cognitive Theory

Critical to cognitive explanations of behavior is the concept of knowledge structures or organized internal (mental) representations of idea complexes, including event

complexes (e.g., scripts, plans). Since the 1970s, it has been common to refer to knowledge structures that deal with recurring events as *scripts* (Schank & Abelson, 1977). Developmental cognitive psychologists appeal to scripts or generalized event representations (Nelson, 1986) to explain people's orderly behavior in well-rehearsed action situations, and also their orderly behavior in relatively novel situations, in the latter case guided by relatively abstract scripts (or schemas) that allow for considerable flexibility in novel situations. Complete scripts (e.g., restaurant scripts, doctor visit scripts, job-specific vocational scripts, and many more) include as components places where the events occur, the sequence of events and actions, objects or "props" that are typically included in the script, people along with the roles they play in the script and the rules governing those roles, and the language typically associated with events and actions in the script.

At the most concrete level, the internal representation of an event complex is an internalized routine—a cognitive version of specific behavior chains described by behavioral psychologists. For example, toddlers' evening routines, complete with the order of bath, pajamas, book, prayers, and goodnights along with the people, places, objects, and dialogue associated with each event in the routine, become internally represented and guide the toddler's actions and talking during that routine. Because their internal representation of the script is specific and concrete, toddlers have difficulty accepting deviations within the routine (e.g., when rubber ducky is missing in action, or somebody other than mom or dad is assisting).

As children age and mature cognitively, their scripts become increasingly general— the cognitive analogue of what behavioral psychologists refer to as growing response and stimulus *classes* within behavior chains. This increasing generality explains children's ability to remain organized and appropriate in their actions and talking during routines, but in varied places and with varied people, varied objects and activities, and varied language. For example, unlike toddlers, older preschoolers typically possess a *general* representation of the bedtime script, enabling them to remain organized and self-controlled during bedtime in a variety of settings and with a variety of people (see Figure 1–2). With cognitive development and increasing experience, scripts evolve into very abstract cognitive schemas. For example, experienced travelers have more than a concrete script for negotiating the typical demands and interaction in a typical airport in their home country. Their knowledge is represented in a sufficiently general way that they are able to guide themselves successfully through extremely varied airports and train stations in diverse countries. In contrast, inexperienced travelers with relatively concrete and inflexible scripts naturally feel anxious in unfamiliar

settings in which the demands exceed their script knowledge, and therefore they may need a guide to help them succeed.

Many studies of young children have shown that they are adept at identifying the general structure in a routine and that they use this knowledge to guide their behavior (Hudson, 1993; Hudson & Nelson, 1986; Nelson, 1986). Indeed, developmental cognitive psychologists have effectively used the script concept to explain important aspects of memory development (Hudson, 1990); comprehension, recall, and organized expression of stories and other types of narrative (Hudson & Nelson, 1983); development of increasingly effective social interaction (Furman & Walden, 1990); and development of executive functions, including planning. Studies of adult cognition similarly suggest that event knowledge is stored in the form of general scripts which serve as a guide to behavior, including language in social context (Abelson,

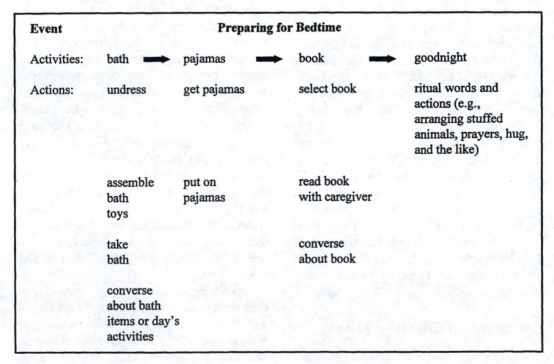

Event		Preparing for Bedtime		
Activities:	bath ➡	pajamas ➡	book ➡	goodnight
Actions:	undress	get pajamas	select book	ritual words and actions (e.g., arranging stuffed animals, prayers, hug, and the like)
	assemble bath toys	put on pajamas	read book with caregiver	
	take bath		converse about book	
	converse about bath items or day's activities			

Figure 1–2. General representation of a typical bedtime story script for a young child. (Based on "Understanding Events: The Development of Script Knowledge," by J. E. Hudson, 1993. In M. Bennett [Ed.], *The Development of Social Cognition* [pp. 142–167]. New York: The Guilford Press.)

1981). Just as developmental language specialists and early childhood educators have increasingly advocated the teaching of language and other social behaviors within the context of well-rehearsed scripts (Ratner & Bruner, 1978), we propose that much of the teaching and support for people of all ages with TBI is effectively implemented within the context of scripts or, to use our term, positive everyday routines.

Increasingly, cognitive neuroscientists have sought to explain script knowledge, its development in children, and its vulnerability following brain injury from a neuropsychological perspective. Perhaps the best developed theory is that of Grafman (1989, 1995), who argues that Managerial Knowledge Units (MKUs), including plans, scripts, schemas, themes, and mental models, are stored in the frontal lobes. Grafman's definition of the MKU is similar to that of script, given above, except that it is more general (including other knowledge structures such as plans, themes, and mental models) and highlights their storage as single units in memory. MKUs underlie organized thinking, acting, and talking, as well as fantasizing. Grafman proposes that the MKU hypothesis is capable of explaining not only disorganized behavior, but also socially inappropriate behavior, attentional weakness, and poorly regulated overt and covert behavior in general (i.e., impaired executive functions) following prefrontal lobe lesions.

The storage system proposed by Grafman, illustrated in Figure 1–3, explains the common and perplexing phenomenon of people with frontal lobe injury scoring well on tests of static knowledge and skill (e.g., language tests, intelligence tests), but evidencing debilitating disability in the real world, given the assault on plans, scripts, and schemas needed to perform successfully in everyday contexts that are not thoroughly structured, externally controlled, or habitual. Within this neuropsychological framework, rehabilitation within everyday positive routines can be interpreted as an attempt to rebuild and reactivate MKUs, if possible, and provide the type and amount of external support needed in the event of ongoing disruption in the neural architecture of MKUs. Experiments with frontal lobe patients have yielded some evidence supporting Grafman's hypothesis (Sirigu et al., 1995).

Organized, Positive Routines and TBI

Readers with experience in TBI rehabilitation should recognize a striking resemblance between the developmental contributions of script knowledge listed in the previous paragraphs (memory, comprehension, and expression of organized discourse, positive social interaction, and executive functions) and the most commonly reported chronic disabilities after TBI. In addition to the common organically based impairments in the areas of memory, social interaction, executive functions, and organized thinking, language, and behavior (see Chapter 2), many people with TBI are required to master new scripts in a sequence of novel environments after the injury. Children may be required to move through a rehabilitation hospital, home tutoring combined with outpatient therapies, a special education class, and finally a general education class, but possibly different from their classroom placement before the injury. Each of these settings is defined in part by scripts different from those of the other settings and from the child's familiar preinjury scripts. In the case of adults, varied medical and vocational settings, along with new peers and social activities, are added to this list of novel script environments.

Our general point here is that there are many threats to successful behavior after TBI; some are directly related to the injury and some are environmental. Unfortunately, many of these individuals—faced with a need to deal with considerable novelty in their lives—have primary damage to the part of the brain specifically designed to negotiate novel, nonroutine tasks. Helping people reestablish positive scripts—positive everyday routines—presents itself un-

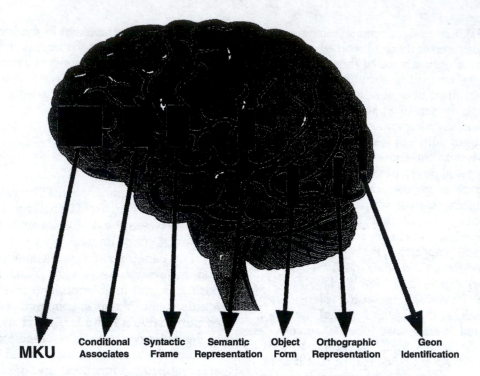

| MKU | Conditional
Associates | Syntactic
Frame | Semantic
Representation | Object
Form | Orthographic
Representation | Geon
Identification |

Figure 1–3. Growth of the "size" of a unit of memory across the cerebral cortex. The MKU framework explicitly suggests that evolution has allowed for memory units that encompass many events on a time scale of minutes to hours. This evolutionary trend appears to take a posterior-to-anterior gradient. This increasing time scale for knowledge stored in memories allows humans to be much more aware of the consequences of their current behavior in relation to behaviors previously emitted or seen or to behaviors that are forthcoming. This awareness (which can be conveyed to others through pictorial or verbal communication or demonstrated through procedural demonstration) has obvious survival value. (Reprinted with permission from "Similarities and Distinctions Among Current Models of Prefrontal Cortical Functions," by J. Grafman, 1995. In J. Grafman, K. Holyoak, and F. Boller, [Eds.], *Structure and Functions of the Human Prefrontal Cortex* [pp. 337–368]. New York: New York Academy of Sciences.)

der these circumstances as a most worthy enterprise for rehabilitation specialists. Furthermore, a deteriorating sense of self, understandably common after a life-altering brain injury, is most effectively addressed by helping people reestablish positive roles within positive scripts within generally satisfying life circumstances.

REHABILITATION IN THE SPIRIT OF VYGOTSKY

The preceding discussion of cognitive development and socially acquired scripts leads almost ineluctably to the theoretical foundation laid by the great Russian psychologist, Lev Vygotsky. Much of the recent research on cognitive development in children—including script development (Nelson, 1981, 1986)—has occurred within and has amassed considerable evidence in support of a vygotskyan social-interactionist developmental framework. In addition to the spirited and widespread revival of Vygotsky's theories in developmental cognitive psychology (e.g., Bruner, 1985; Daniels, 1996; Nelson, 1986; Rogoff, 1990; Rogoff & Misty, 1990; Wertsch, 1985), applied professions are increasingly finding his framework to be fertile soil for growing effective teaching practices. Vygotsky's views have shaped recent work in educational psychology (e.g., Brown, Campione, Weber, & McGilly, 1992; Campione & Brown, 1990), reading instruction (e.g., Palinscar & Brown, 1984, 1989), early childhood education (e.g., Bodrova & Leong, 1996; Berk & Winsler, 1995), special education (e.g., Evans, 1993; Ashman & Conway, 1989), speech-language pathology (e.g., Schneider & Watkins, 1996; Westby, 1994), and other professions.

Our goal in this section is to motivate rehabilitation professionals to consider Vygotsky's framework as a theoretical foundation for much of the enterprise of brain injury rehabilitation, to briefly describe key concepts within this framework, and to suggest rehabilitation applications of these concepts. It is far beyond the scope of this chapter to address details or conflicts in interpretation and application of this comprehensive psychological theory. However, a word of caution is in order. We do not wish to associate our approach to rehabilitation with the views of extreme social constructivists who often invoke Vygotsky's legacy in supporting their psychology of learning and education.

Luria and the Impact of Vygotsky on Neurological Rehabilitation

Vygotsky's theories of cognition and cognitive development have rarely been applied in publications that specifically deal with brain injury rehabilitation. (For an exception to this rule, see Ylvisaker & Szekeres, 1998.) For example, in a recent issue of *Neuropsychological Rehabilitation* (Vol. 6, No. 4) devoted entirely to the history of neuropsychological rehabilitation, there were no Vygotsky citations in the six essays that reviewed the history of brain injury rehabilitation in Europe and the United States. This neglect in the rehabilitation literature is surprising in light of the status among many rehabilitation professionals of Vygotsky's colleague, Alexander Luria. (In the same journal, Luria's work was cited 18 times.) Luria himself was very clear about the importance of Vygotsky's work, not only for Luria's professional development and the formation of a comprehensive psychology of mental function, but for brain injury rehabilitation as well. In his semiautobiographical work, *The Making of Mind* (Luria, 1979), Luria offered these and other extraordinary appraisals of Vygotsky and his work:

> My own work was permanently changed by my association with Vygotsky and by the ingenious studies of our students .... The general conception that organized these pilot studies laid the methodological foundation for Vygotsky's general theory and provided a set of experimental techniques which I was to use throughout the remainder of my career. (p. 51)

> I was to spend my remaining years developing various aspects of Vygotsky's psychological system. (p. 56)

With this high praise from no less an authority on neuropsychology, brain injury, and rehabilitation than Luria, rehabilitation professionals are well advised to seriously consider the usefulness of a vygotskyan framework for cognitive and psychosocial rehabilitation. Furthermore, our repeated call for rehabilitation to be contextualized within everyday routines and our frequent use of developmental analogies in discussing brain injury rehabilitation for adults as well as children both have precedent in Luria's interpretation of Vygotsky. The following quotations are also taken from Luria's *The Making of Mind*:

> One of the many characteristics of Vygotsky's work that was important in shaping my later career was his insistence that psychological research should never be limited to sophisticated speculation and laboratory models divorced from the real world. The central problems of human existence as it is experienced at school, at work, or in the clinic all served as the contexts within which Vygotsky struggled to formulate a new kind of psychology. (p. 53)

> The kindergarten and the clinic were equally attractive avenues of approach to the difficult analytic problems. (p. 57)

...nteraction and Cognitive
...pment:
...cation of Vygotsky's
Theories to TBI Rehabilitation

According to Vygotsky, cognitive functions, beyond those that are instinctive or purely sensorimotor, are derived from internalization of interaction with others, that is, of social-communication routines. "Higher mental functions evolve through social interactions with adults; they are gradually internalized as the child becomes more and more proficient and needs less and less cuing and other support from the adult" (Vygotsky, 1981). That is to say, cognitive processes like remembering, organizing, and problem-solving first exist as *interpsychological processes*—as interaction between a child or other "apprentice-in-thinking" and a more mature thinker. Gradually, the processes are internalized and become internal or intrapsychological processes. Described in Chapter 5, Dave's development of memory, thought organization, and discourse organization serves as an excellent illustration of this vygotskyan theme applied to development of cognitive processes after brain injury.

In the same way, executive functions like self-awareness, goal setting, planning, self-monitoring, and strategic thinking can be understood as gradual internalizations of interaction routines. The 16-year-old whose tenth grade English paper opens Chapter 8 illustrates this process with respect to self-examination. In his view, hundreds of everyday conversations at the dinner table during his elementary school years about what he had learned in school that day were gradually transformed into an internal voice that routinely called on him to evaluate his actions and their outcome.

Finally, within a vygotskyan framework, social self-regulatory processes also begin in childhood as interaction with adults, including adult instructions, praise, and reprimands directed to the child as well as adult modeling of self-regulatory talk (e.g., "I've got to think about this; this is a difficult decision"). Self-regulatory processes are then rehearsed as the child issues regulatory commands and feedback to pets, dolls, other children, and even adults, which are finally internalized as internal, self-regulatory self-talk (Leont'ev, 1978). We have applied this developmental principle in TBI rehabilitation by making active use of group work wherein peers help one another identify important challenges and strategies for dealing with those challenges. In addition, peers are an ideal source of advice and feedback for one another because adolescents and young adults, in particular, receive advice and feedback from peers more readily than from professionals and because the cognitive process of guiding another's choices and behavior is good practice for guiding one's own choices and behavior.

Bill, described in Chapter 6, illustrates this process. His life had been dominated by destructive conflicts and bad decisions until he came to agree that his decisions were often self-defeating and daily conversations with a therapist and peers in a TBI peer-support group—conversations that included the repeated mantra, "You've got to check it out, man"—gradually created a habituated internal self-instruction, "check it out, man." With Bill, the therapist and peers played a necessary mediational role until the process was sufficiently internalized and habituated that Bill could regulate his own behavior and independently seek appropriate assistance. In Luria's (1979) words, "the mediated responding to the world becomes an intrapsychic process. It is through this interiorization of historically determined and culturally organized ways of operating on information that the social nature of people comes to be their psychological nature as well" (p. 45). Language, which is initially a means of social communication, becomes internal speech and thereby comes to organize the individual's thought and volition. Many of the verbal routines described in this book were designed and repeatedly practiced—in some cases hundreds of times—with the goal of ultimately becoming internal, self-regulatory speech.

We have attempted to capture important aspects of Vygotsky's social-interactionist theory of cognitive and social development in Figure 1–4. In this diagram, the roots of

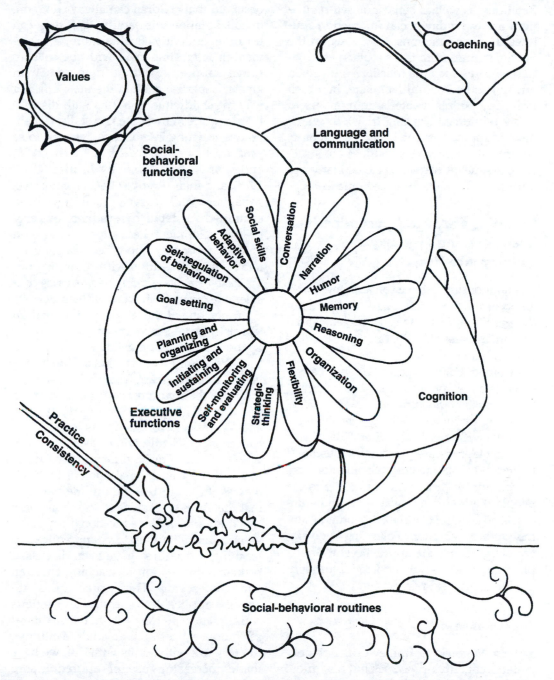

Figure 1–4. Development of cognitive and related executive and communication functions out of everyday interactive routines. In environments in which the functions are valued, coaching and supported practice are liberally provided. This is a graphic representation of Vygotsky's interactionist view of cognitive and communication development. (Copyright M. Ylvisaker, Ph.D. Reprinted with permission from "Cognitive Rehabilitation: Executive Functions," by M. Ylvisaker, S. Szekeres, and T. Feeney, 1998, p. 240. In M. Ylvisaker, [Ed.], *Traumatic Brain Injury Rehabilitation: Children and Adolescents.* Boston: Butterworth-Heinemann.)

cognitive, executive, and communication functions, as well as behavioral self-regulation, are everyday social interaction routines. Higher functions, the petals on the flower, mature from these roots in an environment in which the functions are valued (or, to use behavioral language, in which everyday people create large numbers of richly reinforced learning trials), in which there is appropriate mediation or coaching, and in which everyday routines are structured in such a way as to create many opportunities for contextualized practice.

Learning Through Apprenticeship: Transforming Vygotskyan Theory into Practice

The relationship between an apprentice and an accomplished craftsperson is distinctly different from that between a surgeon and a patient, and equally different from that between an animal trainer and the animal being trained. Each of these relationships can serve as a metaphor for the relationship between rehabilitation professionals (or everyday people playing a helping role) and individuals with disability after TBI. These three metaphors are graphically illustrated in Figure 1–5. In medical rehabilitation, it is customary for professionals to relate to the people they serve in a way that can be understood as a mix of the surgeon and animal trainer metaphors. Following Vygotsky, we suggest that the apprenticeship metaphor can be powerful and fruitful throughout life following brain injury.

Collaboration

Within Vygotsky's framework, not only general cognitive processes but also more specific academic skills (e.g., reading comprehension, scientific investigative skills) and content knowledge are most efficiently acquired by children working in collaboration with adults or older children with greater expertise than the learner. Rogoff (1990) characterizes this as an apprentice-ship model of teaching. Vygotsky (1987) observed that children can always do more in collaboration with adults than they can do independently. Furthermore, engagement in interesting tasks with the collaborative support of adults or others with greater expertise is often the most efficient way for children (and adults with disability) to acquire knowledge and skills. Collaborative teaching interactions, referred to as *joint involvement episodes* by Shaffer (1996) and *joint action routines* by Bruner (1975, 1978), and their positive effect on cognitive, social, and verbal development have been examined in detail by students of early child development. Less attention has been paid to apprenticeship-based teaching interactions with adults with disability, but the term *apprenticeship* by itself carries considerable meaning in work with adults.

Bruner, one of the leaders of the modern Vygotsky renaissance, described his investigations of development as an attempt "to find the manner in which aspirant members of a culture learn from their tutors, the vicars of their culture, how to understand the world" (p. 32). According to Bruner, and Vygotsky before him, this learning occurs most efficiently within teaching interactions that are quite different from those prescribed by traditional operant methodologies. In Table 1–1, we outline paradigmatic features of teaching tasks within these two traditions. In the educational psychology and disability literature, apprenticeship teaching procedures have been discussed primarily in relation to teaching children and adolescents. These procedures are equally applicable to adults, an obvious consequence of the fact that in a literal sense apprenticeship is an adult institution. In our work with adults with TBI, we have made increasing use of apprenticeship tasks. A major difference between working with young children and adults is that teachers and parents contribute the goals as well as the instruction and supports when teaching children. In contrast, professionals must work hard to think of themselves as playing a consultant role in relation to

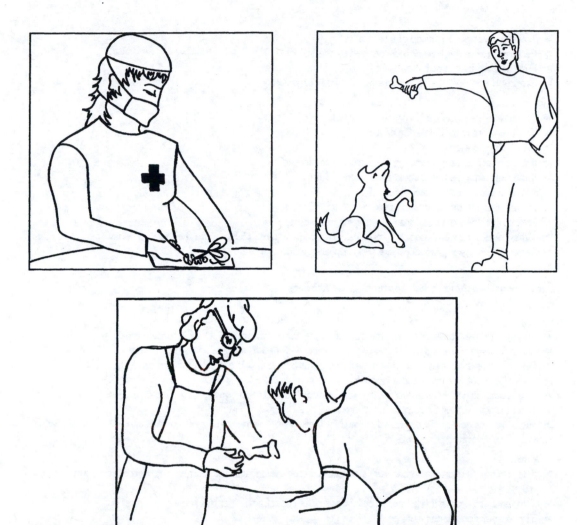

Figure 1–5. Graphic illustration of three metaphors or models of clinician-client relationship, capable of motivating importantly different approaches to rehabilitation after brain injury. The physician-patient metaphor, or medical model, emphasizes cure of the underlying impairment by means of expert application of technical treatments in specialized settings. The animal trainer metaphor, or traditional behavioral model, emphasizes mastery of discrete behaviors by means of massed learning trials. The apprentice model, often associated with the work of Vygotsky, emphasizes collaboration, support, and meaningful tasks and settings. (Reprinted with permission from "Everyday People as Supports: Developing Competence Through Collaboration," by M. Ylvisaker and T. Feeney, 1998, pp. 448, 449, 451. In M. Ylvisaker, [Ed.], *Traumatic Brain Injury Rehabilitation: Children and Adolescents.* Boston: Butterworth-Heinemann.)

TABLE 1–1. Contrast between traditional training procedures and apprenticeship procedures.

Features of Teaching Tasks: Traditional Training Model

Context
- Training takes place outside of a natural setting
- Performance of the learner is demanded by the trainer
- Performance is solo, not social
- Tasks and components of tasks are hierarchically organized

Task structure
- The trainer requests performance of a specific task
- The trainer may model performance
- The learner performs
- If the performance is adequate, the learner is reinforced
- If the performance is inadequate, the trainer either
  - requests a hierarchically easier task
  - reduces the difficulty of the task
  - provides needed cues, prompts, shaping procedures
- When performance is adequate, repeated practice is required to habituate the learned behavior
- Systematic transfer procedures are then applied (see below)

Features of Teaching Tasks: Apprenticeship Model

Context
- Learning (ideally) takes place in a natural setting for the behavior or skill that is to be learned
- Learning takes place within the context of projects designed to achieve a meaningful goal
- Performance is not demanded from the learner; rather the task is completed collaboratively
- Completion of the task is social, not solo
- The learner is not expected to fail; the collaborator is available to contribute whatever the learner cannot contribute to successful completion of the task
- Tasks are not necessarily organized hierarchically; the learner can learn aspects of difficult tasks by participating with a collaborator

Task Structure
- The teacher (facilitator, collaborator) introduces a task and engages the learner in guided observation (not necessarily task specific)
- The teacher engages the learner in collaborative, functional, goal-oriented, project-oriented work
- The learner contributes what he or she can contribute
- The teacher coaches (including suggestions, modeling, brainstorming, cues, feedback, and encouragement) and continues to collaborate as the learner accomplishes more components of the task
- As the learner improves, supports are systematically withdrawn or the task is made more difficult or both
- The teacher continues to provide ongoing incidental coaching
- Transfer is guaranteed because it is part of the contextualized teaching process from the beginning

---

adults with disability who set their own goals, but may need considerable support to achieve them.

Scaffolding

When learning takes place through apprenticeship,

The tutor or the aiding peer serves the learner as a vicarious form of consciousness until such time as the learner is able to master his own action through his own consciousness and control. When the child achieves that conscious control over a new function or conceptual system, it is then that he is able to use it as a tool. Up to that point, the tutor in effect performs the critical function of "scaffolding" the learning task to make it possible for the child, in Vygotsky's word, to internalize external knowledge and convert it into a tool for conscious control. (Bruner, 1985, pp. 24–25)

Bruner introduced the popular metaphor of scaffolding to serve as shorthand for the wide variety of supports that may enable a learner to succeed with a task and acquire the knowledge and skills implicit in the task (Wood, Bruner, & Ross, 1976). Bruner's metaphor has had a profound effect on practice in many fields of education and clinical intervention. However, in one important respect, the metaphor is misleading in that real scaffolds are fixed and inflexible, whereas supports within a vygotskyan framework are as flexible as required by the needs of the learner. These supports can include any combination of the following:

➤ accomplishing the task for the learner, with the learner attending to the task and how it is accomplished (e.g., parents reading books with young preschoolers);
➤ within routine tasks, leaving simple components for the learner to accomplish (e.g., parents pausing for the child to add the last word on each page of familiar books, master craftspersons turning over minor tasks to new apprentices);
➤ accomplishing the task with the learner in a conversational manner, expecting only as much participation from the learner as is possible (e.g., parents jointly constructing with their children narratives about past experiences in a conversational manner, direct care staff conversationally reviewing the day with adults with memory problems after TBI);
➤ providing well-rehearsed routines, possibly including graphic organizers, to help individuals accomplish difficult tasks (e.g., engaging individuals with TBI in a planning routine at the beginning of the day, with a form to support organized planning [see Chapter 4]);
➤ providing advance organizers for complex tasks (e.g., in a vocational setting, providing disorganized individuals with

a sequence of photographs or a graphic flow chart to guide them through the task);
➤ modeling (i.e., showing the individual how to complete the task);
➤ providing peer support (e.g., creating cooperative work or learning groups);
➤ giving advance support (e.g., cues and prompts) to prevent the individual from attempting unsuccessfully to complete the task;
➤ providing environmental support (e.g., reducing distractions, increasing familiarity);
➤ modifying the task (e.g., simplifying the task, reducing the amount of work to be completed, increasing the time for completion);
➤ heightening motivation (e.g., increasing the promised reward, identifying intrinsically motivating learning tasks);
➤ planning for changes in expectations.

Determining the ideal combination of supports for an individual at any given time and in relation to specific tasks involves a dynamic assessment process, which is described in Chapter 3.

Our discussion of Vygotsky's theory of instruction and cognitive growth is intended to apply to the domains of functioning addressed in this book, executive functions, cognition, communication, and behavior. Apparently competing approaches to instruction, such as Direct Instruction (Engleman & Carnine, 1991), may be most appropriate for teaching academic skills to students with significant learning impairment after TBI (Glang et al., 1992). It should be noted that the principles underlying Direct Instruction—thorough task analysis, teaching by means of a carefully designed set of systematically varied examples of the target concept or skill, criterion-based decision making about progress through a hierarchy of educational objectives, and extensive, errorless practice—are equally applicable to a vygotskyian approach to teaching and learning. The differences might lie in the amount of teacher mediation that is provided and in the personal meaningfulness of the tasks selected as the context for instruction.

Summary of Vygotsky's Impact

Our goal in this brief discussion of Vygotsky's legacy was to motivate a highly contextualized and collaborative approach to rehabilitation, and to describe this approach using concepts that are familiar to practitioners in many domains of theoretical, experimental, and applied psychology and education. We have found Vygotsky's work to be a rich source of rehabilitation wisdom and also a framework within which unproductive conflicts between behaviorally and cognitively oriented clinicians can be resolved and within which the often yawning chasm between theory and practice can be bridged. However, we do not recommend exclusively theory-driven rehabilitation practices, allegiance to any particular leader, or unyielding commitment to any existing body of psychological theory and principles. Indeed, we had been working within the framework presented in this book for some years before we noticed striking parallels between this framework and the theoretical formulations of Vygotsky. Clinicians have the luxury of milking theories, even opposing theories, for what they have to offer clinical practice; they also have an obligation to measure their work by the gold standard of meaningful, real-world improvements in the people they serve.

CONVENTIONAL VERSUS FUNCTIONAL APPROACHES TO REHABILITATION

We believe that the approach to rehabilitation illustrated throughout this book deserves the honorary title *functional* and can be contrasted with a conventional approach that has long dominated rehabilitation discussions. In Table 1–2, we summarize functional and conventional approaches to rehabilitation for individuals with disability in the domains of executive functions, cognition, communication, and behavior. What we refer to as conventional and functional approaches are more appropriately understood as classes of approaches that exist toward opposite ends of several rehabilitation dimensions. We operationally define functional approaches as those that:

➤ are driven by the fundamental goal of helping individuals with disability achieve success in academic, vocational, personal, and social life;

➤ maintain a commitment to collaborative assessment and intervention,

➤ focus on individuals' strengths in attempting to address the effects of ongoing impairment;

➤ identify real-world settings, activities, and routines as the primary context for intervention efforts;

➤ recognize the critical role of everyday people as deliverers of rehabilitation services and supports;

➤ strive to facilitate the individual's development of internal control; and

➤ highlight proactive, antecedent-focused intervention procedures within a general apprenticeship model of teaching.

We understand that many clinicians who find their professional practices grouped under the heading *conventional* in Table 1–1 consider those practices highly functional. Indeed, it is likely that all rehabilitation professionals would argue that their services are functional for the individuals they serve; inability to mount such a defense would indisputably stand as an indictment of those services. Therefore, a value judgment—some might say a begging of the question—is implicit in our use of the term *functional*. Our goal is surely not to win an empty victory by merely attaching an honorific label to our approach to rehabilitation for the intended group. Rather, we hope that the theoretical and practical considerations, arguments, and case illustrations presented in this book will lead readers to agree that attention to everyday routines is at the core of functional rehabilitation for people with chronic cognitive, behavioral, and communication disability after TBI.

TABLE 1–2. Conventional versus functional approaches to intervention after brain injury: Communication, behavior, and cognition.

I. Scope of Intervention
  A. Conventional approach
    1. *Speech-language pathology:* The focus is on speech and specific aspects of linguistic competence (semantics, syntax, morphology).
    2. *Behavioral psychology:* The focus is on management of specific problem behaviors in a narrow sense.
    3. *Cognitive rehabilitation:* The focus is on neuropsychological assessment and intervention that sequentially targets separate components of cognition, arranged in a hierarchy for treatment purposes.
  B. Functional approach
    1. The focus of each profession is on helping individuals with brain injury achieve their real-world goals in real-world contexts, including academic, vocational, and social success.
    2. Correctly understood, applied behavior analysis in psychology, pragmatics in speech-language pathology, and social-cognitive intervention in cognitive rehabilitation are essentially the same service, necessitating close collaboration among service providers.
    3. Each profession recognizes the overarching importance of executive or self-control functions for academic, vocational, and social success.

II. Integration of Intervention: Collaboration
  A. Conventional approach
    1. Cognition, communication, and behavior are targeted for assessment and intervention by separate professionals working in relative isolation.
    2. Evaluation reports, including proposed goals, objectives, and plans to achieve the objectives, are separately produced by three professionals.
  B. Functional approach
    1. Although behavioral psychologists, cognitive rehabilitation specialists (including special educators), and speech-language pathologists are recognized as possessing special and unique expertise, the important overlap in their services is frankly acknowledged.
    2. Assessments are conducted and plans for intervention are developed in an integrated manner. Ideally, reports are written as integrated, cross-disciplinary documents.
    3. Individuals with disability and significant everyday people in their lives are included as contributing members of the collaborative assessment and intervention teams.

III. Orientation of Intervention: Deficits and Strengths
  A. Conventional approach: deficit orientation
    1. The cognitive rehabilitation specialist attempts to remediate cognitive deficits and restore specific preexisting cognitive skills in areas of impairment.
    2. The speech-language pathologist attempts to remediate communication deficits and restore specific preexisting speech and language skills in areas of impairment.
    3. The behavioral psychologist attempts to eliminate undesirable behaviors (e.g., noncompliance, agitation, combativeness) and increase specific desirable behaviors (e.g., participation, "socially appropriate" behaviors).
  B. Functional approach: strength orientation
    1. Each professional begins with existing strengths and builds upon them with (a) attempts to ensure success in functional activities at the individual's current level of capacity, (b) apprenticeship procedures (including chaining and shaping), and (c) compensatory strategies, using strengths to compensate for weaknesses.
    2. Success is a goal throughout intervention, using whatever antecedent supports may be necessary to succeed at functional tasks at the individual's current level of ability.
    3. Undesirable and challenging behaviors, including explicitly communicative behaviors, are never *simply* extinguished without an attempt to substitute a positive alternative that achieves the same goal.
    4. Preservation and enhancement of the individual's self-esteem is a background goal for all professionals.

continued

TABLE 1–2. *continued*

IV. Service Delivery: Settings and Activities
A. Conventional approach
1. The speech-language pathologist uses repetitive drill and practice in isolated settings that bear little resemblance to real-world communication settings (e.g., pull-out therapy). Activities in therapy settings are not necessarily related to real-world communication activities.
2. The cognitive rehabilitation specialist uses repetitive drill and practice in isolated settings that bear little resemblance to real-world settings (e.g., pull-out therapy using decontextualized workbook or computer exercises). Activities in therapy settings are not necessarily related to real-world activities that require the targeted cognitive skill.
3. The behavioral psychologist delivers targeted behavioral services on a behavior unit, in a neurobehavioral rehabilitation facility, or in a behavior classroom, with little opportunity to facilitate transfer of training to real-world settings and tasks.

B. Functional approach
1. Each profession focuses on real-world needs in real-world contexts. This focus includes supports for achieving real-world goals in real-world contexts and practice of functional communication, social, and cognitive skills in real-world contexts. Specific aspects of the individual's environments and demands in those environments are considered in choosing objectives.
2. As much as possible, communication and behavioral services are delivered in meaningful social groups, in settings that resemble settings in which the skills will need to be used, and in the context of meaningful activities.
3. Pursuit of cognitive, executive function, communication, and behavioral goals is largely in the context of everyday routines, involving modification of those routines with supports that are gradually withdrawn as the individual's skills improve.

V. Providers of Service: Involvement of Everyday Communication Partners
A. Conventional approach
1. Professionals are considered the primary agents of change in the individual with disability.
2. Each profession primarily focuses on remediation of deficits in the individual; that is, the intervention is impairment-oriented.

B. Functional approach
1. Each profession focuses on improvement of function within everyday routines. Therefore, everyday communication partners (e.g., family members, paraprofessional aides, supervisors, teachers, coworkers, friends) are critical deliverers of rehabilitation services and supports.
2. A primary role of rehabilitation specialists is to train and provide ongoing supports for everyday communication partners. Within a rehabilitation facility, evening and weekend staff are recognized as particularly critical to the development of a positive and therapeutically efficient rehabilitation environment.

VI. Source of Control
A. Conventional approach
1. There is near total reliance on external control of behavior. Little emphasis is placed on helping the individual to set goals and make good choices, plan how to achieve selected goals, monitor and evaluate behavior in relation to those goals, and make strategic decisions in the face of failure. Professionals assume responsibility for most executive dimensions of behavior.
2. The individual with disability is *not* included as a member of the team of people who perform assessments, select goals and objectives, plan intervention, monitor and evaluate performance, and create strategic solutions to problems as they arise over the course of intervention.

B. Functional approach
1. The ultimate goal is to ensure that the individual controls his or her behavior as much as possible by means of effective decision making, strategic thinking, self-regulation of behavior, and self-regulated control over environmental contingencies.
2. The individual with disability *is* included as a member of the team of people who perform assessments, select goals and objectives, plan intervention, monitor and evaluate performance, and create strategic solutions to problems as they arise over the course of intervention.

VII. Intervention Procedures

A. Conventional approach

1. Prescriptive behavioral objectives specify isolated targets; for example, specific language behaviors are selected for training.

2. Modification of behavior is largely a result of the manipulation of the *consequences* of behavior. Within training tasks, correct performance of the target behavior is consequated with presumably desirable objects or events; failure to use the target behavior is followed by a withholding of rewards, a cost of some kind, removal from the situation, or some other neutral or undesirable consequence.

B. Functional approach

1. The goal is an acceptable *range* of behaviors (versus a specific behavior) that may vary in their effectiveness in achieving the communicative objective.

2. Modification of behavior (including cognitive and social behavior) is considered a result of manipulating the consequences as well as antecedents of the behavior, but the focus is on *antecedents*. Antecedent control procedures include creating environmental supports, avoiding triggers for negative behavior, inducing positive setting events, generating positive momentum, creating opportunities for choice and control, establishing familiar, positive routines and effective procedures for deviating from routines, providing advance organizers for difficult tasks, teaching scripts for negotiating difficult social situations, and ensuring that the individual has maximal self-management skills.

3. Contingency management (i.e., manipulation of consequences of behavior) focuses on positive consequences for desirable behavior (versus punishing consequences and time out for negative behavior) and on natural contingencies (versus artificial rewards).

   a. As much as possible, rewards are internally related to the action performed (e.g., when people request something appropriately, they get it; when people initiate social interaction, they are rewarded with a pleasant interaction; when people use strategies, they succeed in their endeavors).

   b. Feedback (positive or negative) is given as much as possible by natural communication partners (e.g., peers or family members).

4. As much as possible, teaching and learning take place within an apprenticeship relationship. The teacher and the learner are jointly engaged in projects designed to achieve meaningful goals. Initially the teacher assumes much of the responsibility for achieving the goal, but turns over responsibility to the learner/apprentice as soon as possible.

Interdependent Themes and Collaborative Professionals

Table 1–1 addresses approaches to intervention for at least three distinct professions: speech-language pathology, behavioral psychology, and cognitive rehabilitation. The authors of this book represent two of these professions, speech-language pathology and behavioral psychology, but we have also spent much of our professional lives delivering a service that most would label, at least in part, cognitive rehabilitation. Despite our distinctly different educational backgrounds and professional titles, we have found over many years of collaborative clinical work that the problems we face and our approaches to dealing with these problems are almost identical—and that they are shared by many people in other professions, including special education, neuropsychology, occupational therapy, vocational rehabilitation, and others.

Furthermore, we have long since abandoned the fruitless and pointless task of surgically dissecting behavioral issues from communication issues from cognitive issues from executive system issues. For similar reasons, it is equally difficult to separate problems that are directly related to brain injury from those that are psychoreactive from those that grow over time as a result of untoward life circumstances and poorly conceived management. Rehabilitation specialists are called on to help people with brain injury who have difficulty with cognitively demanding tasks, difficulty managing their behavior and communication in some contexts, and difficulty with general executive dimensions of behavior and cognitive processing. More to the point, they have difficulty achieving the goals that they set for themselves in life, and we are asked as clinicians to assist them in this pursuit. Often these difficulties, whether they are labeled cognitive, behavioral, communicative, or "executive," have a similar source in types of brain injury that are very common in head trauma, especially damage to the frontal lobes and limbic regions of the brain, and affect functioning in each of these domains (see Chapter 2).

For purposes of presentation, we have chosen to write chapters that separately emphasize executive function themes, cognitive themes, behavioral themes, and communication themes. This separation of themes runs the serious risk of justifying a fragmented and noncollaborative approach to intervention. However, as we repeatedly point out in those chapters, the individuals we selected as case illustrations could have appeared in any of the four intervention chapters. The difficulties that interfered with their successful pursuit of goals were an inseparable mix of the four categories of disability addressed in this book and the interventions that proved useful for them necessitated an integrated and collaborative approach to that inseparable mix.

Sources of Support for the Approach

The perspective on rehabilitation that we present in this book has been shaped by many experiences and considerations. Most influential have been our direct experiences with more than a thousand individuals with TBI, ranging in age from infants to older adults. We have both worked in acute rehabilitation facilities, but more recently have served children and adults in the chronic stages of their disability, from several months to several years after the injury. In addition to acute rehabilitation hospitals, we have worked with individuals with TBI in schools, homes, on the job, in community residences, psychiatric hospitals, jails and prisons, residential substance

abuse programs, and adult day programs. In many of these settings, our efforts have largely been directed at equipping everyday people in those settings, including family members, direct care staff, work supervisors, educational staff, peers, and others, with the knowledge, skills, and attitudes needed to support and facilitate ongoing improvement in the individuals they serve. The case illustrations and single subject experimental designs described later in this book are derived from these experiences.

Second, without the illumination of comprehensive theories, everyday clinical experience can easily be a guide without vision. The unifying cognitive and behavioral theory supportive of our approach derives from the extraordinary work of Vygotsky. The neuropsychological theories that support and add depth to the approach derive historically from Vygotsky's follower and collaborator, the great Russian neurologist Alexander Luria, and, more recently, the elegant account of frontolimbic systems and of consequences of damage to these systems developed by Antonio Damasio and his colleagues.

Rich clinical experience supported by current theory is still not an infallible guide to effective practices in rehabilitation. The third major support for the approach to rehabilitation offered in this book is found in the large and growing body of experimental work on transfer of training (generalization and maintenance). An impressive body of research in cognitive and behavioral science and in many applied fields has consistently supported the observation of teachers and clinicians working with people with cognitive disability: *Behaviors or skills acquired in a laboratory or training context are unlikely to transfer to functional application contexts and be maintained over time without heroic efforts to facilitate that transfer and maintenance* (Durand, 1990; Haring & Kennedy, 1990; Horner & Budd, 1985; Horner et al., 1988; Martin & Pear, 1996; Morris, 1988; 1992; Singley & Anderson, 1989). This bedrock principle is not restricted in its application to people with disability. For example, experienced university teachers of logic and composition are well aware of the limited transfer and maintenance of reasoning and writing skills from the classroom in which they were acquired to the classrooms and other settings in which they should be used, even in the case of bright students. Similarly, those involved in training teachers and clinicians understand that *functional competence as a clinician is not achieved in classrooms* (Meyer & Evans, 1989), but rather through patient modeling and coaching in real-world practicum and internship experiences. Mothers know that it is inefficient at best to attempt to train young children in social competence outside the context of real social interaction or to teach safety judgment outside the context of potentially dangerous situations. These are among the many common everyday observations that should alert rehabilitation professionals to the necessity of placing the notion of *real-world context* at center stage in their work with people with TBI.

A fourth support for our approach, intimately tied to issues of transfer of training, can be identified by examining positive trends in a variety of fields of disability work. Increasingly, helping professionals have become aware of the advantages of delivering services and supports as much as possible in the contexts in which improvement is desired and to focus intervention in large part on antecedent supports in those contexts. For example, the supported work movement in vocational rehabilitation is based in part on this premise: Deliver services on the job, provide sufficiently intensive supports to enable the individual to succeed, and withdraw the supports as indicated by the individual's growing independence (Wehman et al., 1993, 1995). Inclusion of special education students in general education settings, with sufficient supports to ensure success, has been defended in part by the same logic (Giangreco, Cloninger, & Iverson, 1993). At the same time, advance organizers—proactive supports—have become a staple in special edu-

cation and vocational rehabilitation because of the relative inefficiency of teaching mainly by means of manipulating consequences (Deshler & Schumaker, 1988). In special education, investigators have found that peers, mobilized as a circle of friends or as specifically trained confederates in the delivery of intervention, can positively affect students with disability in their development of social and academic skills (Johnson & Johnson, 1992). Collaborative planning processes, including Personal Futures Planning (Mount & Zwernik, 1986; O'Brien & Lyle, 1987) and the McGill Action Planning System (Forest & Lusthaus, 1990), have been developed to assist professionals and everyday people in their design and implementation of community-based supports for individuals with disability of various ages and levels of disability.

Similarly, behavioral specialists have increasingly promoted the use of general case training—using varied natural environments as the stimulus conditions and varied natural consequences as reinforcers—and involvement of everyday communication partners to address historic problems of generalization and maintenance (Carr, Levin, McConnachie, Carlson, Kemp, & Smith, 1994; Horner et al., 1988; Kern, Childs, Dunlap, Clarke, & Falk, 1994; Reichle & Wacker, 1993). Furthermore, antecedent management focusing on proactive procedures, including manipulation of setting events, has recently received the lion's share of attention in many clinical discussions of behavior management, as opposed to the traditional reliance on contingency management (Carr et al., 1994; Carr, Reeve, & Magito-McLaughlin, 1997; Horner et al., 1990; Horner, Vaughn, Day, & Ard, Jr., 1997; Kennedy, 1994; Kennedy & Itkonen, 1993). Inefficiency of decontextualized training has been a primary motivator in the movement toward more naturalistic forms of intervention for individuals with disorders of language and social skills (Fey, 1986; Koegel & Koegel, 1995; MacDonald, 1989; Nelson, Camarata, Welsh, Butkovsky, & Camarata, 1996; Walker et al., 1994). Scores of studies of the effectiveness of social skills intervention yield the conclusion that skills acquired in training tasks rarely generalize to real-world social interaction (McIntosh, Vaughn, & Zaragoza, 1991; Zaragoza, Vaughn, & McIntosh, 1991). Finally, specialists in rehabilitation for people with TBI have increasingly advocated the use of natural contexts for delivery of behavioral services (Feeney & Ylvisaker, 1995, 1997; Finset & Andresen, 1990; Ylvisaker, Feeney, & Szekeres, 1998) and cognitive rehabilitation (von Cramon & van Cramon, 1994; Ylvisaker & Feeney, 1996; Ylvisaker, Szekeres, & Feeney, 1998).

A fifth and final source of support for the perspective offered in this book is presented by the crisis in funding for rehabilitation. Managed care and other economic forces have dramatically shortened lengths of inpatient stay for rehabilitation and, at the same time, reduced access to outpatient services for many clinical populations, including people with TBI. For example, in the rehabilitation hospital in which the first author worked for 10 years, average length of stay for the TBI program was reduced by 75% between 1983 and 1993. Rehabilitation facilities around the country and in other countries have reported similar reductions. Under these generally unhappy circumstances, it is critical for rehabilitation specialists to creatively design ways to accomplish more with less, to achieve positive outcomes with fewer resources. The proposal stated and illustrated throughout this book—namely, that specialists in rehabilitation can extend their effectiveness by empowering everyday people to be effective deliverers of services and supports—is one positive approach to the crisis of funding for rehabilitation.

EVERYDAY ROUTINES AND GENERALIZATION

Generalization and maintenance—or transfer of training—is the cross on which many apparently appealing interventions have been crucified. Clinicians and teachers have long recognized that it is far easier to

improve performance on training tasks in laboratory or clinical settings than to improve everyday routine behavior in the real-world contexts in which improvements are needed and make a difference in the individual's life (Dunlap, Johnson, & Robbins, 1990; Durand, 1990; Durand & Carr, 1991; Halle, 1989; Halle & Spradlin, 1993; Singley & Anderson, 1989). Reviews of the effectiveness of neuropsychological rehabilitation after brain injury have increasingly stressed this timeless truth (Glisky & Schacter, 1989; Thöne, 1996; Toglia, 1991; Wilson, 1992, 1995). Ultimately, intervention must have an impact on everyday life or it is useless. To achieve that goal, either training must occur and supports implemented in precisely the contexts in which improved functioning is desired, or generalization across settings, across tasks, and across behaviors is necessary. Furthermore, when training occurs in specific everyday contexts, generalization remains a highly desirable outcome (Carnevale, 1996; Mayer, Keating, & Rapp, 1986; Meyer & Evans, 1989). Only in the case of people with severe cognitive limitations is it appropriate to set as a rehabilitation goal improved functioning in a small set of specific real-world settings and activities with no effort to effect transfer or generalization.

The Fallacy of Decontextualized Cognitive Retraining

In light of the long history of optimistic appraisals of novel interventions gradually giving way to disillusionment when generalization and maintenance are seriously measured, it is quite astonishing that many clinicians continue to deliver services on the untested assumption that generalization and maintenance will occur as a consequence of improved performance on training tasks. In our experience, this blind optimism is most frequently observed in the field of cognitive rehabilitation. In many facilities in which we have consulted, we repeatedly hear clinicians make statements like "I am using such and such software (or workbook or game or other training activity) with John because it does a good job of getting at attention (or perception or organization or memory or problem-solving or some other cognitive process). And he's doing a lot better on these tasks than when he started, so we're very pleased." The line of reasoning implicit in this optimism is so pervasive and fallacious that we have named it the Fallacy of Decontextualized Cognitive Retraining:

1. Performance of task T involves use of cognitive process P.
2. Repeated performance of task T results in improved performance of task T.
3. Therefore, repeated performance of task T will result in improvement in process P.
4. Therefore, performance will improve in all tasks that engage process P.

It is not difficult to recognize the fallacy in this reasoning. Were it valid, dogs who regularly and successfully chase frisbees would be masters of physics and geometry! Unfortunately (or, perhaps, fortunately) for those two noble fields of inquiry, dogs who chase frisbees only get better at chasing frisbees. Similarly, by this logic, teenagers who spend hours a day playing videogames at the mall should be masters of quick problem-solving across a wide domain of problems, capable of charging premium fees for their consulting services. Unfortunately, teenagers who endlessly practice problem-solving with videogames are often successful with very little other than videogames.

In a somewhat more serious vein, students who work hard at their Latin studies learn Latin, but do not thereby become proficient in varied domains of organized thinking, as was the promise of the doctrine of formal discipline associated with the faculty psychology of the 19th century. And students who master geometry are not thereby improved reasoners in varied domains of reasoning—another promise of the 19th century psychology of education that assumed broad transfer of cognitive skill after the *faculties or forms of the mind* had been adequately *disciplined or trained by exercises* like lessons in Latin and geometry. A super-

ficial approach to cognitive exercises for people with cognitive disability after TBI appears to be based on these 19th century assumptions of general mental faculties and broad transfer of cognitive skill, assumptions that have long since been discredited (Singley & Anderson, 1989). We are again reminded of Santayana's (1905) wise observation, "Those who cannot remember the past are condemned to repeat it" (p. 284).

We choose to highlight this important point about generalization because its neglect is observed not only in the clinical work of some inexperienced rehabilitation professionals, but also in the experimental work of several respected investigators. For example, Ruff and colleagues (1989) concluded their report of a controlled study of the efficacy of a cognitive rehabilitation regimen by saying,

> Do the improvements found on posttreatment testing generalize to everyday life activities? Although this is an essential question, it cannot be directly answered within the context of the present experimental paradigm. It seems reasonable to *assume* (emphasis added) that improvements on neuropsychological measures do correspond to an enhancement of everyday capabilities. (p. 31)

Based on over 100 years of study of the phenomenon of transfer or generalization in several fields of investigation, including special education for people with neurologic impairment, we must insist that it is *never* appropriate to *assume* that generalization and maintenance will occur after improvements in decontextualized exercises and associated improvements on standardized testing (Kavale & Mattson; 1983; Mann, 1979).

Two Analogies for Understanding Generalization: The Wimbledon Approach Versus The Mom-and-Pop Approach

Clinicians committed to using relatively contentless training tasks in settings that bear little resemblance to real-world settings—or exercises that have content that is not related to personally meaningful tasks—have a ready response to the challenge of the preceding section, namely that they do not *assume generalization*; rather they build generalization into their treatment plan as a specific stage of intervention that follows acquisition and stabilization of new skills on training tasks. Furthermore, according to this view, it is easier to focus on specific aspects of cognitive functioning, and therefore acquire skills, *outside* of the often complex and stressful context of skill application in functional, real-world tasks. We will call this the Wimbledon Approach, because central to the approach is mastery of isolated behaviors or skills before beginning to apply them functionally in everyday tasks—just as expert tennis players devote thousands of hours and tens of thousands of learning trials to mastering the strokes of the game before they apply these skills in Centre Court Wimbledon.

Very few people would argue against the Wimbledon Approach as applied to teaching skilled motor activity. Nobody would recommend learning a forehand volley at centre court Wimbledon with a prestigious championship on the line and royalty intently observing the play. Similarly, golfers do not practice a new punch-and-run approach shot at the Masters in Augusta. Sopranos do not work on executing a difficult trill during a performance of *Cosi Fan Tutte* at the Met. Applied to brain injury, the common sense implicit in the Wimbledon Approach dictates, for example, that people do not relearn driving skills behind the wheel of a school bus filled with children. In addition to motor skills, academic skills that must become automatic and that exist as skills independent of reference to any specific context or content would similarly seem to be candidates for decontextualized practice to mastery. Multiplication tables in arithmetic come to mind as the best exemplar of this category.

An alternative to the Wimbledon Approach to generalization is what we call the Mom-and-Pop Approach. We speculate with great confidence that there has never been a mother who has taken her toddler into a training setting and used a simulated stove burner as the context for drilling the child in the correct self-protective response to "Hot!! Don't touch!" Mothers teach this critical danger signal to toddlers beside the stove and in a context in which the child could actually be hurt. In this case, the context obviously carries much of the meaning, and the learner—in this case, a toddler—is a concrete thinker who would not be expected to see the point of decontextualized practice or, in behavioral terms, to form a response association with the correct elements of the stimulus array present during the training exercise. Thus, decontextualized practice for a toddler easily creates confusion and even greater effort when the time comes for transfer to functional application. Older children with mental retardation often experience similar confusion when they learn a functional skill or behavior in a simulated setting quite different from the application setting—for example, learning safe street crossing in the school gym with masking tape representing the curbs and chairs representing cars and trucks. Subsequent learning of the skill with real roads and real cars may be rendered inefficient because of the associations (i.e., competing events) created during the simulation practice in the gym. That is, the original training lacked sensitivity to the need for discrimination learning.

In general, parents teach skills to young children in the contexts in which they are needed. For example, parents generally teach language and social skills in the context of meaningful verbal exchanges and real social interaction; they help their children learn how to organize objects and events in the context of practical activities, play, and conversation when organizing becomes necessary; and they facilitate problem-solving skill in the context of problems that arise over the course of their child's day. Thus we find ourselves again in the domain of Vygotsky's social-interactionist theory of cognitive and language development. Applied to controversies about transfer, the Mom-and-Pop Approach would come down on the side of contextualizing intervention from very early in the process.

Critique of the Mom-and-Pop Approach

The typical criticism of the Mom-and-Pop Approach to generalization in the field of cognitive rehabilitation is that, although it might be helpful for individuals to acquire highly specific skills or behaviors that are useful to them in specific real-world settings, this type of training does not hold the potential to facilitate *general* improvements in functioning because it does not target the underlying skill or behavior deficit (Sohlberg & Mateer, 1989; Sohlberg & Raskin, 1996). Genuine deficit reduction, so this line of reasoning goes, mandates carefully designed hierarchies of exercises that, in the initial stages of training, are designed to address specific aspects of cognition, but with tasks that are as "contentless" as possible—much as the early practice of specific components of tennis takes place outside of the context of the game. Furthermore, using natural contexts, it is difficult to generate the number of learning trials needed by individuals who learn slowly. We return to this criticism later.

Critique of the Wimbledon Approach

In the field of cognitive rehabilitation, the Wimbledon Approach has frequently been referred to—sometimes approvingly, often derisively—as mental muscle building. The classical critique of mental muscle building as applied to memory rehabilitation was offered by Schacter and Glisky (1986), who found experimental support for memory retraining by means of memory exercises to be woefully lacking. A similarly strong criticism of mental muscle building as applied to *attention* training after TBI was presented by Ponsford (1990), who found that im-

provement after intensive training with customized computer-based attentional exercises was not superior to that associated with spontaneous neurologic recovery alone. However, in the domain of attention training after TBI, there continue to be proponents of what we refer to as the Wimbledon Approach to training and generalization. For example, Mateer and Mapou (1996) recently reviewed the experimental literature on attention training after TBI, suggesting that, despite sharply opposing findings, the available body of evidence supports the effectiveness of process-specific attention training, at least when psychometric tests are used as the outcome measure. However, unambiguous evidence is not yet available to support the conclusion that decontextualized process-specific training has a substantial and positive impact on everyday functioning superior to that produced by functional, contextualized practice. In special education, the history of this type of process-specific training is not encouraging (Kavale & Mattson, 1983; Mann, 1979).

Support for the Mom-and-Pop Approach

In declaring the Mom-and-Pop Approach fundamentally limited in its ability to address underlying cognitive processes and therefore necessarily incapable of facilitating generalized improvements in functioning, Sohlberg and Raskin's (1996) criticism, summarized earlier, simply begs the theoretical question at issue. Let us again use parents and children as an analogy: When parents use highly concrete routines to facilitate organized behavior around bath time for a toddler, they do not thereby consign the toddler to a life of dependence on that rigid bathtime routine. In contrast, the parent is doing what parents for centuries have done instinctively, namely helping the child to act, talk, and think in an organized manner, systematically broadening and loosening the organizational routines as the child gradually progresses from being a highly concrete and dependent thinker to being an increasingly abstract and independent thinker. That is, parents systematically facilitate the development of their child's internal representations of event sequences (and other knowledge structures) from concrete routines to increasingly abstract scripts—and they use appropriate scaffolding procedures to achieve this goal. This is cognitive development from a social-interactionist perspective and at no point is decontextualized, process-specific training required. In behavioral terms, parents use natural general case training, promoting rapid acquisition of associations between stimulus *classes* and response classes within natural environments.

Figure 1–6 presents horns of another dilemma. Unlike the dilemma represented in Figure 1–1, this a happy dilemma, indicated by the smile on the bull's face. The bull is smiling because both of its horns are positive outcomes. Using the Mom-and-Pop Approach in cognitive, behavioral, and communication rehabilitation, either transfer occurs or it does not (or, more properly, either there is very little transfer, or there is considerable transfer). If there is very little transfer, at least the individual has something positive to show for the hours of intervention, namely a skill or behavior that is useful in the specific functional contexts

HORN #1:
Minimal generalization
is possible

HORN #2:
Significant generalization
is possible

However, the individual gains functional skills in meaningful specific contexts

The individual gains functional skills in many meaningful contexts

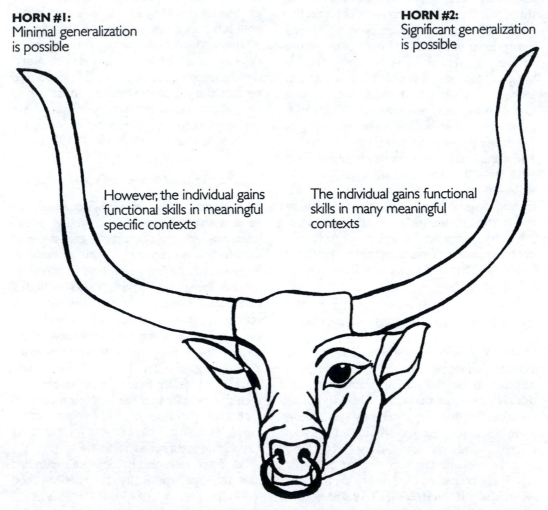

Figure 1–6. A constructive dilemma: positive rehabilitation outcomes with contextualized intervention regardless of the individual's potential for generalization. This bull is smiling because both horns of the dilemma represent positive outcomes.

in which it was acquired. This is a good thing. If there is considerable transfer, or if considerable transfer can be facilitated with effort, so much the better.

With the Wimbledon Approach, if there is very little transfer, or if transfer essentially requires starting over in the natural environment, nothing positive has been accomplished with the decontextualized intervention. This is precisely the unfortunate situation we observe with many of the individuals with chronic cognitive, social, and behavioral disability we serve in community settings. Reports from rehabilitation programs typically describe the individual's positive responses to treatment, based on improved test scores or improved performance of training tasks in those medical settings. Unfortunately, in our work we observe graduates of excellent rehabilitation programs who are failing in school, in social life, or on the job and who require services and supports in those settings, including training and support for everyday people in those settings. The tragic reality is that resources may be exhausted before this need is recognized.

Managed Care: Economic Forces Mandating the Mom-and-Pop Approach

An *apparently* reasonable resolution of these conflicting approaches to generalization in cognitive and behavioral rehabilitation after TBI would be to provide intensive process-specific cognitive retraining, using specialized training tasks, and intensive behavior training in analog training settings, followed by intensive generalization training in natural settings with personally meaningful tasks and routines. Unfortunately, the fierce and growing constraints on funding for rehabilitation rule this option out for most people. Except in rare cases, extensive, labor-intensive decontextualized retraining exhausts available funding, leaving few resources for the critical job of establishing supports in real-world contexts and expertly improving knowledge, competence, and skills within those con-

texts. Schmidt (1997) described a response to the challenge of managed care, outcome-oriented rehabilitation, which is consistent with the themes of this book in its call for early consideration of the patient's discharge destination, identification of skills and supports needed in the discharge environment, functional assessment and intervention in relation to those identified situation-relative skills, and early and ongoing training of the primary support people in the patient's eventual setting.

The Mom-and-Pop Approach Versus Wimbledon Approach in Other Fields

The Mom-and-Pop versus Wimbledon conflict persists in many areas of intervention. In the field of autism, for example, heated controversies rage between those who promote the use of massed, decontextualized, discrete learning trials to teach behaviors such as isolated components of language comprehension and expression (e.g., Lovaas, 1977) and those who promote a contextualized approach. Koegel and Koegel (1995), former colleagues of Lovaas, rejected his discrete trial approach and developed their Natural Language Paradigm approach largely because of their observation of chronic failure of generalization and maintenance using decontextualized practice. Similarly, many authorities among behaviorally oriented specialists in developmental disabilities promote the use of natural communication contexts as the proper setting for teaching communication alternatives to challenging behavior, again because of the positive impact on generalization and maintenance (DePaepe, Reichle, & O'Neill, 1993; O'Neill & Reichle, 1993). In Chapter 7 we summarize some of the research that has led authorities in the field of social skills training to intensify their efforts to contextualize intervention in the interest of increasing the likelihood of an ecologically meaningful outcome. Increasingly, specialists in language disorders in children have found intensive use of natural communication routines with natural communication partners to be an effective approach to intervention for children with language delays and disorders (Nelson et al., 1996; MacDonald, 1989).

In vocational rehabilitation, the supported work movement was motivated in large part by the frequent failure of generalization to actual work sites of gains made as a result of intensive vocational training not associated with the setting or tasks of the individual's actual work. For adults with TBI, promising results have been reported when the focus of intervention switches to supporting the individual at the work site (Wehman, West, Kregel, Sherron, & Kreutzer, 1995). For example, Curl and colleagues (1996) reported positive and cost-effective results using coworkers as the source of job site support for adults with TBI. The parallel "supported education" or inclusion movement in special education has a similar research foundation in the difficulties of generalization and maintenance. In our discussion of cognitive rehabilitation as *supported cognition* (Ylvisaker & Feeney, 1996), we capitalize on these analogies in describing and illustrating an approach to cognitive rehabilitation that begins with intensive supports in context, with the goal of ultimately withdrawing the supports as the individual becomes independent, or increasing the difficulty level of tasks, or both.

Although difficulties with generalization are especially pronounced among people with disability, especially those with general cognitive weakness or specific frontal lobe injury and its associated concreteness and inflexibility, there is mounting evidence of surprising limitations in generalization and maintenance among people with no disability, including bright college students. For example, Singley and Anderson (1989) presented pessimistic results of careful studies of transfer of cognitive skill among college students learning calculus. Similarly, the Writing Across the Curriculum movement on college campuses, analogous in important ways to the supported employment movement in vocational rehabilitation, is based on evidence that writing

skills acquired in freshman composition are frequently not maintained over time and transferred to writing tasks in other aspects of the college curriculum. Within this framework, appropriately trained professors of history, philosophy, economics, and other subjects become facilitators of improved writing just as appropriately trained everyday people become facilitators of improved skills in contextualized rehabilitation, sensitive to human limitations in generalization and maintenance.

Functional Intervention Respectful of Mom-and-Pop's Advice on Generalization

In our work with children and adults with TBI, we have become increasingly convinced of the value of contextualizing intervention from the earliest possible stages and collaborating as much as possible with individuals in identifying their functional needs and solutions to their problems. Context includes the settings in which intervention is provided, the people in those settings, and the intervention activities themselves (Fey, 1986). This book is rich in illustrations of intervention provided within natural contexts or everyday routines. When we worked in pediatric inpatient rehabilitation, for example, we made every attempt to deliver cognitive, behavioral, language, and academic intervention in classroom settings, using materials and tasks natural to those settings. Furthermore, we attempted to create partnerships with everyday people, including parents, so that everyday interaction, during inpatient rehabilitation and beyond, could be as therapeutic as possible. When specific cognitive processes were targeted, such as selective attention or speed of processing, we sought to contextualize the intervention with relevant content, such as educational software or other natural academic tasks. Analogous efforts were made with adults, but in the context of vocational, social, and daily living activities relevant to the adults in question.

In their discussion of generalization in TBI rehabilitation, Sohlberg and Raskin (1996) presented five principles, largely derived from the classical work of Stokes and Baer (Baer, 1981; Stokes & Baer, 1977) on the subject of generalization in behavioral training. In our judgment, these principles are sound, but need to be expanded and can be used to support an approach to rehabilitation with a greater focus on context than that advocated by Sohlberg and Raskin. Their five principles are: (1) "Actively plan for and program generalization from the beginning of the treatment process" (p. 67). Clinicians of varied theoretical persuasions agree that it is no longer acceptable to provide training in a laboratory or clinical setting and hope for the best. (2) "Identify reinforcements in the natural environment" (p. 68). Using a functional, contextualized approach from early in rehabilitation, reinforcements (and consequences generally) are natural and logical consequences of the individual's behavior. (3) "Program stimuli common to both training environments and the real world" (p. 68). Others have highlighted the need for meaningful activities in training as a prerequisite for generalization in brain injury rehabilitation (Toglia, 1990). When training tasks *are* real-world tasks—that is, when intervention occurs largely within everyday routines—this requirement is necessarily met. General case training in natural environments meets conditions for both stimulus and response generalization. When stimuli are allowed to vary within reasonable limits, as they do in everyday contexts, the likelihood is increased that the individual will learn to respond to a meaningful *stimulus class*, rather than a restricted stimulus. Similarly, when varied responses are encouraged, as they tend to be in everyday routines, a *response class* is trained, rather than a single rigid response.

(4) "Use sufficient examples when conducting therapy" (p. 69). People with impaired learning, including many with TBI, require a great deal of practice to master a skill or acquire information. Within a discrete trial, decontextualized training paradigm, sufficient numbers of learning trials are ensured because specialized trainers create the needed number of learning trials in their training sessions. This demand for large numbers of learning trials is one of the justifications frequently offered for using computer training in cognitive rehabilitation. Within a contextualized approach, achieving the needed number and variety of practices depends largely on the level of training and support provided to the everyday people in the life of the person with disability. This book contains several case illustrations in which the thousands of needed learning trials were built into daily routines, thereby creating effective and cost-effective rehabilitation. However, collaboration with everyday people is a necessary component of this approach. (5) "Select a method for measuring generalization" (p. 70). Within a functional, contextualized approach to rehabilitation, the only valid measure of success is meaningfully improved performance of real-world tasks in real-world settings.

Sohlberg and Raskin's (1996) application of Stokes and Baer's principles of generalization to brain injury rehabilitation is useful, but insufficient. Beyond its rather timid embrace of everyday routines as a context for training, their discussion misses the rich history of educational and clinical research associated with the development of metacognitive knowledge and cognitive strategy intervention. Beginning with the seminal work of Flavell and his colleagues in the 1960s, a major field of inquiry has evolved over the past 30 years, emphasizing the learner's understanding of the need for learning, active engagement in the process of learning and development, and correct attribution of the locus of responsibility for success or failure in task completion (Flavell, Miller, & Miller, 1993). Early studies of the effectiveness of strategy training in regular and special education typically showed improved performance on training tasks, but little generalization and maintenance. An approach to strategy instruction that emphasizes the need to contextualize the intervention, to provide intense and long-term intervention, and to help learners understand their limitations, the value of being strategic, and their responsibility in achieving success with strategic behavior has evolved out of these early experiments (Pressley, 1993, 1995).

In brain injury rehabilitation, a similar evolution of intervention paradigms from clinic-based training to contextualized training with a problem-solving or metacognitive focus, seems to have been made about 20 years later and for similar reasons (Thöne, 1996). For example, Lawson and Rice (1989) taught memory strategies to an adolescent with TBI who successfully used them when cued, but never used them spontaneously. However, after an executive system training program, in which he was taught to analyze task demands, select an appropriate strategy, and evaluate its effectiveness, he began to use strategies spontaneously and continued to do so 6 months later. We return to this executive function theme in Chapter 4.

Summary of Generalization and Maintenance

Success of rehabilitation for people with chronic disability in the areas of functioning addressed in this book is meaningful improvement in performance of everyday tasks within the context of a generally satisfying life chosen by the individual with TBI. A review of issues and trends in the study of generalization, from both cognitive and behavioral perspectives, leads us to an approach supported also by the vygotskyan theoretical principles reviewed earlier, by the funding constraints within which rehabilitation professionals now operate, and by our experience with large numbers of children and adults with chronic disability after TBI.

FORMULATING A NEW PERSPECTIVE ON IMPAIRMENT, DISABILITY, AND HANDICAP IN THE CONTEXT OF ROUTINE-BASED INTERVENTION

The approach to rehabilitation presented in this chapter and illustrated throughout the book yields a fresh formulation of rehabilitation in relation to the World Health Organization's classification system (WHO, 1980). An *impairment* is the reduction in ability directly tied to the physical injury. For example, language impairment associated with damage to the dominant hemisphere may include severely restricted ability to retrieve words on command or when needed to express a thought. *Disability*, which may be associated with the impairment, refers to reduced ability to successfully perform functions that are important in life. For example, people with impaired word-retrieval systems may have difficulty reciting in class and maintaining a fluid conversation. In this sense, disability results from the relation between the impairment and the demands of the person's everyday tasks.

Handicap refers to the individual's social loss as a result of the disability, including loss of work, friends, living situation, avocational pursuits, community mobility, and the like. For example, an individual with word-retrieval problems would be severely handicapped if he or she wished to resume work as a trial attorney or sales representative. In contrast, this impairment and associated disability may not be handicapping for a laborer or craftsperson whose job requires minimal verbal expression and whose chosen avocational and social life is relatively devoid of language-intensive activities. Thus, handicap results from a complex relation among the underlying impairment, the associated functional disability, and the expectations and reactions of—and supports provided by—people in the environment.

The Tradition in Rehabilitation

The tradition in cognitive and communication rehabilitation has been initially to engage people in remedial exercises designed to reduce their primary, neurologically based impairment, with the ultimate goal of reducing disability and handicap as a result of the elimination of or reduction in underlying impairment. For example, if cognitive exercises are effective in substantially reducing attentional impairment, or if language exercises are effective in substantially reducing verbal impairment, the individual may be able to succeed in school, at work, on the job, and in social life with no need to direct intervention efforts to specific behaviors in those specific contexts. Theoretically, this is an ideal approach to rehabilitation, because reduction in the underlying impairment holds the potential to reduce associated disability and handicap in every setting and every functional task the individual may face. Unfortunately, cumulative experience with individuals with TBI as well as with other disability groups suggests that chronic cognitive and language impairments are not so easily overcome.

In cases in which the impairment stubbornly resists remedial efforts, the focus in traditional rehabilitation then shifted to some combination of two intervention approaches designed to reduce the disability and associated handicap without necessarily affecting the underlying impairment. (a) In some cases, individuals can be trained to use strategies to compensate for the residual impairment. For example, people with persisting memory impairment may learn encoding strategies or may use external memory systems to succeed in functional tasks despite their ongoing impairment. (b) In some cases, individuals can acquire specific functional skills needed to succeed in school, work, or daily living, again without necessarily influencing the severity of the impairment.

Finally, when disability and associated handicap in important functional domains persist after intensive training in compensatory strategies and specific functional skills, as they often do, efforts are then made to overcome the disability and accompanying handicap by modifying the individual's tasks, the environment, and possibly also others' expectations for the individual's performance, thereby reducing handicap, without necessarily affecting disability or impairment.

A New Perspective

As we see it, an advantage of the perspective we present in this book is that it provides a framework within which impairment, disability, and handicap can be addressed simultaneously. That is, when routine performance of everyday tasks is appropriately supported by others (thereby reducing handicap and disability) and by the strategic behavior of the individual (further reducing disability), the individual is afforded rich opportunities to practice performance of important tasks and, at the same time "exercise" cognitive, executive system, communication, and behavioral self-regulation processes and systems. This contextualized exercise holds the promise of reducing impairment, if reduction of impairment is possible, while also reducing disability and handicap. In this respect, rehabilitation parallels normal development in that young children "exercise" cognitive, executive system, and language processes, like memory, planning, and organization, as well as strategic behavior, in everyday interactions and performance of everyday tasks, particularly when good coaching and mediation is provided by their everyday communication partners.

For example, when preschoolers pleasantly chat with their parents about interesting past events, all of the following occur simultaneously: (a) The parents understand the child's limitations and carry much of the burden for remembering events, organizing them in some reasonable way, and providing explanations for events that need explaining. In these respects, environmental compensations are present for the child, which eliminate the potential *handicap* that would otherwise be present because of the young child's weakness in the areas of memory and organization. (b) The parents model retrieval strategies, helping the child learn that it is useful to throw special effort into remembering and that there are specific procedures (strategies) that are helpful. Furthermore, the practice inherent in daily conversations about the past helps a child become better at this specific task. In these ways, *disability* is reduced by helping a child succeed at a specific task despite immaturity in the cognitive processes of organization and memory. (c) Finally, these conversations are ideal contexts within which to improve the underlying cognitive processes themselves, thereby reducing the *impairment*—that is, improving the child's neurologically based processes so that he or she is able to deal more effectively with a broad domain of tasks that engage organization and memory (see Chapter 5).

In summary, it is not necessary to proceed in a sequential and, in our judgment, inefficient manner, from impairment-oriented to disability-oriented to handicap-oriented intervention. Within the vygotskyan framework that we have described and illustrated throughout this book, intervention within everyday routines has the immediate effect of reducing handicap, but may also be as efficient as any alternative intervention at reducing disability and impairment, that is, at building functional skills, facilitating strategic behavior, and improving underlying cognitive, communication, and self-regulatory processes. This theme is not necessarily applicable to sensory and motor rehabilitation, where it is often useful to block compensations and force the use of the impaired function or body part.

PUTTING THE PIECES TOGETHER: A REVIEW OF INTERVENTION PREMISES

Having described a functional approach to intervention for people with combined executive, cognitive, behavioral, and communication disability after TBI, placed it in a theoretical context, and considered it from the critical perspective of generalization and maintenance, we present in this section a summary of the premises that drive our work in rehabilitation. These guiding principles are derived from our experience with several hundred children and adults with brain injury, from relevant theoretical work, including that of Vygotsky, from the limited efficacy research in TBI rehabilitation, and from the larger efficacy literatures with other disability groups.

General Intervention Premises

Several of our premises apply equally to intervention directed at executive function, cognitive, behavioral, and communication issues.

PREMISE 1: *A critical component of assessment for planning intervention is that which occurs in natural contexts, is ongoing and collaborative, and involves testing hypotheses regarding the individual's performance and what can be done to improve it.* In Chapter 3 we define and illustrate an approach to assessment that is closely associated with a functional, everyday routine-based approach to intervention.

PREMISE 2: *The most effective intervention occurs in meaningful contexts and is designed to influence routines in those contexts.* Several of the theoretical and practical considerations presented in this chapter support this premise, a corollary of which is that everyday people in the individual's environment, including direct care staff, family members, and friends, are critical providers of services and supports. Therefore, rehabilitation specialists have as one of their primary responsibilities the job of teaching everyday people how to provide supports, enough to maintain the individual's success, not so much as to produce learned helplessness (see Chapter 8).

PREMISE 3: *Brain injury rehabilitation requires an integrative, collaborative approach to intervention.* Although we have divided the intervention section of this book into four chapters, addressing executive functions, cognition, communication, and behavior, we repeatedly remind the reader of the dangers inherent in arbitrarily separating the four identified domains. The individuals who serve as case material in each of the intervention chapters clearly illustrate the necessity of integrating professional perspectives and collaborating with other professionals and everyday people alike.

PREMISE 4: *Effective intervention simultaneously addresses impairment, disability, and handicap.* In the previous section, we suggest a way of understanding our approach to rehabilitation as simultaneously addressing impairment, disability, and handicap.

PREMISE 5: *In the absence of meaningful engagement in chosen life activities, all interventions will ultimately fail.* Rehabilitation in the areas of function addressed in this book is more than the mechanical application of intervention procedures designed to improve isolated components of function. Effective rehabilitation requires that specialists play the role of consultant to people seeking satisfying lives. In the absence of reasonable satisfaction and the motivation associated with achieving personally meaningful goals, rehabilitation efforts amount to very little.

PREMISE 6: *Professionals must move beyond narrow medical and training models of intervention.* Many of the rehabilitative practices described in this book will seem foreign to professionals who understand their contribution as analogous to the curative treatments delivered by surgeons or the training regimens of animal trainers. In Chapter 8 we outline a variety of metaphors capable of illuminating aspects of the work of rehabilitation professionals, including coach, consultant, and master craftsperson. Our point is not that there is one metaphor that is correct, but rather that rehabilitation professionals should be conscious of the power of typically unconscious metaphors and flexibly construct their posture in relation to the needs of the people they serve to best meet those needs.

Specific Intervention Premises: Behavioral and Psychosocial Intervention

PREMISE 1: *There are three main categories of reasons for people behaving in ways that are unacceptable to others: Can't do, won't do, and don't do.* (1) Some people do not know how to do what is expected of them ("can't do because they don't know"). (2) Some people are oppositional and defiant (perhaps justifiably) and refuse to do what they know is acceptable to others ("won't do"). (3) Some people simply don't do what they know is acceptable to others because of a lack of inhibition, lack of initiation, or misreading of the social situation ("don't do"). Many people with developmental social skill deficits fall into a mix of categories 1 and 2. Many people with TBI, particularly those with frontal lobe injury, fall into category 3, possibly mixed with 1 and 2.

PREMISE 2: *Behavioral intervention begins with a functional analysis of the target behaviors.* The following questions must be answered: What antecedents seem to be associated with the behavior? What consequences seem to be associated with the behavior? What purpose does the behavior seem to serve for the individual? Is the behavior of others, including their communication behavior, designed to increase or decrease the unwanted behavior?

PREMISE 3: *Effective intervention for individuals with TBI focuses more on antecedents than on consequences.* For reasons described in Chapter 6, traditional consequence-oriented intervention must give way to antecedent-focused intervention for many people with TBI. Antecedent-focused interventions include ensuring generally positive setting events, generating positive behavioral momentum before introducing difficult or stressful tasks, providing people with ample opportunities for choice and control, eliminating provocation for negative behavior (including unreasonable demands), ensuring orientation to setting and task (e.g., making plans, having a daily routine), teaching functional alternatives to negative behavior (including escape communication), establishing alternative scripts, helping the individual to control his or her own antecedents, reducing stress by ensuring that tasks can be accomplished, helping the individual identify and manage levels of anxiety (e.g., teach relaxation), and helping the individual to decrease sensitivity to stressors.

PREMISE 4: *Behavioral rehabilitation after brain injury is designed to facilitate progress from external control to internal self-control of behavior.* Like young children, people in the early stages of improvement after severe brain injury require substantial external control of their behavior. Also like children, the goal is to reduce external control and increase internal control as quickly as possible. When intensive external controls persist beyond the period of their usefulness, the likely result is learned helplessness or oppositionality or some combination of the two.

PREMISE 5: *Changing behavior after the early stages of recovery often requires teaching communication alternatives to unacceptable behavior.* Challenging behavior that begins as reflexive behavior may become part of the individual's communication repertoire if it results in desirable consequences (e.g., escape from aversive situations). In such cases, the individual should be helped to substitute a more acceptable communication alternative for the challenging behavior.

PREMISE 6: *Effective intervention occurs in social-communicative contexts and is designed to influence routines in those contexts.* This premise is supported by all of the considerations elaborated in this chapter.

PREMISE 7: *Behavior problems and cognitive problems are often inseparable after TBI; behavioral intervention requires attention to cognitive supports.* When challenging behavior is associated with reactions to failure and frustration due to cognitive limitations, appropriate management addresses the primary cognitive problems and the supports needed to turn failure into success.

PREMISE 8: *Crisis management is not behavior management.* Staff and everyday people must know how to manage behavioral crises. However, it is a serious mistake to confuse crisis management with behavior management, the latter referring to procedures designed to facilitate positive and successful behavior rather than procedures designed to react to negative behavior.

PREMISE 9: *The best behavior management after TBI is prevention of long-term behavioral consequences.* Because behavior problems after TBI are often a result of growing failure and frustration or unnecessary restrictions on choice making, they are often preventable with proactive measures.

Specific Intervention Premises: Cognitive and Executive System Intervention

PREMISE 1: *Executive system consequences of TBI are often delayed and may grow over time.* Delayed onset of disability associated with executive system impairment is particularly common in children, due in part to slow maturation of prefrontal parts of the brain.

PREMISE 2: *Cognitive problems after TBI (e.g., problems with attention, perception, organization, memory, reasoning, problem-solving) are often interrelated and closely associated with executive system impairment.* Although components of cognition are often separated for analytic and assessment purposes, they function in an integrated and interactive manner in everyday life and develop in an integrated and interactive manner in normal child development. These realities recommend an integrative approach to cognitive rehabilitation apparently inconsistent with the recent fascination with disassembling cognition and targeting components separately and in a hierarchical manner.

PREMISE 3: *Normal development of executive functions in children yields insights for intervention.* Development of executive control over cognitive and other functions begins early (in infancy), continues into adulthood, and is an inextricable component of the development of those functions. These developmental principles recommend an early and growing focus on executive functions in rehabilitation. Furthermore, just as development of executive self-regulation of behavior in childhood can be understood as occurring within apprenticeship relations between children and adults, so redevelopment after TBI can also be understood within everyday apprenticeship relations with clinicians and everyday people.

PREMISE 4: *In related areas of disability intervention that have a longer history than TBI rehabilitation, there has been a steady move away from an exclusive specific skills focus toward an integrated executive system orientation.* In the fields of developmental disabilities and learning disabilities, investigators have increasingly recommended addressing components of chronic disability within the context of personally relevant everyday academic, vocational, social, and self-care activities. For reasons outlined earlier, this book is filled with illustrations of comparable interventions for people with chronic disability after acquired brain injury.

SUMMARY

Our primary goal in this book is to describe and illustrate a functional and richly contextualized approach to intervention for children and adults with cognitive, executive system, communication, and behavioral impairment after TBI. The case illustrations, drawn from our work in a variety of settings, concretely show how the approach is implemented within the routines of everyday life. In this introductory chapter, we have described the principles underlying our approach to intervention and suggested a theoretical rationale for embracing these principles. In our judgment, good clinical decision making is exactly this process of creatively applying important principles to individual people with individual needs in specific contexts of life. This creative process results in slightly different intervention plans for each individual. We hope that readers will gain insight from the application of principles to the individuals we describe, thereby putting themselves in a position to apply the same principles to the unique circumstances of the individuals with whom they work.

CHAPTER 2

Traumatic Brain Injury: Functional Outcome and Its Neuropsychological Basis

I n this chapter, we discuss common consequences of TBI in the areas of executive functions, cognition, behavior, and communication. In addition, we suggest a pathophysiologic basis for many of the types of disability associated with TBI. Several qualifying comments are in order. First, the totality of damage to the brain caused by external trauma is notoriously difficult to localize (Brazzeli et al., 1994). Thus, in individual cases, neurodiagnostic information from computed axial tomography (CT) or magnetic resonance imaging (MRI) scans may not give a completely accurate picture of tissue damage, making a knowledge of brain-behavior relationships a partial guide at best to outcome (Diamond, 1991; Kertesz, 1994). Second, in several areas crucial to understanding the consequences of TBI, research remains at an early stage. For example, neuroscientists continue to work with a variety of competing models of prefrontal lobe and frontolimbic functioning (Grafman, Holyoak, & Boller, 1995).

Third, consequences of brain injury are rarely direct. The phrase *brain-person-world-relationships* invites more fruitful reflection on the consequences of brain injury than the more common and superficial phrase *brain-behavior relationships*. For example, it is well established that identical brain lesions in different people can have importantly different consequences, due to individual differences in neural architecture and to potentially major differences in the individuals themselves, including their age, preinjury knowledge, skill, personality, and resilience, and their support systems after the injury (Asarnow, Satz, Light, & Newmann, 1991; Brown, Chadwick, Shaffer, Butler, & Travis, 1981; Cockrell, 1991; Eames, 1988; Eslinger et al., 1997; Fletcher, Ewing-Cobbs, Miner, & Levin, 1990; Gaultieri & Cox, 1991; Hart & Jacobs, 1993). Similarly, a given lesion in one individual can have importantly different consequences in the context of different life circumstances. Thus, wisdom dictates caution in predicting outcome from knowledge of the lesion alone.

Fourth, knowledge of brain function and pathophysiology is neither necessary nor sufficient for implementing highest quality rehabilitation services and supports. Some of the most effective rehabilitationists with whom we have worked over the years had little knowledge of brain function and dysfunction, but were experienced teachers and great problem solvers, with an abundance of the attributes that define effective helping professionals: intuitive, optimistic, charismatic, respectful, and enthusiastic about collaborating with other professionals and everyday people. Conversely, thorough knowledge of brain function and consequences of damage is no guarantee of insight regarding how to help the injured person improve functioning and achieve meaningful goals. To paraphrase Kant, scientific knowledge and theoretical models without clinical experience and insight are hollow.

Having made these qualifications, we urge those involved in the rehabilitation and education of people with TBI to acquire a rich understanding of brain function and impairment. Generally, understanding central tendencies in outcome after TBI and, more importantly, understanding probable issues associated with specific lesions alerts clinicians to possibilities that must be thoroughly explored. For this reason, professionals with specialized insight into the consequences of specific types of injury can be invaluable contributors to collaborative teams of people seeking to provide effective and efficient interventions for people with TBI.

EPIDEMIOLOGIC AND PATHOPHYSIOLOGIC FACTORS

Brain injury is the leading cause of death and disability in children and young adults in industrialized countries. About 500,000 people are hospitalized each year with brain injury in the United States of America, and probably several times that number experience concussion with no hospitalization, but possibly transient neurologic symptoms that could interfere for a time with daily activities. It is estimated that between 50,000 and 100,000 people each year in the United States of America have a traumatic brain injury that results in persisting disability, with roughly one-third of the total children or adolescents (Annegers, 1983; Annegers, Grabow, Kurland, & Lewis, 1980).

Epidemiologic and pathophysiologic information is of marginal relevance to clinicians or teachers seeking to effectively serve one or two or a small number of unique individuals. For example, the common TBI profiles described later in this section are of little use to staff serving a 5-year-

old female who was precocious before her injury, who was being raised in advantageous social and economic circumstances, and whose brain injury resulted from a lawn dart that penetrated into the posterior sections of her brain. Features of her case deviate from important central tendencies in the population in virtually every respect. Rehabilitation and education specialists must construct their services and supports around her unique needs, circumstances, and goals. Indeed, this prescription (or metaprescription) holds for every individual with TBI. There is and can be no such thing as a TBI curriculum. However, knowledge of population central tendencies at least creates a general conceptual map that may assist practitioners in their exploration of potentially unfamiliar territory.

Preinjury Factors

Not everyone has an equal probability of having a brain injury. The classic profile is that of an adolescent or young adult male who was something of a risk taker before the injury (and therefore more likely to place himself in harm's way), may have overused or abused alcohol and recreational drugs, may have had academic, social, and vocational difficulties before the injury, and more likely than not can be found toward the lower end of the socioeconomic spectrum. Younger children are also at greater risk for injury than are middle-aged adults, although the ratio of male to female is less lopsided in children than in young adults (roughly 4:1 male-to-female ratio in 20-year-olds, Annegers et al., 1980).

Many clinicians and researchers have reported that close to 50% of their patients with TBI had been identified as having academic difficulties or weak social adjustment before their injury (Haas, Cope, & Hall, 1987). It is possible that a mild, possibly undiagnosed underlying neurologic impairment accounts in some cases for preinjury academic, social, and vocational difficulties and also predisposes the individual to injury. Roughly half of the patients admitted to hospitals after TBI are intoxicated on admission (Brismar, Engstrom, & Rydberg, 1983; Corrigan, Rust, & Lamb-Hart, 1995; Rutherford, 1977), suggesting a high rate of alcohol abuse in this group. In many cases, young people with TBI were impulsive, hyperactive, and oppositional before the injury (Dalby & Obrzut, 1991; McKinlay & Brooks, 1984; Pelco, Sawyer, Duffield, Prior, & Kinsella, 1992). Previous brain injury also increases the risk of subsequent injury; those with two injuries increase their risk for a third eightfold over the general population (Annegars et al., 1980).

In adolescents and young adults, car and motorcycle crashes account for the vast majority of head injuries in most localities during peacetime. In specific high-risk communities, assault may play a leading role. Older adults and young children have an increased risk of TBI from falls, and disproportionate numbers of very young children are injured as a result of abuse.

Clinicians must take care not to overinterpret risk factors and central tendencies in the population of people with TBI. In clinical practice, for every adolescent or young adult male with a history of substance abuse, academic failure, and family conflict, there is a person with TBI who deviates in many important ways from this stereotype. Nevertheless, it is well to underscore the important point that most people with TBI are young, thereby often requiring some type of services or supports for decades after the injury. They also often bring a set of personal or family needs with them into the injury, needs that are often exacerbated by the injury. When legal responsibility for an injury is to be parceled out, Herculean efforts are expended in dissecting preinjury characteristics from consequences of the injury. In contrast, clinicians whose sole concern is intervention are free to assist the individual without needing to distinguish between problems and disability present before the injury and those created by the injury.

Injury Factors

Damage to the brain in traumatic injuries is a function of more than the magnitude of the force applied to the skull. Pathophysiology varies as a function of (1) penetration or nonpenetration of brain tissue; (2) movement or lack of movement of the skull; (3) linear and rotational inertia of brain tissue in relation to skull movement; (4) destructive events secondary to the initial trauma, including hemorrhage, swelling, hypoxia, and other pathologic phenomena unleashed by the primary injury; and (5) complicating injuries elsewhere in the body. Figure 2–1 includes three views of the brain, highlighting areas most vulnerable in TBI: orbitofrontal, medial and anterior-temporal, and dorsolateral frontal. Figure 2–2 depicts the basic anatomical divisions in the cortex.

Mechanisms of Injury

Penetrating and Nonpenetrating Injuries. Injury to the brain acquired sometime after birth (i.e., acquired or noncongenital brain injury) can result from a wide variety of events and conditions. The broadest distinction is that between injuries caused by forces *external* to the skull and those caused by *internal* conditions, such as stroke, tumor, encephalitis, meningitis, toxic encephalopathy, and the like. In this book, we use the term *traumatic brain injury* to refer to injuries with an external etiology, although the assessment and intervention procedures that we describe may be appropriate for individuals with brain injury associated with other causes as well. Among traumatic, or externally caused brain injuries, the major distinction is between *open head injury* (or penetrating brain injury) and *closed head injury* (CHI, or nonpenetrating brain injury). In penetrating brain injuries, the dural lining (the tough outer sheath that protects the brain) is penetrated by a missile (e.g., a bullet) or by a depressed skull fracture. If the individual survives, outcome is largely a function of the trajectory of the missile and the amount of tissue damaged in that trajectory.

Technically, closed head injuries are those in which destructive forces are deliv-

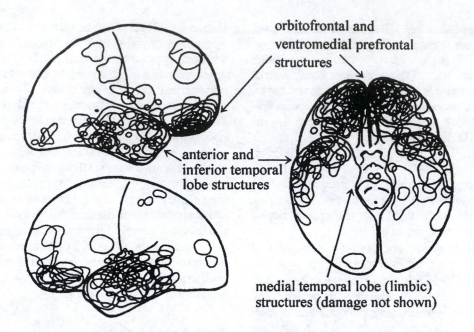

Figure 2–1. This drawing of contusions after traumatic brain injury based on 40 consecutive cases clearly depicts the tendency for maximum pathology in the orbital frontal and temporal regions. (Reprinted with permission from *Pathology of the Central Nervous System*, by J. Courville, 1937, Mountain View: CA: Pacific Publishers.)

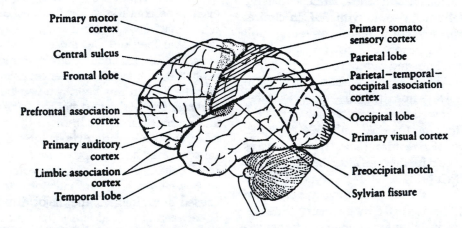

Figure 2–2. The lobe divisions of the human brain and their functional anatomy. (Reprinted by permission of Oxford from *Brain Biochemistry and Brain Disorders*, by P. G. Strange, 1992. Oxford, UK: Oxford Press.)

ered to the brain without penetrating the dura. In a somewhat looser but more helpful sense, closed head injuries are those in which the primary mechanism of damage is a blunt blow to the skull (Levin, Benton, & Grossman, 1982). The primary reason that TBI is a useful diagnostic category is that certain regions of the brain are vulnerable in CHI regardless of site of impact (see later in this section). In peacetime, most traumatic brain injuries are nonpenetrating, and the epidemiologic and outcome profiles currently associated with TBI tend to be those of individuals with CHI.

Nonacceleration and Acceleration Injuries. Nonacceleration injuries, which are relatively rare, occur when a moving object strikes a stationary, restrained head. For example, such an injury occurs when a jack holding a car in position slips and the car falls on a mechanic working below. Although apparently devastating, particularly if the result is a depressed skull fracture, nonacceleration injuries tend to cause much less severe brain injury than acceleration injuries, which paradoxically may have no external sign of injury whatsoever (Pang, 1985).

Acceleration (or acceleration-deceleration) injuries occur when the movement of the skull contributes to destructive forces within the brain. Although in most cases the head strikes or is struck by an object

(e.g., the head hits the windshield, the pavement, or the basement floor), serious damage can occur with no contact whatsoever, as in the case of shaken baby syndrome. When a stationary skull is suddenly accelerated or a moving skull is suddenly decelerated, the brain, which is not affixed to the inner surface of the skull and is subject to its own inertia, compresses against the skull at one side or the other, depending on the acceleration or deceleration force. When acceleration of the skull results from an external blow, the compression of brain tissue and consequent damage at the site of the blow is called a *coup* injury and damage at the opposite side of the brain, caused by the brain's inertia as the skull suddenly stops and the brain continues to move, compressing into the skull, is called a *contrecoup* injury (see Figure 2–3). Impairment associated with such injuries obviously de-

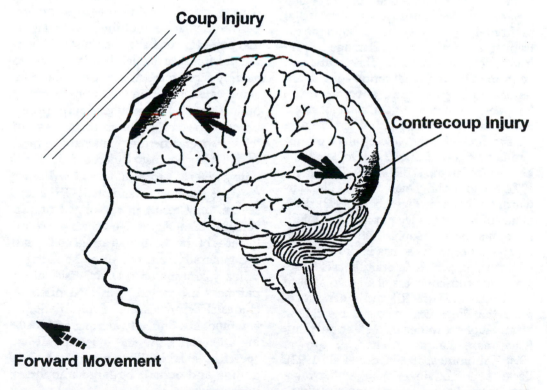

Figure 2–3. A representation of coup injury (i.e., contusion and cavitation at the site of impact) and contrecoup injury (i.e., contusion and cavitation at the opposite side of the brain). (Adapted with permission from *Best Practices in Assessment and Programming for Students with Traumatic Brain Injury*, by William Walker and the North Carolina State Board of Education, 1997. Raleigh, NC: State Board of Education.)

pends on the site of impact and, as such, cannot explain the great many commonalities among people with severe TBI.

More ominous than the linear acceleration forces producing coup and contrecoup injury are *rotational* acceleration forces, which account for many of the common sites of focal injury in CHI and also for diffuse axonal injury (DAI), a hallmark of CHI. Most head injuries are associated with acceleration and deceleration forces that create rotational inertia. For example, at the moment a person's head strikes the windshield in a car crash, he or she is likely turning reflexively from the point of impact. Thus, when the movement of the skull is abruptly halted by that impact, the brain continues to rotate within the skull.

These rotational inertial forces create vulnerabilities where brain tissue is adjacent to sharp ridges or other bony prominences on the inner surface of the skull (e.g., the sharp wings of the sphenoid bone separating frontal from temporal cortex; the crista galli separating right from left ventromedial prefrontal cortex). Figure 2–1 shows the extraordinary frequency of damage to prefrontal cortex—especially orbitofrontal and ventromedial prefrontal cortex—and to anterior and inferior temporal cortex. It has long been known that the frontal lobes are the most vulnerable parts of the brain in CHI in both children and adults (Adams, Graham, Scott, Parker, & Doyle, 1980; Levin Goldstein, Williams, & Eisenberg, 1991; Mendelsohn, Levin, Bruce, Lilly, Harward, Culhane, & Eigsenberg, 1992). Estimates of the frequency of prefrontal injury have increased as sophistication of neurodiagnostic procedures has improved from CT scanning, which notoriously fails to detect some consequences of CHI, to MRI to functional MRI (fMRI) and other procedures that dynamically measure blood flow or metabolism rather than static anatomy (Chapman, Kairiss, Keenan, & Brown, 1990; Cummings, 1993; Oder et al., 1992). Because most of the serious executive function, cognitive, behavioral, and communication problems after TBI are associated with prefrontal or frontolimbic damage, it

is critical for clinicians to understand the pathophysiologic basis for the extreme vulnerability of these critical structures. As representatives of the population of people with TBI, most of the individuals described in this book had some combination of frontal lobe and limbic area damage. A comparison of the composite diagram of vulnerable areas in CHI (see Figure 2–1) with the CT scans indicating the lesion location of Damasio's patient Elliot (Figure 2–4) underscores the critical importance of the TBI dilemma and its resolution discussed in Chapter 1.

Rotational inertia also causes widespread stretching and tearing of tissue, especially to subcortical tissue in vulnerable frontal and temporal regions, to the brain stem and reticular activating system, because of its anchoring position as the brain rotates around the axis, and to structures made vulnerable because of differential movement as a function of differential tissue density in adjacent structures (e.g., fornices, periventricular zone of the hypothalamus, and superior cerebellar peduncles). Figure 2–5 illustrates an axonal shearing plane created by rapid rotational acceleration of the skull causing differential movement of brain tissue in areas where bony prominences carry surface brain tissue forward, while deeper structures remain momentarily stationary because of inertia. This type of injury, referred to as *diffuse axonal injury* (DAI), is extremely common in CHI and, if severe, may result in prolonged or irreversible coma. Figure 2–6 shows the consequences of the twisting, tearing, and breaking generally referred to as shearing, a primary contributor to DAI. Persistent impairment associated with DAI often includes slow processing of information in any modality, difficulty alerting and focusing attention, slow and labored gait and speech, easy fatigability, and difficulty integrating and organizing large amounts of information.

Secondary Brain Injury. Emergency treat-

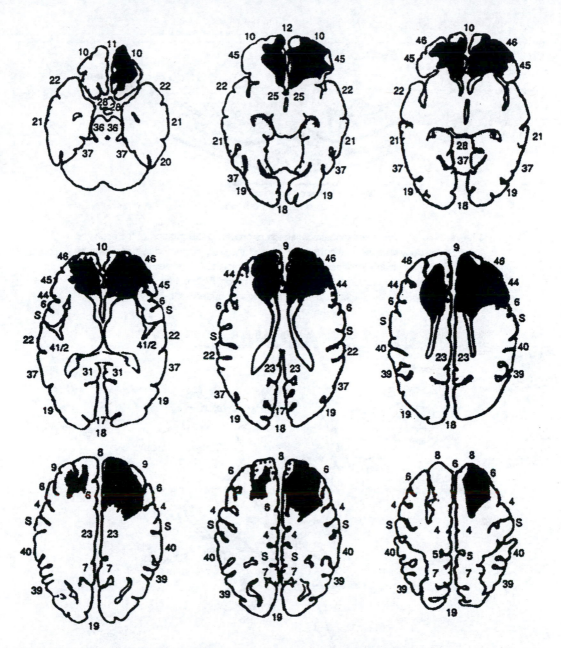

Figure 2–4. Transverse sections through the lesion in the brain of the patient EVR. The most ventral section is at the top left, the most dorsal section at the bottom right. (Reprinted by permission of Lippincott-Raven from "Severe Disturbance of Higher Cognition Following Bilateral Frontal Lobe Ablation: Patient EVR," by P. J. Eslinger and A. R. Damasio, 1985, *Neurology, 35,* 1731–1741.)

ment for people with severe TBI is often focused on monitoring and treating elevated intracranial pressure (ICP). Pressure within the skull, a nonexpandable enclosed space, increases with increases in cranial contents, including blood from ruptured vessels, intracellular water associated with general swelling, and cerebral spinal fluid that does not circulate properly because of swelling (traumatic hydrocephalus). If severe, elevated ICP can cause death. Survivable levels of elevated ICP can cause brain damage and

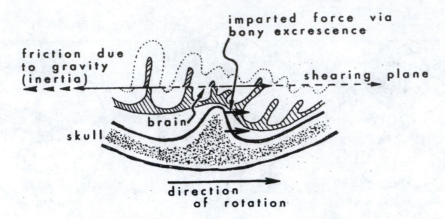

Figure 2–5. Surface shearing occurs when forces propelling the rotation of the brain are imparted by bony prominences in the inner table of the skull. (Reprinted by permission of Butterworth-Heinemann Publishers from "Pathophysiological Correlates of Neurobehavioral Syndromes Following Closed Head Injury," by D. Pang, 1985, p. 14. In M. Ylvisaker, [Ed.], *Head Injury Rehabilitation: Children and Adolescents.* Boston: Butterworth-Heinemann.)

DIFFUSE AXONAL INJURY

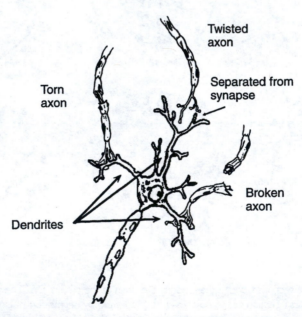

Figure 2–6. Diffuse axonal injury: twisting, tearing, and breaking of axons associated with primary impact damage in traumatic brain injury.

impairment secondary to compression, distortion, and stretching of tissue.

Second, a cascade of negative events typ-ically produces some degree of hypoxic-ischemic damage after severe TBI. The flow of blood to the brain can be disrupted and reduced by elevated ICP, hemorrhages within the brain, and cortical vasospasm. To compound this set of infelicitous conditions, the blood that does manage to reach the brain may be poorly oxygenated because of apparently unrelated respiratory problems associated with the injury. Taken together, these possibilities create a near inevitability of some level of hypoxic injury in severe CHI (Graham, Adams, & Doyle, 1978). Experimental evidence from a variety of sources suggests that the basal ganglia and hippocampus are particularly vulnerable to hypoxic-ischemia injury (Bigler, 1990), with an estimate of hippocampal involvement in approximately 80% of cases of ischemia (Miller, Pentland, & Berrol, 1990). Hippocampal damage secondary to

hypoxia is the likely cause of pervasive explicit and declarative memory problems after TBI (see section on cognitive disability).

Figure 2–7 shows brain structures traditionally considered parts of the limbic system, including the hippocampus, although recent work has questioned the usefulness of the concept of a unified limbic system (LeDoux, 1991, 1993, 1995; Morgan & LeDoux, 1995). LeDoux and others have proposed functional, behavior-regulating subsystems (see later under Behavioral Outcome) that include limbic structures along with specific prefrontal areas and their interconnections (Adolphs, Tranel, Damasio, & Damasio, 1994; Bechara et al., 1995; Cohen & Eichenbaum, 1993; Devinsky & Luciano, 1993; McClelland, McNaughton,

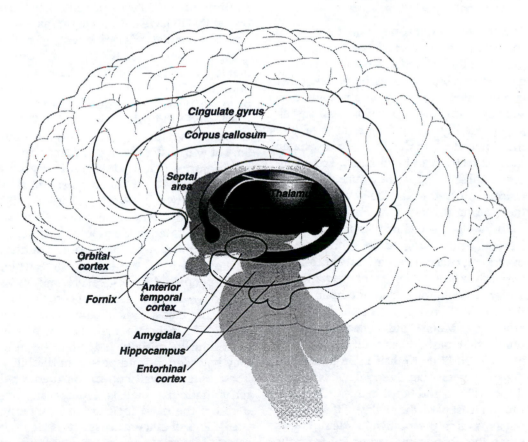

Figure 2–7. The limbic lobe of the cerebrum and structures of the limbic system. (Reprinted by permission of Singular Pubilshing Group from *The Speech Sciences*, by R. D. Kent, 1997, p. 255. San Diego: Singular Publishing Group, Inc.)

& O'Reilly, 1995). For example, the amygdala (traditionally classified as part of the limbic system) has major interconnections with orbitofrontal areas, anterior insula, and temporal poles via the uncinate fasciculus (Aggleston, 1992; Cummings, 1993). This subsystem appears to be involved in interpreting visceral responses to novel stimuli and in inhibiting responses that are not adaptive in specific contexts (Adolphs, Tranel, Damasio, & Damasio, 1995; Allman & Brothers, 1994). This subsystem, like the other major frontolimbic subsystem involving the hippocampus (Eichenbaum & Otto, 1992; Eichenbaum, Otto, & Cohen, 1994; O'Keefe, 1989), is vulnerable in TBI because of the vulnerability of the prefrontal structures to contusion and laceration, of axonal connections to shearing, and of the limbic structures to secondary hypoxic injury (Bigler, 1990).

Other Injuries. People with severe TBI commonly incur other injuries as a result of the event that injured the brain. Internal organ injuries, broken bones, burns, and other complications not only sap physiologic resources during the recovery process, they also potentially create long-term disability that interacts with the disability associated more directly with brain injury. For example, facial scars, apparently minor in importance compared to the life-threatening and life-altering damage to the brain, can profoundly affect social reintegration for adolescents and young adults who have an overriding concern for physical appearance. Similarly, a crushed leg might mean more to a high school athlete than the brain injury that modestly reduced his or her cognitive efficiency. Moore and colleagues (1990) found that individuals with multiple injuries in addition to their brain injury had generally poorer psychosocial outcome than those with no additional injuries. Clinicians must at least place the totality of the individual's losses in perspective in attempting to grasp the phenomenology of TBI from the perspective of the person with the injury.

Other Losses. It is not uncommon for the event that caused the individuals' injuries (e.g., a car crash) to injure or kill others, possibly including family members or friends. Such losses interact with direct consequences of the injury in ways that are difficult to untangle. For example, when children tragically lose one or both parents in the crash, their recovery is inevitably clouded in a way that is different from that of comparably injured children whose parents are available to nurture and support them through the difficult weeks and months after the injury. The same reasoning holds for young adults who lose a friend in the accident, a husband who loses his wife, and a mother who loses her son or daughter.

Severity of Injury

Approximately 10% of patients hospitalized with TBI have a severe injury, as measured by an initial index of severity (e.g., the Glasgow Coma Scale [GCS], length of coma, length of posttraumatic amnesia). Another 10 to 15% of the injuries are judged to be moderate, with the remaining 75 to 80% considered mild (Miller & Jones, 1990). In the case of children, proportions are similar, but with a slightly higher percentage of mild injuries (Kraus, 1995). Although investigators have identified a general relationship between severity of injury and severity of outcome, with more severe injuries associated with more severe long-term disability, there are important outliers on both ends of the severity spectrum. Some people with very severe injuries as judged by extended length of coma or low GCS score enjoy a remarkably positive recovery of function, whereas some people with injuries initially judged to be mild may have serious and persistent disability. These outliers, well known to experienced rehabilitation specialists, dramatically underscore the need for caution in making predictions of outcome based on early indicators of severity.

Miller and Jones (1990) estimated that up to a third of those with mild TBI experience prolonged posttraumatic sequelae (e.g., headache, dizziness, memory and attention problems, irritability, fatigue). In most cases, neurologically based problems resolve within a few weeks. However, if the individual has in the meantime experienced serious educational, vocational, or social failure, real-world problems may long outlive their original neurologic basis. The frequency of such secondary consequences of mild TBI calls for adequate education and counseling of the injured person, family, and possibly other significant people and a safety net system present in the environment to identify problems if they arise and to provide useful accommodations. Ylvisaker, Feeney, and Mullins (1995) described such a system for school-age children and adolescents.

Postinjury Factors

Long-term outcome is influenced by preinjury factors, injury-related factors, and postinjury factors, including the availability of effective early medical treatment, the quality of acute rehabilitation, and long-term supports, including supportive families, schools, work places, and social networks (Alberst & Binder, 1991; Asarnow et al., 1991; Bijur, Haslum, & Golding, 1990; Brooks et al., 1987; Brooks & McKinlay, 1983; Condeluci, 1992; Eames, 1988; Fletcher, Ewing-Cobbs, McLaughlin, & Levin, 1985; Fletcher, Miner, & Ewing-Cobbs, 1987; Goldstein & Levin, 1989; Jacobs, 1990; Jaffe et al., 1993). Studies of children and adolescents have shown that the quality of the family and social environment to which the child returns profoundly influences long-term outcome, particularly in the area of social and behavioral adjustment (Asarnow et al., 1991; Brown et al., 1981; Lucyshyn, Nixon, Glang, & Cooley, 1996; Perrot, Taylor, & Montes, 1991; Taylor et al., 1995). Similarly, adults who return to highly supportive families, friends, and employers enjoy a profound advantage in outcome over those who return to challenging and nonsupportive life circumstances that would place them at risk without the added com-

plication of disability caused by the injury (Hall et al., 1994; Jacobs, 1990; Kaplan, 1990, 1991; Klonoff, Costa, & Snow, 1986; Lezak, 1988; Oddy et al., 1984).

Finally, the individual's psychological reactions and coping style influence outcome in obvious ways (Hinkeldey & Corrigan, 1990; Moore & Stambrook, 1992). Those who manage to retain a resilient and optimistic orientation toward their life and its possibilities are likely to achieve a level of personal success beyond the grasp of those whose persistent anger or depression compound their social and vocational vulnerability and place them at risk for suicide or other serious psychiatric consequences (Klonoff & Lage, 1995).

Delayed Consequences

Researchers and clinicians alike have highlighted the frequency with which disability, particularly in the areas of behavior and psychosocial adjustment and of academic functioning in children, increases over the years following TBI, particularly if frontal lobe injury is involved (Benton, 1991; Eslinger, Damasio, Damasio, & Grattan, 1989; Feeney & Ylvisaker, 1995, 1997; Grattan & Eslinger, 1992; Ylvisaker, 1993; Ylvisaker & Feeney, 1995). Some investigators have emphasized the neurobiological contributors to delayed onset of behavioral symptoms after frontal lobe injury in children (Eslinger, Damasio, Damasio, & Grattan, 1989; Grattan & Eslinger, 1990, 1992; Marlowe, 1989, 1992; Mateer & Williams, 1991). According to this account, the slow anatomic and physiologic development of the frontal lobes provides the biological foundation for gradual maturation of executive or self-regulatory functions (Goldman-Rakic, 1987). This anatomic development of the frontal lobes continues (at a decelerating rate) through the adolescent years, possibly paralleling the ongoing biological development of prefrontal neural systems over that period of development (Diamond, 1991; Thatcher, 1991). Thus it is possible for early damage to yield no observable consequences until the function specifically associated with the injured part of the brain is expected to mature (Case, 1992; Stuss, 1992). For example, a 3-year-old with prefrontal injury who is impulsive, disinhibited, egocentric, labile, volatile, and concrete may be indistinguishable from normally developing peers. However, the same child may appear to have a serious disability at age 6 or 7 if adequate maturation in these areas of functioning has not occurred in the intervening years. Ylvisaker and Feeney (1995) described analogous delayed consequences when the injury occurs in early adolescence.

Delayed consequences of brain injury may also represent a psychological reaction to failure, frustration, and severe restrictions on personal choice (Hart & Jacobs, 1993; Jacobs, 1990). In either case, clinicians must be alert to this possibility and provide early supports in an attempt to prevent growing disability over time. Successful efforts to reverse serious long-term behavior problems in adolescents (Feeney & Ylvisaker, 1995) and to prevent them in children who are known to be vulnerable (see Chapter 6) support a multifactorial explanation of delayed consequences and give reason for optimism in relation to preventing behavior problems before they arise and to reversing downward behavioral spirals that are allowed to begin.

OUTCOME

In this chapter and generally in the book, we have not addressed outcome or rehabilitation from the perspectives of specific medical, motoric, perceptual, or linguistic impairment. In choosing areas of focus, our intent was not to minimize the importance of disability in these areas when such disability exists. Rather, our decisions about content were based on frequency, chronicity, and long-term significance of problem areas across the population of children and adults with TBI, leading to our focus on executive functions, cognition, behavior, and social communication. Furthermore, rehabilitation professionals have available to them an extensive literature in the areas of disability not covered in this book, litera-

ture associated with developmental problems in children and with focal brain injury (e.g., stroke) in adults. Because we only indirectly address academic and vocational themes, we encourage readers to consult texts on TBI-related educational issues (e.g., Glang, Singer, & Todis, 1997; Mira, Tyler, & Tucker, 1988; Rosen & Gerring, 1986; Savage & Wolcott, 1994; Ylvisaker, 1998) and vocational issues (e.g. Kreutzer & Wehman, 1991; Wehman et al., 1993, 1995; Wehman & Kreutzer, 1990). Finally, we say nothing in this chapter about family outcome and we address family services and supports only in a general way in Chapter 8. This omission is probably most problematic, in light of the extraordinary importance of families in shaping long-term outcome and ensuring ongoing positive supports for people with chronic disability (Taylor et al., 1995). In Chapter 8, we underscore the importance of creating a working alliance with families and offer some suggestions to achieve this important goal. Williams and Kay (1991) and Singer, Glang, and Williams (1996) have addressed family reactions, intervention, and support after TBI in a loved one.

EXECUTIVE FUNCTIONS

Executive Functions From a Neuropsychological Perspective

Most generally understood, the executive system includes mental functions involved in formulating goals, planning how to achieve them, carrying out the plans, and revising those plans in response to feedback (Lezak, 1982; Luria, 1966). In this broad sense, the same set of control functions directs deliberate cognitive behavior (e.g., paying attention in the presence of distractions), communication behavior (e.g., planning an effective way to express a complex or sensitive thought), social behavior (e.g., inhibiting aggressive behavior when provoked), academic behavior (e.g., studying for an exam), and vocational behavior (e.g., planning a day at work to complete a large number of assigned tasks). Some investigators restrict their consideration of executive functions to those that relate directly to cognition (i.e., the "cold" aspects of self-regulation; Denckla, 1996). As we use the term, executive functions are those responsible for regulating all aspects of deliberate, nonautomatic, nonroutine behavior.

Recent attempts have been made to organize otherwise unsystematic lists of components of executive functioning. For example, Levin and colleagues (1996) applied factor analytic procedures to results of purported tests of executive functions in a population of children and adolescents with TBI. They derived five factors: conceptual/productivity (e.g., word fluency), planning/execution (e.g., number of broken rules on the Tower of London task), schema (e.g., number of constraint-seeking questions on a 20-question task), cluster (e.g., use of organizational strategies in memory tasks), and inhibition (e.g., false alarm errors on a Go/No-Go task). In contrast, Taylor and colleagues (1996) derived three factors, using similar factor-analytic procedures, but somewhat different tests and a different clinical population: response speed, planning/sequencing, and response inhibition. The weakness of factor analysis, of course, is that results depend entirely on the tests and other tasks selected for administration. Therefore, it is not surprising that critical components of executive functioning, such as self-awareness of strengths and weaknesses, initiation, ongoing monitoring and evaluation of performance, and problem solving in stressful social situations, are not included in either of these lists of factors.

Other investigators have attempted to create organized models of executive functioning directly based on lesion studies and the distinctive profiles of executive system deficits associated with distinct frontal lobe lesions. Several of the authors included in the stimulating collection edited by Grafman, Holyoak, and Boller (1995) presented such attempts. Although groundbreaking studies are underway, agreement regarding the structure and function of the human prefrontal cortex and associated models of executive functioning is not yet at hand.

Executive Functions From a Rehabilitation Perspective

As clinicians whose primary responsibility is to help people with brain injury achieve their goals and ultimately achieve satisfying lives, we choose to operationalize the concept of executive functions in a way that ties it in a direct and practical way to the real world of deliberate, controlled behavior. The question that motivates our interest is this: Beyond building-block perceptual, motor, and linguistic skills and domain-specific knowledge, what enables a person to succeed at tasks that require more than automatic or routine behavior, particularly when there are competing goals and obstacles to achieving those goals? From this perspective, we propose that executive functions be understood as including:

➤ self-awareness of strengths and limitations, and associated understanding of the difficulty level of tasks;
➤ ability to set reasonable goals;
➤ ability to plan and organize behavior designed to achieve the goals;
➤ ability to initiate behavior toward achieving goals and inhibit behavior incompatible with achieving those goals;
➤ ability to monitor and evaluate performance in relation to the goals; and
➤ ability to flexibly revise plans and strategically solve problems in the event of difficulty or failure.

Sources of Executive System Impairment

Executive functions are so closely associated with prefrontal regions of the brain that the two terms, *executive functions* and *prefrontal functions*, are often used interchangeably. This is probably a mistake in that other parts of the brain, notably the limbic regions, contribute in essential ways to executive self-regulation of behavior (Cohen & Eichenbaum, 1993; Cummings, 1993; Pribram, 1986). Nevertheless, damage to prefrontal tissue is known to interfere with executive functioning. Because prefrontal cortex, limbic regions, and interconnections between these areas are among the most common sites of injury in TBI and because executive functions are critical for successful, mature strategic behavior, executive system impairment tends to be the dominant theme in rehabilitation after TBI. Indeed, the overarching theme of this book—positive everyday routines—is based in part on the premise that if behaviors can become routine, however complex or abstract they may appear, they will then make systematically decreasing demands on the parts of the brain most vulnerable in TBI. This thesis is consistent with the observation that even relatively routine tasks place some demands on the executive system.

It would be a mistake, however, to focus exclusively on the neurologic contributors to outcome in the domain of executive functions. The extreme variability in self-regulation of social and cognitive behavior in normally developing children and in adults suggests that experience, culture, teaching, and expectations play an important role in development of these aspects of human functioning. Similarly, studies of learned helplessness (Peterson & Seligman, 1985; Seligman, 1974), on the negative side, and of the effectiveness of a strategic focus in education (Pressley, 1993, 1995; Pressley & Associates, 1990; Pressley & El-Dinary, 1992), on the positive side, demonstrate that environmental factors play a leading role in development of executive self-regulation of behavior in people with and without disability. Rehabilitation professionals and others who interact with individuals with disability are often inclined to assume responsibility for the executive dimensions of behavior: assessing the person's strengths and weaknesses, setting his or her goals, planning how to achieve them, initiating appropriate behavior and inhibiting inappropriate behavior, monitoring and evaluating the individual's performance, and creating strategic alternatives in the event of failure. Our experience is that when this persists, learned helplessness beyond the

disability produced by the injury is the likely result. In Chapter 4, we describe everyday routines designed to facilitate maximal redevelopment of executive functions within the general context of everyday executive system routines.

What follows is a brief indication of the neuropsychology of these executive functions relevant to understanding the consequences of TBI.

Self-Awareness of Strengths and Weaknesses

Historically, *anosagnosia* has been used to describe denial of illness or disability (Heilman, 1991), a possible consequence of TBI. The use of the word *denial* is importantly misleading, suggesting that the problem has psychological roots. It is, of course, natural and common for people who are intellectually aware of the consequences of a life-altering brain injury to attempt to maintain hope that they will recover their preinjury abilities and to resist frank acknowledgment of the injury's effects on their lives. Nevertheless, anosagnosia has organic, not psychoreactive, roots. Anosagnosia is commonly associated with damage to the parietal lobe of the right hemisphere, including deep, subcortical structures and white matter that includes interconnections among somatosensory centers (Heilman, Watson, & Valenstein, 1993). Such injuries are accompanied by unawareness of the associated left-sided hemiplegia and a more general neglect of the individual's altered life situation. Furthermore, the prognosis for improvement in this condition is often guarded (Anderson & Tranel, 1989).

In contrast to the specific and dramatic unawareness associated with large right hemisphere lesions, individuals with diffuse, including bilateral prefrontal, injury often acknowledge specific difficulties with tasks when those difficulties are brought to their attention, but fail to integrate this awareness into a revised understanding of themselves, their educational, vocational, and social potential, and their need to compensate for residual disability with extraordinary effort (Prigatano, 1986; Prigatano, Altman, & O'Brien, 1990). In this sense, unawareness of the implications of the injury creates substantial frustration for rehabilitation professionals seeking to help the individual maximize residual functioning and compensate for ongoing deficits. Within the framework of everyday rehabilitation described in this book, unawareness is addressed, not with confrontational counseling procedures, although these may be helpful in selected cases, but rather within the context of executive function routines in which the individual is routinely expected to set goals, predict performance on tasks, and later review that performance, comparing prediction with outcome (see Chapter 4). Confrontation can be added, but is often not needed if the daily routine over time reveals the need to modify goals or accomplish important tasks in a better way.

Goal Setting

Executive functions have been identified as those necessary to achieve goals when automatic, routine behavior is inadequate for the task (Lezak, 1982, 1993). Realistic goal setting is a notoriously problematic area after TBI, in part for natural, psychoreactive reasons. From a neuropsychological perspective, in contrast, weakness in this area may be a secondary consequence of unawareness of deficits, leading to unrealistic goals, of initiation impairment, leading to a general reduction in activation of behavior, and of self-monitoring impairment, leading to a failure to modify goals (Levin, Benton, & Grossman, 1982; Lhermitte, 1983; Luria, 1966, 1973a, 1973b; Shallice & Burgess, 1991a, 1991b). Weakness in goal setting may also be a consequence of psychoreactive denial or of confusion regarding possibilities after the injury. Finally, in circumstances that result in an active helper-dependent helpee relationship, individuals may develop a habit of waiting for others to set their goals for them. The everyday executive system routines described in Chapter 4 begin with the individual articulating a goal and end with a review of performance in relation to the goal. Within this framework, goal setting becomes a routine focus of attention throughout all aspects of the individual's rehabilitation program and life.

Planning and Organizing

Organization is discussed later in this chapter as a specific cognitive function, although that discussion could as easily have been included under executive functions. Planning is a type of organizing, namely organizing future behavior in relation to goals that have been set (Miller, Galanter, & Pribram, 1960). Disorders of planning and execution of plans can occur at a variety of levels. In some cases following brain injury, individuals lack content knowledge necessary for formulating effective plans (Schwartz, Mayer, Fitzpatrick DeSalme, & Montgomery, 1993). If this lack of knowledge is related to brain injury, the damage is likely to posterior structures, which are not especially vulnerable in TBI. Frontal lobe injury can disrupt planning in a variety of ways (Cicerone & Wood, 1987; Levin, Eisenberg, & Benton, 1991). Indeed, planning deficits are a hallmark of frontal lobe injury (Grafman et al., 1989; Shallice, 1982). First, many people with frontal lobe injury (specifically those with large dorsolateral prefrontal injuries) who have adequate world knowledge nevertheless have difficulty assembling a plan, possibly because script structures, critical for effective planning and possibly stored prefrontally, are lost or fragmented (Sirigu et al., 1995). Individuals with frontal lobe injury have historically been found to have difficulty with the sequential order of event complexes, conceivably because of damage to a contentless prefrontal sequencing operator, but more likely because of damage to complex knowledge structures that are the basis for orderly, sequential progression through complex sequences of events (Duncan, 1986; Fuster, 1989; Grafman, 1995; Grafman, Sirugu, Spector, & Hendler, 1993; Sirigu et al., 1995).

Second, people with frontal lobe injury often have difficulty monitoring their behavior over time, maintaining a focus on their goal, and sustaining engagement with the script specifically designed to achieve that goal (Fuster, 1989, 1990). In this sense, the same underlying executive system weakness can interfere with sustained attention, planning, and any other goal-directed behavior that occurs over time (Graham & Harris, 1996). Third, individuals with frontal lobe injury may be successful in the intellectual aspects of planning but fail to execute the plans (Lhermitte, 1983, 1986). This failure may result from impaired initiation, associated with dorsolateral and dorsomedial prefrontal injury (discussed in the next section) or from specific decision-making impairment, associated with ventromedial prefrontal injury (discussed in Chapter 1 and later in the section on Behavior).

Initiating

Blumer and Benson (1975) introduced the now classic personality syndromes associated with frontal lobe injury, *pseudopsychopathic syndrome* and *pseudodepressive syndrome*, terms that are often descriptive despite their suggestion of an overly gloomy prognosis. The latter, sometimes referred to as adynamia, initiation/activation impairment, excessive passivity, or, in extreme cases, pathologic inertness, includes apathy, empty indifference, loss of initiative, automatic responding, and slowness. This syndrome has been associated with dorsolateral prefrontal injury (Luria, 1965), but is more commonly associated with dorsomedial prefrontal injury (Holst & Vikki, 1988). Although reports of initiation impairment have generally been restricted to the adult neuropsychology literature, Daigneault and colleagues (1997) described a 7-year-old child with adynamia and associated pseudodepressive characteristics following a focal left hemisphere frontomedial lesion.

Individuals with initiation impairment may have adequate knowledge of social rules and expectations, but nevertheless not act on that knowledge unless prompted by others. Similarly, they may possess adequate cognitive skill and strategic abilities to succeed at tasks presented to them, but not use those skills unless prompted (Lhermitte, 1983, 1986). In mild to moderate cases, this organic disorder may be misdiagnosed as laziness (Bijur et al., 1990). Initiation impairment must also be carefully distinguished from true depression and associated social withdrawal, another common consequence of a life-altering injury. In the absence of careful differential diagnosis, individuals with adynamia may receive counseling for depression when their real need is for everyday routines that facilitate initiation with enough support to ensure that the person acts, but not so much that helplessness or oppositionality is threatened. In our discussion of initiation in Chapter 4, we emphasize the need to create initiation supports that avoid the pitfall of excessive verbal cues and prompts from authority figures, which are often received as nagging and easily elicit oppositional responses.

Inhibiting

The so-called *pseudopsychopathic personality*, described by Blumer and Benson (1975), includes as symptoms disinhibition, hyperactivity, episodic anger and euphoria, tactless behavior, sexual acting out, irritability, and generally unrestrained behavior. Most investigators associate this complex with orbitofrontal injury (Malloy, Bihrle, Duffy, & Cimino, 1993; Stuss & Benson, 1986). Although most readily observed and troubling in the context of social behavior, difficulties with inhibition create a variety of problems, including those that are classified as cognitive and communicative. For example, Stuss and Benson (1987) described difficulty maintaining a focus of attention and inhibiting irrelevant thoughts or stimuli as associated with dorsolateral prefrontal injury. Both Levin and colleagues

(1996) and Taylor and colleagues (1996) identified inhibition as one of the critical factors to emerge from analysis of performance on tests of purported frontal lobe functioning in children with brain injury. Furthermore, Barkley (1997) identified weak response inhibition as being the core of the executive system impairment traditionally referred to as Attention Deficit/Hyperactivity Disorder. In a communication context, weak inhibition results in socially inappropriate language as well as disorganized, wandering, and tangential discourse as the individual fails to filter out thoughts and observations that are not germane to the topic at hand.

In everyday life, the best illustrations of disinhibited behavior are presented by normally developing preschoolers who say and do strange and sometimes inappropriate things that we readily understand, and sometimes but not always excuse, because we know that the children lack the developmental wherewithal to inhibit impulsive responses. Common sense management of preschool impulsiveness is through a combination of "childproofing" the environment to eliminate triggers for undesirable impulsive behavior, preparing the children for difficult times, teaching and rehearsing scripts so that responses are increasingly dictated by the script as opposed to a socially inappropriate impulse, and generally understanding the limitations on the child's inhibition ability so that normal impulsiveness is not punished. The everyday inhibition routines described in Chapter 6 are based on similar common sense management principles, with the addition that older children and adults can learn—as part of their routine—to anticipate situations in which they will not be able to inhibit negative behavior and therefore avoid those situations.

Self-Monitoring and Self-Evaluating

Luria (1966) argued that critical frontal lobe functions include programming activity, regulating execution of the activity, and monitoring or verifying the activity. Individuals with frontal lobe injury often fail to detect errors in task performance or, more generally, fail to notice and integrate the knowledge that what they are doing or failing to do at any given time is interfering with achievement of goals that they have explicitly embraced. This self-monitoring and self-evaluative function has been associated with a variety of prefrontal areas as well as the anterior cingulate gyrus and connected subcortical nuclei, considered by some anatomists as part of the prefrontal system (Damasio, 1994; Dehaene & Changeux, 1995; Devinsky & Luciano, 1993). The role of limbic structures in identifying value for and threats to the organism suggests that self-monitoring and self-evaluating should probably be considered a frontolimbic function (Allman & Brothers, 1994; Bechara et al., 1995; Cummings, 1993). Alternatively, self-monitoring difficulty may be due to working memory impairment, that is, an inability to simultaneously engage in ongoing activity and the evaluation of that activity (Damasio, 1989; Schwartz et al., 1993; Shallice & Burgess, 1991a, 1991b).

Because of the frequency and importance of self-monitoring and self-evaluation impairment after TBI, the everyday executive system routines described and illustrated in Chapter 4 include a monitoring/evaluating component, in most cases consisting of a general self-evaluation of performance and a brief consideration of what worked and what did not work.

Problem Solving/Strategic Thinking

In an important sense, problem solving and strategic behavior encompass most of what are referred to as executive functions. Understood as planned, self-regulative behavior required when automatic or habitual behavior is insufficient to achieve goals, executive functioning and problem solving or strategic thinking are virtually synonymous. Therefore, all of the considerations presented in this section are relevant to a discussion of TBI and problem solving. Furthermore, the frequency of problem-solving or strategic-thinking impairment after TBI makes sense in light of this connection to general executive functioning (Eslinger & Damasio, 1985; Shallice & Burgess, 1991b). We have created a special category for problem solving and strategic behavior because of their practical importance after TBI.

We also wish to highlight the fact that strategic behavior is not always time and energy consuming reflection of obstacles, consideration of possible strategic solutions, and choice of the best (Grafman, 1989). Strategies can themselves be stored along with other content components as large MKUs (Grafman, 1995). What master chess players bring to the game is not massive raw intellectual power that enables them to think through each play and the thousands of possible implications of each move, but rather a stored representation of many strategy complexes that dictate successful play under varied game conditions. One of the lessons to be derived from studies of expert strategic performance, such as that of chess masters, is that individuals with disability must be encouraged to rehearse well-conceived strategies in the context of the academic, vocational, and social routines that make a difference in their lives. This recommendation is in sharp contrast to the frequent use of decontextualized "what would you do if . . ." exercises in traditional cognitive rehabilitation, exercises that can be expected to have little effect on everyday functioning.

Because of the many roles played by the frontal lobes in organized problem solving and strategic thinking, it is easy to understand the frequency of problem-solving and strategic-thinking impairment after TBI. Unfortunately, because of the dramatic increase in problems and obstacles posed by the injury, people are called on to be better problem solvers and strategic thinkers than they would have been required to be without the injury. For this reason, attention to contextualized problem-solving and strategic-thinking routines, of the sort de-

scribed in Chapter 4, is critical for individuals with TBI.

COGNITION

In Table 2–1 we present one among many ways to classify components or aspects of cognitive functioning. This classification scheme is not intended to suggest that each of its components is conceptually or neuropsychologically distinct from the others. Nor do we wish to suggest a model of cognitive processing. Rather, we present the scheme as one way to organize clinical discussions of cognition and to ensure that no cognitive stone is left unturned in assessing and providing intervention and supports for people with cognitive impairment (Ylvisaker & Szekeres, 1998). We discussed executive functions separately because of their special importance in TBI rehabilitation and because executive functioning in relation to social behavior takes that concept beyond the domain of cognition.

In the following discussion, we attempt to highlight areas of particular clinical importance after TBI and to identify the neuropsychological basis for impairment in each key area.

Component Systems of Cognition

Working Memory

After TBI, the structural capacity of working memory—formerly referred to as short-term memory and measured by digit span—is less vulnerable than most other aspects of memory (Brooks, 1983). However, its functional capacity, the heart of working memory as it is currently conceived (Baddeley, 1986), is often impaired. People with frontal lobe injury may have difficulty keeping several thoughts active at one time because they are ineffective at organizing their thoughts, fail to execute efficient allocation procedures to make maximal use of working memory, or experience unacceptable levels of stress with increases in demands on their processing resources.

TABLE 2–1. Aspects of cognition.

Component Systems
 Working Memory
  Structural capacity versus functional capacity
  Phonological and visual holding space versus supervisory control system
 Knowledge Base (Long-Term Memory)
  Episodic versus semantic memory
  Declarative versus procedural memory
  Explicit versus implicit memory
  Remote memory (retrograde amnesia) versus recent memory (anterograde amnesia)
 Executive System
 Response System

Component Processes
 Attention
  Arousal and alertness
  Preparing attention
  Maintaining/sustaining attention
  Selecting a focus of attention (concentrating attention)
  Suppressing/filtering distractions
  Shifting/switching attention
  Dividing/sharing attention
 Perception
 Memory and Learning
  Encoding, storage, and retrieval
  Involuntary (incidental, Type II) versus deliberate (strategic) memory
  Retrospective versus prospective memory
  Verbal and nonverbal memory
  Sensory modality-specific memory
 Organization
  Feature identification
  Classifying/categorizing
  Sequencing
  Analyzing
  Integrating into main ideas, themes, and scripts
 Reasoning
  Deductive versus inductive versus analogical reasoning
  Evaluative reasoning
  Convergent versus divergent thinking

Functional-Integrative Performance
 Efficiency
  Rate of performance
  Amount accomplished
 Scope
 Manner
 Level

Working memory has been associated with large bilateral expanses of dorsal prefrontal cortex, including dorsolateral and mesial dorsal cortex, with the left hemisphere associated with manipulation of verbal information and the right hemisphere with visual information (Awl, Smith, & Jonides, 1995; Petrides, 1995). These prefrontal regions appear to be somewhat less vulnerable in CHI than ventral, orbital, and frontal polar regions. However, because efficient use of working memory requires effective executive decisions, efficient organizing, and a reasonable threshold of tolerance for stress, working memory deficits are common in TBI. People with impaired working memory have difficulty managing more than one task at a time and therefore tend to have relatively extreme difficulty in real-world, nonautomatic tasks in which it is necessary to hold a variety of considerations in mind at once in order to succeed (Grafman et al., 1993). One of the many advantages of focusing rehabilitation on the development of positive everyday routines is that the more routine a task is, the lower the demand on the resources of working memory.

Knowledge Base (Long-term Memory)

Information stored in the knowledge base has been categorized in a variety of ways by memory theoreticians. Some of these categories and distinctions are useful for rehabilitation professionals. Declarative memory (memory for facts, remembering that such and such is the case) is importantly different from procedural memory (memory for procedures or routines, remembering *how* to do something). Episodic memory (remembering events in one's life) and semantic memory (context-free memory for abstracted information, word meaning, scripts, and much more) are both types of declarative memory. Explicit memories are those that are stored along with a consciousness of having acquired the information, whereas implicit memories are traces that have the potential to influence behavior, but without a conscious awareness of having been exposed to the information.

Declarative and Explicit Memory. Investigations of memory impairment suggest that declarative and explicit memory systems rely on medial temporal lobe structures (particularly the hippocampus) (Izard, 1992; Squire, 1992) and are therefore quite vulnerable in TBI, given the frequency of damage to the hippocampus, often as a result of secondary anoxic brain injury (Pang, 1985). Declarative and explicit memory problems are easiest to detect, for example difficulty remembering on command events from earlier in the day (explicit, declarative, episodic memory problem) and difficulty remembering on command information presented in an earlier instructional situation (explicit, declarative, semantic memory problem). Studies of adults with CHI, routinely report that memory problems of this sort are among their most common residual problems (Bachman, 1992; Hunkin et al., 1995).

Procedural and Implicit Memory. In contrast, procedural and implicit memory systems appear to be less dependent on vulnerable medial temporal lobe structures. For example, the hippocampus appears not to be involved in learning new motor sequences (Squire, 1992; Squire et al., 1992). Implicit memories for emotionally charged events appear to rely on the activity of the amygdala (Adolphs et al., 1995; Aggleton, 1992; LeDoux, 1995). Pascual-Leone and colleagues (1995) suggested that procedural learning relies especially on contributions of the basal ganglia and cerebellum, both of which are richly connected to dorsolateral prefrontal cortex. Therefore, it is often possible to teach even densely amnesic people (with severe medial temporal lobe damage) new skills, procedures, and routines, provided the teaching is consistent with what is known about procedural learning and implicit memory. The method of vanishing cues (a backward chaining teaching procedure; Glisky & Schacter, 1987) has been successfully used to teach a variety of functional skills (e.g., word processing, data entry) to amnesic adults. Errorless learning has been found to be particularly essential for people with severely impaired explicit memory but relatively intact implicit memory (Wilson & Evans, 1996). If errors are rehearsed, but the individual cannot explicitly recall having been exposed to the erroneous information, the errors are likely to be retained and difficult to eliminate (Baddeley & Wilson, 1994). In our experience with people with TBI, it is often possible to teach procedures and routines with repeated practice even in the presence of significant explicit, deliberate, declarative memory problems. Approaching rehabilitation through positive everyday routines relies in part on the relative superiority of procedural learning. However, even procedural learning may be inefficient, requiring a very large number of learning trials and considerable contextualized support in some cases.

Remote and Recent Memory. The term remote memory is often used to refer to memories acquired before the injury, whereas recent memory, in contrast, refers to memory for events experienced and information acquired since the injury (although the term is sometimes used in a more limited sense). Impairment of remote memory (i.e., retrograde amnesia) is probably associated with posterior brain damage because much information is stored in posterior cortical regions. Because posterior cortical damage is less common than frontal lobe damage in TBI, it is not surprising that many such individuals have relatively good recovery of pretrauma information and skill despite serious difficulty learning new information and acquiring new skills. This asymmetry in impairment explains the otherwise curious phenomenon of good scores on tests of knowledge and skill after the injury despite severe learning disability upon return to school or the workplace. Difficulty learning new information (i.e., anterograde amnesia) is particularly debilitating for people, such as students, who return to a world that demands learning efficiency. Whereas there are few investigations of attempts to help people recover remote memories, the literature dealing with attempts to facilitate more efficient new learning is extensive. New learning problems are discussed later in the section on memory as a process.

Component Processes of Cognition

Attention

After severe TBI, disorders of arousal and alertness are initially the salient aspects of cognitive impairment. Damage responsible for early unresponsiveness may include specific and often reversible insult to the reticular activating system within the brain stem as well as bilateral cortical damage. In all but the most severe cases, individuals regain adequate arousal, but may experience persistent fatigue, which negatively affects alertness (Bachman, 1992). Damage to the right parietal lobe is associated with a different form of attentional impairment, namely inattention to space and to body parts contralateral to the site of injury (Heilman, Watson, & Valenstein, 1993).

Following TBI, the aspects of attention most commonly impaired are those identified as executive or supervisory control attentional processes (Shallice, 1988). These components of attention have traditionally been associated with prefrontal structures. Executive control processes are those required when routine responses, whether cognitive, social, or purely motoric, are inadequate to the task at hand. Stuss and colleagues (1995) have proposed seven distinct types of executive attentional control processes:

1. *Sustaining Attention:* Engaged when relevant events occur slowly and vigilance is required, this process has been associated with the prefrontal cortex.
2. *Concentrating (Directing) Attention:* Engaged when the task is demanding and stimuli or required responses occur quickly, this process has been associated with the anterior cingulate cortex, considered part of the prefrontal cortex.
3. *Sharing (Dividing) Attention:* Engaged when two or more tasks must be executed simultaneously, this process has been generally associated with the frontal lobes.
4. *Suppressing Attention (Filtering):* Engaged when relatively automatic responses or

schemata are inappropriate or unhelpful, this process has been associated with the dorsolateral prefrontal cortex (with possible hemispheric asymmetry).

5. *Switching (Shifting) Attention:* Engaged when tasks require shifts among cognitive or perceptual sets (e.g., Wisconsin Card Sorting Test), this process has been associated with the dorsolateral prefrontal cortex (both hemispheres).

6. *Preparing Attention:* Engaged when an individual is alerted to a need to respond in a specific manner later and therefore must maintain this preparatory set, this process has been associated in a few research reports with the dorsolateral prefrontal cortex or the connecting regions.

7. *Setting Attention:* Engaged when an individual mobilizes a task schema that was successful on a previous occasion, this process is closely related to maintenance of learning and has at least a loose association with the dorsolateral prefrontal cortex. Internal self-regulating self-talk, associated with the left hemisphere dorsolateral cortex, may serve as an example of this attentional function.

Each of these aspects of attention is phenomenologically real and important in analyzing the strengths and weaknesses of people with frontal lobe injury. However, we do not wish to suggest that each is neuropsychologically distinct or, indeed, that they are processes at all as opposed to ways in which knowledge and knowledge schemas are managed within the brain (Grafman, 1995).

Attention, Knowledge, and Motivation. In theoretical discussions of attention as a set of neuropsychological processes, it is unfortunately easy to lose sight of practical realities critical to good rehabilitation. First, it is a fact of everyday life that in all areas of attention, people function more efficiently and successfully in domains in which they have knowledge and interest (Bandura, 1977). For example, a football coach's ability to attend to the game is incalculably superior to that of a novice onlooker who has no investment in the outcome.

Second, processing is deeper, learning more efficient, and transfer more likely if training tasks occur in domains of content in which the trainee has some expertise and which are important for the individual to process efficiently (Hecimovic, Fox, Shores, & Strain, 1985; Horner et al., 1988). For example, if a student with TBI neglects the left side of space and has difficulty with visual scanning, exercises involving meaningful reading passages are useful. The meaning implicit in the language helps to drive return-to-left scanning; furthermore, improved performance on this task has an immediate payoff because it is a task on which the student must succeed. Similarly, if a student has difficulty sustaining attention, there is value in using functional tasks, like educational software, that exercise the function in a context in which improvements are particularly critical.

Memory and Learning

Earlier we discussed types of memories stored in the knowledge base (sometimes called *memoria*). In this section, we address memory processes or aspects of the learning process. The memory literature is not consistent in the distinctions drawn and processes proposed. However, some aspects of memory and learning as a process must be understood by clinicians that serve individuals with memory impairment.

Encoding, Storage, and Retrieval. *Encoding,* or the acquisition stage of memory, refers to the internal construction of a representation of a perceived event; *storage* involves holding that representation over time in what is thought to be a highly organized long-term memory system; *retrieval* involves transfer of information from storage to consciousness and can be involuntary or effortful.

Encoding of new information is often impaired in TBI as a result of damage to the hippocampal system responsible for consolidating new memories or of damage to the frontal lobes, resulting in shallow organization and elaboration of information as it is initially being processed (Anderson, Damasio, Tranel, & Damasio, 1988; Brazzeli et al., 1994; Gluck & Myers, 1995; Squire, Knowlton, & Mussen, 1993). Storage is less commonly impaired in TBI; once information is adequately processed and encoded, it is unlikely to decay rapidly, as is the case in degenerative diseases such as Alzheimer's. Retrieval may be impaired in TBI as a result of posterior damage that reduces the number of retrieval routes in the networks of neural connections that compose the storage system (Buschke & Fuld, 1974). Or retrieval can be impaired as a result of frontal lobe injury, which can result in nonstrategic searches of memory (Damasio et al., 1990). Recent positron emission tomography (PET) scan investigations of explicit retrieval of information have isolated important contributions of left lateral prefrontal cortex, right anterior frontal-polar cortex, and anterior cingulate gyrus (Buckner et al., 1995).

Deliberate, Strategic Memory Versus Involuntary, Incidental Memory. Investigators of cognitive development in children draw an important distinction between involuntary (or incidental, type II; Postman, 1964) memory and deliberate (effortful, strategic) memory. When the learner is oriented to learning as a goal of the task, it becomes a deliberate or strategic learning task. College students creatively studying for an exam present the classical illustration of deliberate learning. Considerable cognitive sophistication is presupposed by deliberate learning tasks. One must understand learning as a goal, recognize that certain learning tasks are difficult and require special effort, use special procedures (learning strategies), and monitor and evaluate the outcome of the effort. The ability to profit from the instruction to try to remember develops gradually in childhood. With young children and with others with significant cognitive weakness, deliberate learning tasks interfere with learning rather than helping.

Similarly, when an individual is consciously oriented to retrieval of information or of a word as a goal of the task, retrieval becomes deliberate (effortful, strategic). The same developmental observations can be made about strategic retrieval as were made about strategic encoding. Recent studies using fMRI (Demb, Desmond, Wagner, Vaidya, Glover, & Gabrielli, 1995) and PET (Buckner et al., 1995) have shown that frontal lobe structures are involved in explicit (versus implicit) retrieval of information and that left hemisphere prefrontal cortex is involved specifically in semantic encoding and retrieval. Ste-Marie and colleagues (1996) found a dramatic impairment of controlled memory processing relative to automatic memory processing in a group of brain injured adults, most of whom had a history of CHI. Finally, in his summary of the contribution of prefrontal structures to memory functioning, Petrides (1995) emphasized the important role of prefrontal (ventrolateral) structures in active, explicit, strategic encoding and retrieval of information, which is consciously and effortfully directed by the subject, but not in passive, noneffortful encoding and retrieval.

In contrast to controlled, effortful, strategic encoding and retrieval, if the goal for the learner is internal to the task, or anything other than learning, then the task is an involuntary or incidental learning task. Young children learn efficiently when to-be-learned information is presented to them in the context of functional activities and in such a manner that they must process the information in order to achieve the goal of the task (Hudson, 1993; Hudson & Fivush, 1993). Preschool teachers tend to be masters of designing involuntary learning tasks. Because TBI, and frontal lobe injury in particular, often interferes with deliberate, strategic learning and retrieval, learning tasks for adolescents and adults are ideally designed with age-appropriate activities and materials, but with the structure of involuntary learning tasks. Unfortunately, the opposite is often the case: The greater the memory impairment, the more people are tempted to encourage the individual to try hard to remember, thereby probably exacerbating the impairment.

Metamemory. Understood as including both knowledge of memory processes and deliberate control over those processes, metamemory includes many of the aspects of memory included above in the discussion of strategic learning. Although metamemory is a well-established field in educational psychology (Brown, 1975, 1979; Schneider & Pressley, 1989), it is relatively understudied in neuropsychology. However, in light of the frequency of deficits in self-awareness and strategic thinking among people with frontal lobe injury, it is reasonable to conclude that metamemory in general is a relative weakness in this population and therefore in the population of people with TBI. This weakness is a likely explanation for the common finding that, whereas people with memory impairment after brain injury may improve performance of training tasks with compensatory procedures, they rarely generalize these procedures from training tasks to other tasks and maintain them over time. This was precisely the finding made decades earlier in studies of memory training for students with learning impairment, a finding which stimulated the early development of the field of metacognition (Flavell, Miller, & Miller, 1993). In our view, it is critical for rehabilitation professionals to confront the conclusion from many years of research in educational psychology that compensatory strategy intervention is unlikely to be effective unless it is implemented for extended periods of time (at least several months if not years) and largely in the context of meaningful everyday learning pursuits (Pressley, 1993, 1995).

Free Recall, Cued Recall, and Recognition Memory. For reasons implicit in the discussions of strategic versus involuntary learning and metamemory, free recall (e.g.,

"Tell me as much as you can remember about the story I read you") is likely to be relatively more impaired in patients with frontal lobe injury than is cued recall (e.g., "Where was he? Who was he with?") or recognition memory (e.g., "Was he in New York? Was he with John?") because of its relatively greater demands on consciously controlled searches of memory. In general, people with frontal lobe injury have significant impairment on tests of free recall, some difficulty with cued recall tasks, and relatively little difficulty with recognition memory (compared with patterns of performance of people with no memory impairment) (Petrides, 1995). This pattern suggests that assessment of learning of individuals with frontal lobe injury must include recognition memory tasks; free recall tasks alone may fail to reveal the learning that occurred. If free recall is known to be relatively impaired, teachers and others should use cued recall or recognition memory tasks to assess learning.

Retrospective Versus Prospective Memory. *Retrospective memory* refers to memory for past events, whereas *prospective memories* are those for upcoming events, such as appointments. People with explicit memory impairment after TBI often have impairment in both retrospective and prospective memory. Whereas simply practicing retrospective memory, with no facilitation in the form of deep semantic encoding or other strategies, has been found to be ineffective as a form of intervention (Thöne, 1996), intensive repetitive practice of prospective memory tasks has been shown to improve functioning, at least on training tasks (Mateer & Sohlberg, 1992). Transfer of these slight improvements to everyday prospective memory tasks has not been unequivocally demonstrated. People with prospective memory impairment commonly rely on prosthetic systems, like appointment books, reminders from others, or electronic reminder system such as Neuropage (Hersh & Treadgold, 1994).

Sensory-Modality Specific Memory. In some contexts it is also helpful to divide memory and learning into categories based on the sensory modality in which the information is received (e.g., auditory versus visual memory) and on whether the information is linguistically coded or not (verbal versus nonverbal memory). Because unilateral posterior damage and sensory-specific damage are not particularly common in TBI, we will not elaborate on these aspects of memory.

Organization

Organization problems are among the most common cognitive deficits after TBI (Grafman, 1995; Grafman, Sirigu, Spector, & Hendler, 1993; Schwartz, 1995; Schwartz et al., 1993; Szekeres, 1992). At the most basic level, organizational impairment manifests itself in action breakdowns, including faulty sequencing (e.g., putting on shoes before socks), errors of omission (e.g., brushing teeth without toothpaste), perseveration (e.g., continuing to vacuum long after the rug is clean), and object substitution or misuse (e.g., buttering bread with a fork). From a language perspective, organizational impairment often manifests itself as wandering, tangential discourse in speech or writing, as paucity of language, as slow and disorganized retrieval of words, and as weak comprehension of extended discourse. More generally, any task that has components and is not completely automatic is subject to breakdowns in the event of organizational impairment. Many of the individuals described in this book had serious organizational impairment, in some cases misdiagnosed as an attention deficit, psychiatric disturbance, oppositional behavior, or laziness.

Schwartz and colleagues (1993) described three neuropsychologically distinct types of breakdown in organized action. The first, *ideational apraxia,* is associated with posterior cortical damage (possibly occipitoparietal cortex in the case of disrupted action routines) (Schwartz et al., 1993) and bilateral temporal lobe cortex in the case of disrupted declarative knowledge (Patterson & Hodges, 1995), and results in action breakdowns in real-world contexts as well as on testing under ideal circumstances. People with ideational apraxia have difficulty acting, talking, and thinking in an organized manner because they have lost some or all of the organized neural networks that help to bind connected units of knowledge together. In contrast, *frontal apraxia* refers to a condition that includes a weakened connection between an intention (e.g., I want to get dressed, I want to tell a story) and the organized action schemas needed to accomplish the intention. The appropriate organizational scheme is not selected and activated for the task at hand. Individuals with frontal apraxia may score well on tests of organization (i.e., they have knowledge that may be stored in organized networks), but they nevertheless act, talk, and think in a disorganized manner in the real world. The third source of disorganized behavior is *supervisory attentional system distractibility syndrome*, which is consistent with organized behavior under ideal conditions, but which causes serious breakdowns in the presence of distractors. Frontal apraxia and supervisory attentional system distractibility syndrome are both associated with prefrontal lobe lesions, partially explaining the frequency of organizational problems after CHI. In a more recent publication, Schwartz (1995) used the term *action disorganization syndrome* to replace Luria's term frontal apraxia and proposed that it combines some damage to the posterior knowledge storage system with damage to the frontal control system.

In Chapter 1, we briefly described Grafman's neuropsychological theory of MKUs (including scripts, schemas, plans, themes, and mental models) stored in the prefrontal cortex (see Figure 1–3) (Grafman, 1995). Grafman appears to go further than Schwartz and colleagues in tying organized thinking and behavior to prefrontal function. MKUs regulate attention, social behavior, planning, and other aspects of executive functions. The comprehensiveness of this hypothesis enables it to explain in a parsimonious manner widespread breakdowns in controlled, organized behavior following prefrontal injury. Depending on the MKUs affected by the injury, it is also possible to explain differential impairment of controlled cognitive and social functions (e.g., relatively intact planning, but weak social interaction).

It should be noted that none of these neuropsychological hypotheses supports the remedial approach to rehabilitation commonly observed in many cognitive rehabilitation programs, namely, practicing categorizing, sequencing, and other forms of cognitive organization in the abstract. Current theories in cognitive science and cognitive neuroscience rather emphasize the role of stored organizing schemes, or knowledge structures, which are more or less specifically tied to a domain of knowledge. Thus, one can be a master organizer in a library, but wholly disorganized in a supermarket; one can be a master problem solver in chess, but totally incompetent in marriage counseling. In Chapter 5, we describe appropriately contextualized approaches to helping people with organizational impairment, based on the thesis that there do not exist organizing processes neuropsychologically represented as contentless operations that can be strengthened with exercise and, once strengthened, support improved performance in all domains of organized thinking and acting. These themes are elaborated in greater detail by Ylvisaker, Szekeres, and Haarbauer-Krupa (1998).

Reasoning

As a complex cognitive process, reasoning in any of its forms listed in Table 2–1 depends on the integrity of several brain centers, including posterior cortical areas associated with storage of factual knowledge and word meanings. Reasoning difficulty reported in many individuals with TBI may be a consequence of the critical roles played by prefrontal systems. Because reasoning requires simultaneous attention to a variety of considerations in attempting to achieve a goal or draw a conclusion, weakness in working memory creates difficulty in reasoning. Damage to frontal and limbic regions responsible for attaching value to experiences may interfere with evaluative reasoning. Analogical reasoning, presumably based on a comparison of a well-developed knowledge structure or schema with a less well-developed schema, may be vulnerable to frontal lobe injury if current neuropsychological models that house large MKUs (scripts, frames, themes, mental models, and other large, organized knowledge structures) in the frontal lobes are correct (Grafman, 1995). Divergent reasoning requires flexibility in thinking, a notorious weakness in people with frontal lobe injury. Finally, social perception and social reasoning may be particularly vulnerable in people with a combination of basal forebrain injury and right hemisphere-related social perception weakness (Holyoak & Kroger, 1995).

However reasoning is parsed by cognitive scientists, everyday observations suggest that reasoning skill and content knowledge are not independent. People famous for their reasoning skill in particular domains—for example, master chess players, military strategists, scientists, marriage counselors, athletic coaches, videogame champions—typically reason no better than any other novice when placed in an unfamiliar domain of content. For example, videogame champions are probably not helpful when reasoning about marital conflicts is required; chess masters are unlikely consultants to struggling corporations; great scientists may be completely incompetent if invited to think through complicated military strategy or to help a baseball team mired in a prolonged slump.

The everyday approach to rehabilitation described in this book captures these important insights by addressing reasoning deficits with supported contextualized exercises in reasoning, rather than the more common decontextualized workbook or software exercises. Just as children are encouraged to be more and more thoughtful in their deliberations about everyday activities and employees are encouraged to think with increasing clarity and insight about the complex issues posed by their jobs, so also we engage individuals with TBI in the cognitive dimensions of tasks that are personally meaningful.

Functional Integrative Performance

We highlight aspects of functional integrative performance as components of this classification system to ensure that rehabilitation staff inject an appropriately real-world focus into their exploration of cognitive functioning and intervention plans. As we point out in Chapter 3 in connection with assessment, and throughout the book in connection with intervention, successful or unsuccessful performance of tasks in office-bound assessments or clinical practice settings does not necessarily predict success or lack of success with purportedly comparable tasks in other settings. Furthermore, it is insufficient to know simply that a person fails on a task; rehabilitation professionals must identify the circumstances under which he or she can succeed. Clinicians are well advised to observe real-world performance under varying conditions, tracking that performance with the following four real-world performance variables.

Efficiency refers to the rate at which an individual can perform a task and the amount of work that can be accomplished. Slowed processing and slowed performance are among the most common consequences of TBI. Slowness can result from specific perceptual and motor deficits, from diffuse injury that interferes with efficient neural transmission within the brain, and from frontal lobe injury.

Scope refers to the variety of settings and contexts in which optimal levels of performance can be maintained. Ecologically

valid assessment of people with TBI mandates observation and exploration of important behaviors in a variety of settings and contexts. Effective intervention typically requires services and supports in a variety of functional contexts.

Manner refers to features of the way in which the task was performed, for example, impulsive or reflexive, dependent or independent, flexible or rigid, active or passive. Many people with TBI are impulsive, dependent, rigid, and relatively passive.

Finally, *level* refers to the developmental, academic, linguistic, or vocational level of a task as it is measured on scales such as early to late grade level, simple to complex, concrete to abstract, and low to high language level.

BEHAVIOR

There is no doubt but that TBI can have generally devastating effects on behavior and psychosocial functioning. Furthermore, those effects probably contribute more to negative academic, vocational, social, and familial outcome than medical, physical, and cognitive factors. It is simply hard to live with a family member whose personality has changed in negative ways, to supervise or work with an employee whose behavior is irritating and whose work habits seem to be irresponsible, and to teach a student who acts out in class.

Taken together, the behavioral and psychosocial themes described in this section constitute what are often labeled personality changes after TBI: irritability, frequent loss of temper, impatience, emotional volatility, egocentrism, impulsiveness, anxiety, depression, loss of social contact, lack of interests, fatigue, and loss of initiation (Brooks & McKinlay, 1983; Brown et al., 1981; Filley, Cranberg, Alexander, & Hart, 1987; Fletcher, Levin, & Butler, 1995; Jacobs, 1993; McKinlay, Brooks, Bond, Martinage, & Marshall, 1981; Petterson, 1991; Prigatano, 1986; Thomsen, 1984; Weddell, Oddy, & Jenkins, 1980). Most often, these personality changes present the greatest obstacles to satisfying family and community reintegration (Brooks et al., 1987; Hall et al., 1994; Lezak, 1986, 1987; Livingston & Brooks, 1988). Thomsen (1974) reported that 84% of family members surveyed complained of personality, behavioral, and emotional changes in their loved one with TBI. Furthermore, in adults with TBI, social-interaction challenges are associated with difficulty maintaining employment, living independently, and maintaining satisfying relationships with friends (Bond, 1990; Klonoff et al., 1986; Lezak, 1987b; Livingston & Brooks, 1988; Prigatano & Fordyce, 1986; Thomsen, 1984, 1987).

Preinjury Factors

In discussing preinjury factors earlier in this chapter, we emphasized that TBI does not randomly select its victims. Many children, adolescents, and adults with TBI were at risk before their injury because of challenging social circumstances, high activity levels, excessive risk-taking behavior, and often frank antisocial behavior (Asarnow et al., 1991; Lehr, 1990; Lezak, 1982; Pelco et al., 1992). In these circumstances, persistent behavior problems are typically exaggerated versions of problems present before the injury (Hart & Jacobs, 1993; Prigatano, 1987). In the famous words of Sir Charles Symonds (1937, p. 26), "it is not only the kind of injury that matters but the kind of head." More generally, adjustment problems after brain injury increase with environmental stressors (e.g., family conflict, insufficient resources) and preinjury behavioral challenges. Having highlighted the frequency of preinjury issues, we hasten to add that preinjury challenges are not a reason to deny a person needed services and supports after the injury, as is sometimes argued. Nor are preinjury behavior problems an inevitable indicator of postinjury behavioral challenges. In our view, the goal is to help people who need and want help, even if the source of that need in large part preexisted the injury.

Postinjury Factors Not Directly Related to the Injury

It is natural that changes in ability, levels of success in chosen pursuits, restrictions on choices and activities, and loss of friends and social outlets should negatively affect a person's emotional state and behavior. The negative control cycle, described in Chapter 6, unfortunately flourishes in a situation in which adolescents and young adults with TBI—and with their developmentally natural intense need to govern their own choices and behavior—find themselves in a setting in which professionals or others provide them with little opportunity for choice and control, and allow themselves to be sucked into classic negative control battles. Not surprisingly, depression and social withdrawal are frequently reported in individuals with TBI (Eames, 1988; Katz, 1992; Rosenthal & Bond, 1990). In others, reactions to their changes in life circumstances may be manifested in anger and aggressive behavior. Both withdrawal and acting out may, of course, have organic roots (see injury factors in the next section) but often reflect the individual's ability or lack of ability to cope with significant loss and changes in life.

Van Zomeran and van den Burg (1985) found that neither impairment-related complaints (e.g., complaints by people with TBI that they are forgetful, cannot concentrate, cannot divide attention, and cannot monitor their behavior in social context) nor intolerance-related complaints (e.g., complaints by people with TBI that they have become irritable and overly sensitive) were correlated with severity of injury. That is, psychological reactions play into the individual's perception of the effects of the injury and feed into the complicated mix of factors that determine psychosocial adjustment. In their comprehensive summary of the large literature on psychosocial adjustment after TBI, Kendall and Terry (1996) captured these powerful variables in their model with the categories *primary appraisal* (including subjective severity of injury, perceived stigma, and perceived uncertainty) and *secondary appraisal* (including self-efficacy and perceived control). Negative self-image after TBI is correlated with social deficits (Klonoff & Lage, 1991), while internal locus of control appears to positively influence emotional and behavioral adjustment (Moore et al., 1990). In other disability groups, the attributes, beliefs, and behaviors that compose self-determination are known to contribute in profound ways to successful adult outcome (Wehmeyer & Schwartz, 1997), and efforts are underway to identify intervention procedures that hold the potential to influence self-determination in a positive way.

Earlier we also highlighted the contribution of family style of coping and quality of support—as well as other forms of social support—to behavioral and psychosocial outcome. Taylor and colleagues (1995) found that family variables had a marked impact on long-term behavioral adjustment in children and adolescents with TBI, confirming the classic findings of Brown and colleagues (1981). In a longitudinal study of adults with TBI, Kaplan (1990, 1991) found that levels of social support correlated positively with vocational success during the first year after the injury and with emotional and psychosocial adjustment 3 years post-injury. More specifically, individuals with TBI who described their families as low in cohesion and expressiveness were more irritable, aggressive, anxious, and depressed than those who described cohesive and expressive families (Kaplan, 1990). Highlighting the importance of support and personal resilience, Ponsford and coworkers (1995) found that, adults with TBI who were working 2 years postinjury (contrary to early predictions based on severity of injury) tended to have considerable employer support and to be personally adaptable. Those who were not working contrary to early predictions that they *could* resume employment tended to have behavior problems and lack of employer support.

Injury Factors: Indirect Contribution to Behavioral Outcome

Various investigators have concluded that impairment in higher cognitive functions contributes to compromised psychosocial adjustment (Marsh & Knight, 1991; Martzke, Swan, & Varney, 1991; Vilkki et al., 1994). However, the relationship remains unclear. In some cases, it may be that the same underlying impairment is labeled cognitive or psychosocial, depending on how it is observed and assessed. For example, impaired perception of social cues (e.g., misreading intonation patterns that might signal humor or irony rather than literal meaning) can justifiably be classified as a cognitive or as a psychosocial deficit. Similarly, difficulty taking the perspective of others (i.e., egocentrism) is often a cognitive impairment and is clearly recognized as such in normally developing toddlers, but is typically interpreted as a psychosocial impairment in older children and adults with frontal lobe injury.

In other cases, cognitive impairment may create academic or vocational failure and frustration that naturally triggers negative behavioral reactions. Finally, cognitive impairment may interfere with coping mechanisms and accommodation processes. If psychosocial adjustment requires marshaling relevant information, interpreting it, formulating alternative goals and plans to achieve those goals, and proceeding strategically in this process, then certainly cognitive weakness can and does contribute to poor psychosocial adjustment.

Injury Factors: Direct Contribution to Behavioral Outcome

Behavioral Impairment: Excesses of Behavior

Troubling behaviors, ranging from irritating comments and mildly inappropriate behavior to seriously aggressive behavior, are extremely common after TBI (Ackerly, 1964; Benton, 1991; Eames, 1990). Lezak and

O'Brien (1988) reported that 60% of their sample retained a significant social handicap over the first year postinjury due to disinhibited behavior considered inappropriate in the context. Brooks and colleagues (1986) found that more than half of the adults with TBI they followed were reported by relatives to use frequent threats and abusive gestures, with 20% of the relatives reporting physical assault. In the same group, more than 50% of relatives reported excessive moodiness and tantrums in their relative with TBI. Brown and colleagues (1981) found that socially inappropriate and disinhibited behavior was the primary theme running through the dramatic frequency of new psychosocial problems (i.e., those that did not predate the injury) after TBI in children and adolescents.

As described in the section on executive functions, damage to orbitofrontal regions (among the most vulnerable sites in closed head injury) has frequently been associated with aspects of the so-called pseudopsychopathic personality: transient or persistent disinhibition, impulsiveness, lability, reduced anger control, aggressiveness, sexual acting out, perseveration, and generally poor social judgment (Blumer & Benson, 1975; Stuss & Benson, 1986). Orbitofrontal areas have rich connections with the amygdala, anterior insula, and temporal poles by way of the uncinate fasciculus (which is vulnerable to stretching and tearing in rotational inertial injuries). This subsystem appears to be related to perception of novel stimuli and relationships, and interpretation of visceral responses to them, thereby contributing to the controlled performance of acceptable, positive behaviors in social context. Significant damage to this system may result in dependence on others to direct action in context (Lhermitte, 1983, 1986; Lhermitte et al., 1986).

Some of these symptoms may also be associated with right hemisphere temporoparietal lesions (Bakchine et al., 1989) and, if severe, may indicate Kluver-Bucy syndrome (episodic dyscontrol), associated with bilateral medial temporal lobe damage (Pang, 1985). One must also be alert to the possibility that the symptoms were longstanding personality characteristics before the injury. Finally, in some cases, explosive anger reactions are perfectly understandable responses to intolerably and unjustifiably restrictive treatments and regulations after the injury.

Behavioral Impairment: Deficits of Behavior

In this section, we use the phrase *behavior deficit* as it is often used in the behavioral literature to refer to a reduction in behaviors or levels of activity. From a neuropsychological perspective, such a reduction may be related to what we referred to earlier as the pseudodepressed personality, that is, the phenomenon of adynamia or activation/initiation impairment. Although not consistent, neuropsychological investigations often implicate left hemisphere frontal lobe lesions, particularly dorsolateral or dorsomesial damage, in this disability. These areas have dense interconnections to the mediodorsal nucleus of the thalamus. These structures and their connections may form a prefrontal subsystem associated with activation, set shifting, flexible organization of behavior in context and allocation of priorities.

Correct diagnosis of the phenomenon of initiation impairment is critical. In the absence of an understanding of its organic basis, incorrect and unhelpful diagnoses such as *lazy* and *unmotivated* or, possibly, *depressed* are predictable. Alternatively, true emotional depression may be misdiagnosed, followed by an inappropriate course of psychotherapeutic treatment.

Reduction in levels of activity may also be an indirect consequence of the injury. It is tragically common for individuals with disability after TBI to lose friends and the possibility of engaging in pretrauma recreational activities. Furthermore, physical and cognitive disability may dramatically reduce the domain of alternative social and recreational outlets (Morton & Wehman, 1995). Under these circumstances, the individual simply lacks things to do. Among the most important current developments for people with TBI is the spread of the Club House movement, which offers activities and an opportunity to make an important contribution despite disability that might block return to work and preinjury social life (Jacobs, 1997).

Finally, low levels of activity may indicate genuine depression. Klonoff and Lage (1995) pointed out that the dramatic and permanent changes in work status, income, family life, support network, and general quality of life that often accompany TBI naturally predispose people to depressive reactions, including profound feelings of social isolation, helplessness, and hopelessness. They review the risk factors for suicide and describe what they consider appropriate treatment, including rehabilitation using a milieu-oriented approach and a concerted attempt on the part of everybody involved with the individual to help him or her reestablish personally meaningful roles and a sense of control over important aspects of everyday life.

Initiation and inhibition impairment often coexist after severe frontal lobe injury. For example, Williams and Mateer (1992) described an adolescent with frontal lobe injury associated with TBI that left his superior IQ intact, but that ultimately resulted in disinhibited and often out-of-control behavior at school and complaints of pervasive inactivity at home. The likely explanation for the apparent conflict in behavioral profiles in these two settings is that the demands of the school setting revealed inhibition impairment, a presumed consequence of orbital prefrontal injury, while the absence of demands at home revealed initiation impairment, a presumed consequence of dorsal prefrontal injury.

Behavioral Impairment: Disassociation of Thinking and Acting

In Chapter 1, we described the so-called Gage Matrix (Damasio, 1994), which includes normal performance on most tasks in structured testing situations combined with seriously ineffective decision making and implementation of decisions in the real world. Despite average to above average reasoning ability and knowledge, including social knowledge, individuals who meet this description may experience devastating social and vocational failure in their lives. Also in Chapter 1 we sketched a potential explanation for this striking phenomenon that included injury-related disruption of the decision-guiding somatic marker system in the frontal lobes, critically involving ventromedial prefrontal cortex and interconnected medial temporal lobe (limbic) structures. This system is thought to be central to the neurology of conditioned learning. Individuals with damage to this system may perseverate in highly ineffective actions, including those that routinely result in punishment, despite an intellectual understanding of the folly of the behavior. Initiation and inhibition impairment can and often do add to disability in these individuals with severe, bilateral frontal lobe injury.

COMMUNICATION AND SOCIAL SKILLS

Communication Outcome After TBI

As is the case with cognition and behavior, virtually any combination of communication strengths and weaknesses is possible after TBI, depending on the individual's age and preinjury functioning, the nature and severity of the injury, and treatment and supports available after the injury. A disproportionate number of individuals with TBI had language or communication problems before the injury. A minority of adults with TBI have long-term speech and language profiles that closely resemble those of adults with aphasia associated with focal left hemisphere strokes. Similarly, a minority of children with TBI have profiles of residual speech and language deficits that closely resemble those of children with congenital language disability. However, reviews of studies of communication outcome after TBI in children (Chapman, 1997; Chapman, Levin, Matejka, Harward, & Kufera, 1995, 1997; Ylvisaker, 1993) and adults (Hartley, 1995; Sarno, Buonaguro, & Levita, 1986; Turkstra & Holland, 1998; Ylvisaker, 1992) have emphasized that communication profiles following severe TBI are typically quite distinct from those of adults with aphasia and children with congenital language disability.

With the exception of those with severe global impairment or significant dysarthria, most children and adults with TBI adequately manage the phonological, lexical, and grammatical aspects of language processing. This presentation contributes to gross—and often erroneous—clinical judgments of full recovery of language and to the common finding that verbal IQ tends to recover faster and more completely than performance IQ. However, clinicians and researchers alike have persuasively argued that valid identification of language impairment after TBI necessitates the use of measures that impose cognitive stressors on language processing (e.g., timed tests and tests requiring organization of extended units of language, both expressive and receptive) or social stressors on language processing (e.g., socially effective use of language in varied social contexts) (Chapman, 1997; Groher, 1992; Hartley, 1995; Ylvisaker, 1992, 1993). Standardized tests commonly used to measure verbal intelligence or to diagnose aphasia in adults or language disorders in children rarely include measures of the functions most vulnerable after TBI. The social dimensions of language disability after TBI are described later in the section on communication and social skills and in Chapter 6.

During the past decade, several investigators have made effective use of monologic (i.e., noninteractive) discourse measures to identify subclinical language processing impairment in children and adults with TBI (Biddle, McCabe, & Bliss, 1996; Chapman et al., 1995, 1997; Hartley, 1995; Hart-

ley & Jenson, 1991; Liles, Coelho, Duffy, & Zalagens, 1989; Mentis & Prutting, 1991). Chapman (1997) reported that 75% of children with severe closed head injury demonstrated expressive discourse problems 3 years postinjury, which was frequently undiagnosed and untreated by the children's school staff. Difficulties with discourse are the manifestation in language of underlying cognitive-organizational impairment and are most often associated with frontal lobe lesions. Impaired discourse may be evidenced in expressive language by disorganized and tangential conversations and monologues, imprecise language, or restricted output and lack of initiation. The same underlying organizational difficulty often results in word-retrieval problems. Receptively, organizational impairment may result in difficulty comprehending extended text or spoken language, detecting themes, and following rapidly spoken language. Some of these cognitive-language themes, associated with widespread bilateral frontal lobe injury (Alexander, Benson, & Stuss, 1989), are addressed in Chapter 5. Ylvisaker, Szekeres, and Haarbauer-Krupa (1998) presented a variety of intervention strategies for individuals with language-organizational impairment after TBI.

Just as it is difficult to draw a distinction between linguistic and cognitive phenomena in the case of organizational impairment and associated difficulty with discourse, so also linguistic and cognitive realities blend in the impairment of abstract language, indirect language, and ambiguous language. Many children and adults with TBI interpret language concretely, fail to comprehend all but overlearned figures of speech and metaphors, and have difficulty shifting among alternate meanings of ambiguous words and sentences (Alexander, Benson, & Stuss, 1989; Dennis, 1991; Dennis & Barnes, 1990). Concreteness in language processing can contribute to ineffective social interaction, particularly if the individual misinterprets as negative comments those that were intended to be sarcastic, ironic, or humorous, or in some other way had an intended meaning different from that received by the individual with brain injury.

Communication and Behavior

Behavior problems after TBI, their etiology, and their long-term course were described earlier and are elaborated in Chapter 6. In some cases, challenging behaviors develop as a means of communicating critical messages, such as (a) a desire to escape difficult or otherwise undesirable tasks or (b) a desire to acquire attention, sympathy, activities, objects, people, or other types of stimulation. When well-meaning staff and family members respond in systematically reinforcing ways to the unintentionally negative behaviors characteristic of the early postonset period of agitation and confusion, those behaviors may evolve into learned components of the individual's communication system. In such cases, communication specialists must collaborate with behavior specialists, staff, and family members in facilitating acquisition of a more acceptable substitute communication behavior (see Chapter 7).

Communication and Social Skills

Social skills include the general competencies and situationally relative behaviors that enable a person to be accepted and possibly liked in chosen social settings. Socially skilled people are able to positively affect others with the effect that they intend to have and are capable of being affected positively by others the way others would like to affect them. Given this broad definition, social-interactive competence includes a variety of learned behaviors as well as neurologically based capacities in many areas of functioning. Therefore, possible sources of disruption abound.

The characteristics described earlier under the headings pseudopsychopathic personality (primarily associated with orbitofrontal injury) and pseudodepressed personality (primarily associated with dorsolateral and dorsomesial prefrontal injury) could justifi-

ably reappear here under the heading of communication and social skills. More generally, all of the considerations in the previous section on behavior are relevant here. This nearly complete overlap in issues cries out for intensely collaborative efforts in rehabilitation, in this case among professionals concerned with communication, with behavior, and with psychosocial adjustment.

Traditional social skills training programs are designed to teach knowledge of social rules, roles, and routines, typically using role playing in a training context. Clearly, candidates for this type of intervention are people who lack the knowledge needed to behave in a socially competent manner. In contrast, many people with TBI possessed adequate social knowledge before the injury and retain it after the injury. In such cases, it is unlikely that role playing and discussion in a training setting will substantially improve social interaction. In Chapter 7 we describe an approach to social skills intervention that involves greater use of coaching in context.

Social skills may also appear to be weak for a variety of reasons not related to the injury. These were described in some detail in the previous section on behavioral outcome. Many children and young adults with TBI were at risk for their injuries in part because of checkered and sometimes unsuccessful social lives before their injury. Some experience severe psychological reactions to the injury and changes in life caused by the injury. Others grow progressively less competent socially because they have little opportunity to interact with others in varied social settings.

SUMMARY

Our goal in this chapter has been to orient readers to pathophysiologic and disability themes with which clinicians serving individuals with TBI should be familiar. We summarized in a general way much of the available information about outcome after TBI in our four overlapping domains of interest. Furthermore, we attempted to place common outcome themes in a neuropsychological perspective, while also remaining alert to the reality that many aspects of disability are, at best, indirectly related to the injury. The remaining chapters present what we hope is a coherent and practical approach to serving individuals with the sort of impairment and disability described in the current chapter.

CHAPTER 3

Functional Collaborative Assessment

Our goal in this chapter is to present a perspective on assessment when that assessment is designed to serve one important purpose, namely the development of a functional intervention plan consistent with an understanding of brain injury rehabilitation delivered in large part through positive everyday routines. The chapter opens with a discussion of the varied purposes of assessment and frank acknowledgment of the value of other approaches to assessment given other purposes to be served. We then explore in detail the process of ongoing, contextualized, collaborative, hypothesis-testing assessment (OCCHTA). We include procedures for analyzing everyday routines of interaction and end with a program-monitoring checklist designed to help staff and family members remain focused on critical priorities within the rehabilitation framework presented in this book. We intend this discussion to apply to children and adults with chronic disability in the four domains of functioning addressed in this book: executive functions, cognition, behavior, and communication.

PURPOSES OF ASSESSMENT

Assessments can serve a variety of purposes. The types of assessment related to the domains of function addressed in this book, namely neuropsychological, psychoeducational, language, vocational, and behavioral assessment, can be performed for purposes of:

- ➤ diagnosing a disease, disorder, or injury,
- ➤ deriving epidemiologic information about disability populations,
- ➤ deriving information about brain function,
- ➤ identifying consequences of injury for litigation,
- ➤ establishing that an individual meets criteria for classification or for qualification for services,
- ➤ formulating a prognosis,
- ➤ establishing baseline measures and subsequent measures of progress, and
- ➤ planning rehabilitative and educational intervention.

As a general rule, the purpose served by an assessment places specific constraints on the procedures used to achieve that purpose. For example, if the evaluator is preparing to defend judgments in a legal proceeding, the assessment tools used to support those judgments must possess psychometric properties sufficiently strong to withstand the potentially withering criticism of the counsel for the other party in the litigation. Similarly, if the goal is to derive information about a population of people, one of the constraints on assessment is that all individuals in the study sample are assessed using the same assessment tools.

In general, assessment procedures must be selected that achieve the goals of that assessment and are validated for that specific purpose. Useful and valid assessment is often threatened when several distinct purposes are combined and a procedure validated for one assessment purpose is used to serve a purpose that it is incapable of serving.

In this chapter, our only concern is with assessment for purposes of planning intervention and supports for individuals with executive function, cognitive, behavioral, and communication disability after TBI. When this is the sole purpose of assessment, clinicians are free, indeed mandated, to use procedures that would not meet criteria established for many of the other purposes of assessment. For example, administering tasks in a standardized manner and using the same tasks for all subjects would seem to be critical if the goal is the acquisition of epidemiologic information. In contrast, customizing assessment tasks, embedding them in everyday contexts, creatively modifying them in a hypothesis-testing manner, and possibly even engaging the individual in designing his or her own assessment tasks are critical when the purpose of the assessment is to identify how best to teach, manage, or otherwise support the individual with disability.

CONVENTIONAL ASSESSMENT: DISCIPLINE-SPECIFIC, TIME LIMITED, AND DECONTEXTUALIZED

In Chapter 1 we outlined in broad strokes major differences between what we characterized as conventional and functional approaches to rehabilitation. These differences in intervention have analogs when comparing conventional and functional approaches to assessment. In many clinical professions, including neuropsychology, special education, speech-language pathology, and others, assessment has historically been considered a time-limited activity (e.g., to be completed within the first 2 weeks of an admission or of the school year), is dominated by the administration of standardized, office-bound tests, is conducted separately by professionals who take responsibility for evaluating relatively distinct domains of functioning, and results in a static description of strengths and weaknesses, possibly combined with a diagnosis, prognosis, and recommendations for intervention. Excellent resources are available for those wishing to acquire information about assessment from this conventional diagnostic perspective. Lezak's (1995) *Neuropsychological Assessment* is a comprehensive reference for neuropsychologists; speech-language pathologists can consult Haynes, Pindzoal, and Emerick's (1992) text on assessment; Sattler's *Assessment of Children* (1995) describes issues in educational assessment.

For reasons described in the next section, assessment understood in these terms contributes only a portion of the information needed to create and maintain a functional and effective approach to intervention for people with brain injury. In some cases, test results are critical to planning intervention, for example, in cases in which the assessment leads to important technical interventions, such as pharmacologic management. Furthermore, office-bound tests may be an important component of the hypothesis-testing process described later: Tests can generate hypotheses to be tested in the real world and hypotheses generated in the real world can on occasion be tested using standardized measures (Ylvisaker, Hartwick, Ross, & Nussbaum, 1994). Finally, professionals responsible for office-bound standardized assessments typically supplement the information derived from testing with information from other sources (e.g., interviews with family members), information that may possess a higher degree of ecological validity than test results.

FUNCTIONAL ASSESSMENT: ONGOING, CONTEXTUALIZED, COLLABORATIVE TESTING OF HYPOTHESES

Ylvisaker and Feeney (1994) described a young student, Jim, who had multiple brain injuries as an infant and preschooler. At age 6, Jim had moderate-to-severe motor, cognitive, linguistic, and academic impairment, but was an object of intense concern mainly because of severe behavior problems, including frequent, intense, and prolonged acting out at school. At the first meeting we attended about Jim, it emerged that there were four distinct views about his behavior and its appropriate management. A small number of staff were convinced that Jim's challenging behaviors had been learned as a result of ill-advised management by staff and family in the past. That is, people in Jim's environment had insufficiently attended to his positive behavior and had routinely attended to disruptive behavior, allowing him to manipulate them with generally negative behavior. Therefore, group one argued, Jim needed a prolonged period of intensive, consistent, consequence-oriented behavior management designed to reverse these learned patterns of behavior.

The second group argued, in contrast, that Jim was extremely disorganized and confused and that his negative behavior was designed to inject orderliness and predictability into a world that otherwise was too difficult to understand and therefore produced intense anxiety. They insisted that Jim needed a simpler, more predicable life at school and at home. Group three argued that the issue was control. They observed that Jim had little control over events in his life at school and at home and used his disruptive behavior to wrest control from others, perhaps to escape undesirable activities or gain access to desirable ones, but definitely to experience control. They added that Jim had been abused, had twice been removed from his family to be placed in a new home, and in general had experienced the life of a powerless person who therefore needed a sense of control. He needed a dramatic increase in opportunities for choice and control, they concluded. The final group argued with considerable passion that Jim was depressed, that he had few meaningful activities, was successful at very little that mattered to him, and had no reciprocal friendships. Like many children, Jim was manifesting his de-

pression with oppositional behavior. The goal, they argued, should be to help Jim create more meaningful activities and satisfying peer relationships in his life.

All four opinions were surrounded by the sweet smell of reason; they all made sense and seemed consistent with what everybody knew about Jim. But they yielded different prescriptions regarding the best course of intervention. Therefore, this group had three options. First, they could continue to argue with each other. They had shown themselves to be quite capable of indefinitely continuing and escalating their arguments; unfortunately, this was of no help to Jim, the person they were supposed to be serving. Second, they could implement intervention procedures designed to address all four of the competing views. The primary problem with this option was that their intervention might turn out to be extremely inefficient and unnecessarily expensive. Furthermore, if they were successful, they would not know what contributed to the success, requiring them to continue possibly unnecessary interventions indefinitely.

With some encouragement, school staff and family members chose the most reasonable course, namely to consider each of the four views a hypothesis (versus a revealed truth, as these views were passionately presented at the original meeting) and to subject them to testing. They began with the cognitive hypothesis (confusion and disorganization) because they considered it the easiest hypothesis to test. They created a photograph orientation board that they used to keep Jim oriented and organized in three of his therapy sessions at school—and ensured that these sessions were organized and routine—and then compared behavior under these conditions with behavior with no special attempts to meet Jim's apparent need for orderliness and predictability. Challenging behaviors decreased by about 25% in the experimental condition, not enough to confirm the hypothesis that the issue was largely cognitive.

Next they tested the control hypothesis. They transformed the orientation board into a choice board and gave Jim the opportunity to choose activities (from a somewhat limited set of possibilities) and their order in the experimental settings. Under these circumstances, challenging behavior was reduced to near zero in those settings, but remained at high levels in settings with little or no choice. With this experimental verification in hand, school staff reorganized Jim's routines at school to include the maximum possible amount of choice and control across all of his daily routines. Their experiments enabled them to objectively identify the intervention and supports that would and did make a critical difference for Jim and his regulation of his behavior.

Jim's case vividly illustrates the process of ongoing, contextualized, collaborative, hypothesis-testing assessment (OCCHTA) for purposes of planning intervention. In the real world of complex people and multiply determined activities, this process cannot be experimental in the sense in which experiments in chemistry or physics are experimental. Many variables and complex interactions among them are often involved in determining performance of complex tasks or behavior under complex conditions. In Jim's case, for example, proponents of the depression hypothesis could have argued that they were right all along and that increasing opportunities for choice and control in Jim's life was the appropriate and successful treatment for his depression, thereby reducing challenging behavior as a secondary consequence. This real-world messiness notwithstanding, in our experience with individuals with complex and chronic disability after brain injury, the process of contextualized hypothesis testing is indispensable for identifying effective intervention procedures and for resolving conflicts among staff or between staff and family members.

OCCHTA: History of Dynamic Assessment

In educational psychology, speech-language pathology, and related fields, flexible hypothesis-testing assessment has its roots in the dynamic assessment movement, whose ancestry is generally traced to Vygotsky (Palinscar, Brown, & Campione, 1994). According to Vygotsky, the goal of psychoeducational assessment is to identify the learner's zone of proximal development, which he defined as "the distance between the actual developmental level as determined by independent problem solving and the level of potential development as determined through problem solving under adult guidance or in collaboration with more capable peers" (Vygotsky, 1978, p. 86). In today's terms, the zone of proximal development is the gap between performance on standardized psychological, neuropsychological, educational, vocational, or language tests, on the one hand, and performance supported by an expert collaborator, on the other. In most general terms, the examiner establishes the learner's levels of unassisted ability and then systematically modifies dimensions of the task to identify how much farther the learner can go with modification and assistance and what types of assistance or supports are most helpful.

Several attempts have been made to operationalize the process of dynamic assessment. Feuerstein (1979) created an assessment instrument, the Learning Potential Assessment Device (LPAD), which includes tasks similar to those found on intelligence tests, but with an invitation to the examiner to intervene in the child's performance, ask questions, make suggestions, and stimulate reflective thinking. Feuerstein's procedures have been criticized on grounds that the tasks are far too removed from real-world tasks to identify the learner's strategies with everyday tasks and that successful assessment is highly, perhaps overly, dependent on the insight, skill, and flexibility of the examiner (Palinscar, Brown, & Campione, 1994).

Campione and Brown (1984) have applied Vygotsky's concept of dynamic assessment in a different way. Learners are first pretested to determine their static level of performance on problem-solving or academic tasks (e.g., reading comprehension).

Then more difficult tasks are presented along with a hierarchically organized series of hints—starting with the most general—until the student succeeds with that type of task. The type and amount of help provided is a measure of learning potential. Learners are then given transfer tasks, again with help if necessary. The amount of help needed is a measure of the student's true understanding, or ability to transfer.

Behavioral psychologists have a rich history of using real contexts and systematically varying real-world stressors in their attempts to identify the variables that affect positive and negative behavior. This experimental process is similar in concept to dynamic assessment, although it has different historical and theoretical roots. Dunlap and Kern (1993) described a hypothesis-testing process closely resembling that described here. The goals of functional analysis of behavior are to identify stimuli that elicit and maintain problem behaviors, to identify events that increase or decrease the probability that behaviors will be maintained, and to evaluate the contexts in which behaviors occur, modifying those contexts if necessary. Kern and colleagues (1994) illustrated this process in identifying the cause of disruptive behavior in a classroom context and thereby creating an effective intervention plan. More generally, for many behavioral psychologists, functional analysis of behavior is precisely this process of systematic manipulation of hypothesized variables (Iwata, Vollmer, & Zarcone, 1990). Useful discussions of functional analysis of behavior can be found in Blackman and LeJeune (1990), Fernandez-Ballesteros and Staats (1992), Franzen (1991), and Horner (1994).

Consistent with the general themes of this book, our application of the concept of dynamic, experimental assessment liberates it from the limitations of an office or laboratory setting and opens the entirety of everyday life to the process. The goals remain the same: (a) to identify the individual's ability to succeed in selected tasks without assistance and to regulate behavior

positively without special supports and (b) to identify the types of assistance (supports or types of instruction) that are most effective in improving performance on relevant tasks and increasing the variety of contexts in which behavior is generally positive. We conceive of this process as *ongoing*, involving *collaboration* with a variety of people (including the individual with disability and everyday people in his or her life), occurring in a variety of contexts (including varied tasks, people, and settings), and involving systematic *tests of selected hypotheses*. Similar to Feuerstein's LPAD and unlike Campione and Brown's procedures, functional, dynamic assessment as we practice it is not a prescriptive procedure. However, its collaborative and contextualized nature helps address some of the shortcomings of one-person, office-bound, dynamic assessment with no specific direction for probing the effects of supports, suggestions, or modification of tasks.

OCCHTA: Rationale

Each component of ongoing, contextualized, collaborative hypothesis-testing assessment can be separately justified in its application to individuals with TBI.

Why Ongoing?

In the early months and possibly years after severe TBI, neurologic improvement can alter the individual's profile of strengths and weaknesses, necessitating ongoing monitoring of skills, of performance of everyday tasks, and of the appropriateness of placements, intervention programs, and supports (Benton, 1991; Filley et al., 1987; Hart & Jacobs, 1993). In addition, psychoreactive consequences of injury and disability may grow and change over time, resulting in changed patterns of behavior and performance (Grattan & Eslinger, 1991; Prigatano, 1986). In some cases, especially those involving children, negative consequences of the injury are delayed as the child grows into a disability related to a brain injury that lacks a functional consequence until the injured part of the brain is expected to mature and support a new developmental transition (see Chapter 2).

In a more immediate sense, hypothesis testing, like that described in Jim's case, is ongoing because it may require several weeks or more of systematic manipulation of relevant variables until the contributors to positive and negative behavior are clearly identified and integrated into a successful intervention plan. For all of these reasons, assessment must be considered an ongoing process and not a time-limited process that results in an assessment report and that precedes intervention.

Why Contextualized?

Neuropsychological research has produced considerable data calling into question the ecological validity of office-bound tests for individuals with frontal lobe injury (Benton, 1991; Bigler, 1988; Crépeau, Scherzer, Belleville, & Desmarais, 1997; Dennis, 1991; Eslinger & Damasio, 1985; Grattan & Eslinger, 1991; Mateer & Williams, 1991; Stelling, McKay, Carr, Walsh, & Bauman, 1986; Stuss & Benson, 1986; Varney & Menefee, 1993; Welsh, Pennington, & Groisser, 1991). For example, Dywan and Segalowitz (1996) found that psychometric measures had very little ability to predict real-world behavior problems in a group of adults with moderate-to-severe TBI. The classic situation is illustrated by Damasio's patient, Elliot, described in Chapter 1. MRI revealed a large, bilateral ventromedial and orbital prefrontal lesion. There was every reason to believe that this injury was responsible for pervasive and disastrous consequences in Elliot's life. However, he performed well, in some cases exceptionally well, on every neuropsychological test presented to him, including those specifically designed to reveal the consequences of prefrontal injury.

This pattern of adequate performance on tests combined with serious functional breakdowns in everyday life is well docu-

mented and must be accounted for in making judgments about people specifically with frontal lobe injury and generally with TBI. The frequent, but unacceptable error made by poorly informed clinicians is the judgment that individuals who have adequate scores on tests after TBI should perform at levels predicted by these test results in their real worlds of school, work, and social life. Of course they may do just that; however, the number of documented counter examples to this inference demands professional caution in predicting real-world performance in the basis of test results.

Challenges to the ecological validity of office-bound assessments arise in the opposite direction as well. Many people with frontal lobe injury, possibly combined with damage to other parts of the brain, perform poorly on the unfamiliar tasks included in neuropsychological or other assessments, but nevertheless perform beyond expectations when they return to work or other routine and supported contexts of everyday life. A likely explanation for this phenomenon revolves around the role of the frontal lobes in nonroutine behavior (Fuster, 1989, 1991; Hebb, 1945). If the office-bound assessment tasks require solutions to novel problems and efficient performance of unfamiliar tasks, significant impairment may be revealed. However, adequate real-world performance of *routine* vocational or daily living tasks is fully compatible with this impairment. In either case, whether the potential threat to assessment comes from the side of false positives or false negatives, there is no alternative but to include structured probes of performance of contextualized, real-world tasks, both routine and nonroutine, as part of comprehensive assessment after TBI.

Why Collaborative?

Collaboration in assessment can be supported by a variety of considerations. Most obviously, increasing the number of people who contribute to an assessment increases the number and variety of observations that can be made and contexts in which they can be made. Professionals responsible for coordinating particular types of assessment must, of course, establish the reliability of these observations. Collaborators are also available to enhance the hypothesis-generation discussions and to enrich the hypothesis-testing process by making available a wide domain of contexts for experimentation.

Second, the more that people collaborate in assessment, the greater the likelihood of collaboration in implementing the intervention plan derived from the assessment. Professional colleagues, paraprofessionals, and family members are notoriously lukewarm collaborators in intervention plans that are handed down from on high, with no opportunity to shape the plan or to thoroughly understand it and its rationale (Bailey, 1987). In contrast, when the same people contribute observations, help to test hypotheses, and work with specialists to shape the intervention plan, cooperation increases and with it the likelihood of successful implementation of the plan (Bailey, 1987; Durand, Berotti, & Weiner, 1993).

Third, collaborative hypothesis-testing helps to resolve conflicts among staff, between staff and family, and between staff or family, on the one hand, and the individual with TBI on the other (Carnevale, 1996; Feeney & Ylvisaker, 1995, 1997). That is, differences of opinion about the cause of problems and about the best course of action have the potential to become conflicts or even raging territorial warfare if allowed to fester. In contrast, when staff routinely translate differences of opinion into statements of alternative hypotheses waiting to be tested, potentially destructive conflicts can often be avoided.

Finally, collaboration in assessment is a statement of respect. Individuals with chronic disability are served well if they are served by professionals and everyday people who respect one another. Specialists communicate respect to their colleagues and to everyday people when their posture is captured in a collaborative invitation such as, "I have some ideas about the critical issues, but I would love it if you could help me sort them out and then determine how best to proceed" as opposed to, "I have completed my assessment and have written the treatment plan. Here is what you must do to make this plan successful." As consultants, we find ourselves routinely inviting collaboration in hypothesis-testing, even in cases in which we are quite sure we know how best to proceed. The small investment in time and effort typically yields substantial returns as staff and everyday people set about to implement a coherent program of intervention.

Why Testing of Hypotheses?

Virtually all human behavior is multiply determined. Many variables, in the individual and in the environment, contribute to performance of tasks. Therefore, breakdowns in varied domains, in the individual and in the environment, can disrupt performance. Just as a given task can be performed poorly for many different reasons, a given task can be performed well as a consequences of many different strategic approaches and supports. Ylvisaker and Gioia (1998) used the example of failure on a simple paragraph comprehension task to illustrate this fundamental point. Failure on the task could be explained by any combination of the following:

Physical Problems: The student may be fatigued, hungry, overmedicated, undermedicated, in pain, sick, or experiencing subclinical seizures.

Sensory/Perceptual Problems: The student may be unable to see the print, maintain one clear image, track from left to right, or scan back to the left.

Cognitive Problems: Attention: The student may be unable to sustain attention sufficiently, filter out internal or external distractions, divide attention between the information and the questions, shift attention from the previous task to the current task.

Cognitive Problems: Orientation: The student may be unclear about what is expected of him.

Cognitive Problems: Memory: The student may have difficulty encoding the information for subsequent storage and retrieval, storing information long enough to answer the questions, or retrieving information from storage to answer the questions.

Cognitive Problems: Organization/Integration: The student may have difficulty organizing information to comprehend the text, to understand how details relate to each other, to understand how the questions relate to the text, or to formulate an organized answer.

Cognitive Problems: General Speed of Information Processing: The student may simply be very slow at all tasks.

Language Problems: The student may be unable to comprehend the vocabulary or syntax of the text or questions, or may have difficulty retrieving words to answer the questions.

Academic Problems: The student may be unable to decode printed language efficiently.

Emotional/Motivational/Behavioral Problems: The student may be depressed, anxious, fearful, angry, unmotivated, oppositional, or euphoric.

Clearly, if the evaluator only knows that the student failed on the task, it would be impossible to identify an appropriate intervention to improve relevant skills or to create an appropriate set of compensations. In the case of reading failure, common sense would drive evaluators to rule in or rule out possible contributors to the problem. Possible visual-perceptual contributors could be explored by following up the task with a comparable task, but now with large print or possibly a window to block out all but one line at a time. Possible organizational contributors could be explored by providing an advance organizer or breaking the paragraph into smaller units. The other

possibilities could be explored in a similar systematic manner. If performance increases sharply with one or other of the task modifications, there is reason to believe that an important contributor to failure has been identified.

This common sense activity of systematically teasing out what contributes to failure and what contributes to success is experimentation or hypothesis-testing. In adult neuropsychological assessment, hypothesis-testing is often referred to as *process assessment* (Kaplan, 1988). In child psychoeducational assessment, it is typically referred to as *dynamic assessment*. In applied behavior analytic assessment, it is typically referred to as *functional analysis* (Horner, 1994; Neef & Iwata, 1994). In our everyday framework, it is part of a larger and indispensable process of ongoing, collaborative, contextualized testing of hypotheses. Illustrations of hypotheses and appropriate tests are presented in Table 3–1. Illustrations 2 and 3 in Table 3–1 are actual case material; the hypotheses and tests of hypotheses were generated by collaborative teams attempting to help difficult-to-serve clients.

OCCHTA: Implementation Process

Described in somewhat idealized terms, OCCHTA proceeds sequentially through five distinct stages: identification of the problem, formulation of reasonable hypotheses, selection of hypotheses to test and their order, testing of the hypotheses, and formulation of an intervention plan based on the results of this experimentation. In the case of complex cross-disciplinary issues, such as those addressed in this book, OCCHTA is a process implemented by a team of people, typically including several professional staff members, everyday people, such as paraprofessional aides and family members, and, most importantly, the individual with TBI. Depending on the specific concerns driving the assessment, the process should be coordinated by a specialist in that area who actively collaborates with other members of the team.

TABLE 3–1. Illustrations of contextualized, collaborative hypothesis testing.

ASSESSMENT QUESTION #1

Why does John seem to understand information when I present it to him, but rarely can state the next day what he had learned? What should we do about this?

Collaborative hypothesis generation

John's problem could be a consequence of many cognitive or executive system breakdowns, or combinations of them. For example, (1) Retrieval: John processes, encodes, and stores the information, but has difficulty retrieving it the next day. (2) Storage: He encodes the information, but simply does not retain it. (3) Organization/Encoding: His initial processing of the information is superficial, making it possible for him to answer questions immediately, but not retain the information. (4) Attention: He can remember information, but only when he is not distracted at the time of encoding and at the time of retrieval. (5) Repetition: He can remember information, but only if it is repeated many times.

Collaborative hypothesis testing

Hypothesis 1: Retrieval: John processes, encodes and stores the information, but has difficulty retrieving it the next day.

Test: Systematically compare John's performance on *free recall* tasks (e.g., "Tell me about the story we read yesterday.") versus *recognition memory* tasks (e.g., true/false questions). If John does much better on recognition memory tasks, teachers and others will need to use such tasks in assessing his retention of information.

Hypothesis. 2: Storage: John encodes the information, but simply does not retain it.

Test: Systematically compare John's performance on immediate recall tasks versus delayed recall tasks. Vary the time delay. If storage is specifically impaired, John will need memory prostheses.

Hypothesis 3: Organization/Encoding: John's initial processing of the information is superficial, making it possible for him to answer questions immediately, but not retain the information.

Test: Systematically compare John's performance on memory tasks when given advance organizers versus no advance organizers. If organizers make a substantial difference, he may benefit from a rich assortment of advance organizers for tasks throughout the day.

Hypothesis 4: Attention: John can remember information, but only when he is not distracted at the time of encoding and at the time of retrieval.

Test: Systematically compare John's performance in the presence of distractions versus none. If distractions substantially impair performance, he may need to receive instruction in a nondistracting environment.

Hypothesis 5: Repetition: John can remember information, but only if it is repeated many times.

Test: Systematically compare Jon's performance when given only one or two repetitions versus many repetitions. If repetition makes a substantial difference, staff and family will need to find a way to encourage large amounts of repetition.

ASSESSMENT QUESTION #2

Why does Bill refuse and become aggressive when asked to leave the bus in the morning upon its arrival at school?

Collaborative hypothesis generation

Bill's oppositional and aggressive behavior could be the result of many factors. For example, (1) he may be confused and disoriented when he arrives at school and therefore act out as a result of associated anxiety; (2) he may use aggressive behavior to communicate his need or desire to escape nonpreferred activities at school; (3) he may act out because he enjoys the attention that he routinely gets from many staff members and other students when he is acting out.

continued

TABLE 3–1. *continued*

Collaborative hypothesis testing

Hypothesis 1: Confusion: Because of significant cognitive and organizational impairments, Bill does not understand what is happening and is afraid.

Test: Compare the frequency, intensity, and duration of challenging behavior with no preparation for the bus-to-school transition versus when the bus-to-school transitional routine includes preparation using photographs of school staff and school activities, consistent orientation to the first activity of the day, given while Bill is still on the bus, and a routine welcome from school staff before Bill leaves the bus.

Hypothesis 2: Avoidance: Bill does not like the activities that are expected of him when he arrives at school and he successfully avoids these nonpreferred activities by engaging in challenging behaviors

Test: Compare the frequency, intensity, and duration of challenging behavior with no change in the current routine versus (a) when Bill is given the opportunity to choose the first activities of the day and (b) when activities are systematically altered (e.g., 1 week of math [nonpreferred] upon arrival, then 1 week of physical education [preferred], then 1 week of English [nonpreferred]).

Hypothesis 3: Attention. Bill engages in these problem behaviors because he enjoys the attention that he gets from staff and other students when he is acting out.

Test. Compare the frequency, intensity, and duration of challenging behavior with no change in the current routine versus the following experimental alternative routines:

A. Wait to ask Bill to leave the bus until all the other students are gone and minimize the number of people that are in proximity to Bill during the bus transition time (testing proximity attention).
B. Verbally prompt Bill at the beginning of the bus transition time and then keep verbal interactions at a minimum and only speak in a low voice tone (testing verbal attention).
C. Verbally prompt Bill at the beginning of the bus transition time and only speak in a low tone of voice (testing emotional attention).
D. Increase the frequency of attention that Bill receives while riding the bus (before the transition) and after entering the school and engaging in prescribed activities.

ASSESSMENT QUESTION #3

Why does Charlie, who was pretraumatically obese, continually ask for food and become aggressive when his requests are denied?

Collaborative hypothesis generation

Charlie's uncontrolled eating behavior may be (a) a result of an unknown metabolic or other medical condition, (b) an expression of access-motivated behavior, (c) an expression of his need to control others' behavior.

Collaborative hypothesis testing

Hypothesis 1: Medical: Charlie has an unknown metabolic or medical condition that results in an irresistible drive to eat, which cannot be redirected.

Test: Charlie could be referred for a medical evaluation, including neurology, endocrinology, and gastroenterology consults. If there are positive findings, recommended changes will be made in his program, carefully comparing eating behaviors before and after the change in regimen.

Hypothesis 2: Acquisition: Charlie simply wants to eat and he does whatever it takes to get food.

Test: Compare the frequency and onset of eating-related behaviors under the following conditions:

A. Continue with the current attempts to prevent Charlie from getting food.
B. For a preagreed period of time, give Charlie free access to as much food as he would like to eat.

Hypothesis 3: Control: Charlie has few opportunities to control even the most basic elements of his daily routine. The only thing he can really control is what he eats and he fiercely resists any attempts to control this part of his life.

Test: Compare the frequency and onset of eating-related behaviors under the following conditions.

A. Develop a system in which Charlie is able to make decisions about what activities he will engage in and when he will engage in them, including what he will eat and when he will eat it (within preagreed limits).

B. Use the same system but have the staff make the decisions about what he will do and when he will do it, including eating.

Problem Identification

In some cases, such as Jim's (described earlier), there is no difficulty identifying the problem that mandates a functional assessment. Staff were in conflict about the basis of the problem, but all agreed that the problem was his frequent and intense acting out behavior. In other cases, team discussion is required to clearly identify the problem, which can then be explored experimentally. For example, we once consulted with school staff who were concerned about an 11-year-old with TBI, Beth. Beth's social worker characterized the problem as social isolation; her teacher said that the problem was lack of initiative and motivation; her mother requested help with what she considered the key problem, namely oppositional behavior and angry outbursts. After some discussion, staff and family agreed that they were all focusing on only one aspect of a complex problem that may manifest itself under different circumstances as isolation and withdrawal, apparent lack of motivation, and oppositionality. In other words, their separate identifications of the problem were actually implicit hypotheses about the source of the problem. After experimenting with some supports designed to compensate for a hypothesized organically based lack of activation and initiation, it became clear that Beth had an underlying activation impairment that often appeared as social withdrawal (the social worker's concern), as apparent absence of motivation (the teacher's concern), and as oppositionality when pressed (the mother's concern).

In the case of individuals with behavior problems, it is useful to obtain descriptions of and judgments about the challenging behaviors from a variety of people, including the person with TBI. This screening is the first step of a process that proceeds next to testing hypotheses. In Appendix A we present a screening form that has been successfully used in New York State as part of a major effort to identify individuals with behavioral problems after TBI who are living and receiving services in settings that may be overly restrictive. A major goal of the program is to support these individuals in less restrictive community settings, providing technical assistance and other forms of support to the community-based professionals and others charged with the task of helping the individual to succeed and achieve a satisfying life in that setting. We developed the screening process to identify, in at least a preliminary way, the person's needs and plan community supports to meet those needs. In addition, we have used this screening process in the early phases of hypothesis generation and as a means of orienting each member of the intervention team to the goals and priorities of the other team members.

Hypothesis Formulation

Having identified the problem, team members must formulate hypotheses to be tested. In many cases, neurologic information and results of standardized testing contribute to the goal of this stage. For example, in Beth's case, neurodiagnostic information suggested damage to cortical regions known to be associated with activation and initiation. It is important to note that this information suggested a *hypothesis* about Beth's behavior; it did not necessarily explain that behavior in the absence of further exploration. Even with an injury to that part of the brain, it is possible that her isolation resulted primarily from genuine depression or anxiety, not lack of activation; similarly, it is possible that her inactivity in class was a primary consequence of lack of interest, not brain injury; finally, behavior with her mother could have been preadolescent oppositionality wholly independent of the brain injury. Therefore, hypothesis testing was still needed—and typically continues to be needed after neurodiagnostic information is gathered and interpreted and after standardized office-bound tests have been administered.

Hypothesis formulation is a creative process, with no firm rules to follow. Working collaboratively within a team framework helps to ensure that no stone is left unturned. During the brainstorming phase of this discussion, staff should be encouraged to think expansively and consider all of the possible forces that may be contributing to the identified problem. Especially when staff have already become hardened in their opinion (e.g., "It's all the fault of the crazy mother," "I know that he is a lazy child. He always has been and he always will be," "Adolescents just need more discipline from firm authority figures," "He's been in trouble with the law his entire life. What can we do now?"), the leader of the discussion must urge participants to be flexible and consider alternative possibilities, even if they believe they have good reason to reject them without an extensive assessment.

Hypothesis Selection

Often several hypotheses are offered, each of which has proponents and appears reasonable in light of what is known about the person. Which hypothesis should be tested first? Typically, this question is best answered by balancing three factors: likelihood of confirmation, importance of the hypothesis, and ease of testing. In Jim's case, the team chose the cognitive hypothesis first, in part because it seemed to several team members to be a major contributor to Jim's behavior, but more importantly be-

cause they considered it the easiest of the four hypotheses to test. They correctly judged that they would be able to test the hypothesis within 2 to 3 weeks with very little change of their prevailing routines and no additional resources. In contrast, had they chosen to test the traditional operant hypothesis first, they would have had to train all staff in consistent contingency management practices, probably endure a prolonged worsening of Jim's acting-out behavior (i.e., an extinction burst), wait for weeks or longer to see if the experiment succeeded, and finally, in the event of apparent disconfirmation, argue among themselves about the validity of the results because of predictably inconsistent implementation of the experimental plan.

Hypothesis Testing

In some cases, such as the reading difficulty described earlier, several hypotheses can be tested quickly and efficiently by one evaluator in a testing situation. However, in the case of major issues that have an impact on many dimensions of the person's life, such as Jim's acting-out behavior described earlier, putting hypotheses to the test requires collaboration among several people using several contexts of activity at various times of the day. To create something approaching experimental conditions, each member of the team, often including family members, needs to follow an agreed-upon script and pay close attention to the outcome. This is not to say that individuals are locked into their script come what may, an unreasonable demand that would surely generate staff oppositionality, nor is it to say that data collection becomes the top priority in their lives, another common fear of busy staff. The point is to devise a general framework within which to operate.

It is critical for team members to be on the same page with respect to the scripts that define the experiments and to pay close enough attention to the outcome of the experiment so that something can be made of the results. If they choose to deviate from the script, this must be discussed with the team so that the ongoing experiment can have interpretable results. If the issue is a serious behavior issue, the team must have an agreed-upon crisis plan (i.e., an alternative plan B) and guidelines for shifting from plan A to plan B. Finally, a decision should be made in advance about the length of time that the experimental conditions will be in place and about which team members will be responsible for monitoring various aspects of the experiment.

Compound Hypotheses

In situations in which the problem is serious and must be addressed quickly, and in which team members are convinced that several factors are involved in determining the individual's difficulty, those variables can be packaged and tested as a unit. For example, Feeney and Ylvisaker (1995) described such a situation involving three adolescents whose behavior had deteriorated sharply over several years following severe TBI in early adolescence. Each of the young men had become aggressive, two had been expelled from school, and one had been expelled from a special vocational program in favor of an admission to a locked psychiatric unit. The aggression was of such a frequency and intensity that there was insufficient time to systematically explore hypothesized variables one at a time.

Therefore, working with us, the young men, their families, and staff formulated a complex hypothesis about the adolescents' behavior. First, they proposed that the boys had greater organizational impairment than had been identified, requiring more effective supports to compensate for the organizational impairment. Second, they recognized that these boys were oppositional and needed more opportunities for choice and control than had been allowed them. Third, they recognized that staff who interacted with the boys needed to be better at interpreting their first communications of frustration and anger, rather than nagging

and thereby causing a manageable situation to escalate into a crisis. Finally, they recognized the frequency with which the boys experienced failure and frustration. Therefore, they added an element to daily routines mandating high success tasks before stressful low success tasks were introduced; that is, the boys needed to have positive behavioral momentum established before being invited to attack difficult or stressful tasks. These four components of a compound hypothesis were then packaged together into an experimental intervention—a major modification of daily routines—which proved to be highly successful.

Our point here is not to promote the intervention that proved successful in this case. Rather, this illustration shows how potentially separate hypotheses can be packaged and tested together if decisions about changes in the intervention plan must be made quickly. Once the situation is under control, the combination of supports can be systematically disassembled to determine which components are especially critical. In some cases, disassembly is not possible. There may be multiple and interactive reasons for a particular individual to engage in a particular behavior. Isolating variables in these cases may yield erroneous information.

Formulation of the Intervention Plan

When the results of the hypothesis testing are clear, as they were in Jim's case, formulation of the intervention plan is conceptually rather simple. That is, the team attempts to modify the environment and supports based on results of the experiment so that the individual is as successful as possible and ongoing growth in the area of concern is facilitated. After completing their experiment, Jim's staff created choice and control routines throughout his day at school; similarly, his family did the same, given the constraints of their home routines and the needs of the other children. In some cases, a *series* of plans may emerge, with a criterion for moving from one plan to the next.

There may be conflicts about the plan, as there were in Jim's case. Some staff were more flexible than others in their willingness to create opportunities for choice and control. More generally, the hypothesis-testing process may suggest modifications in the environment, staff behavior, or other supports that are simply impossible to implement. These are important practical and strategic concerns, often necessitating some degree of compromise and balancing of competing values. However, the point remains that the experimental process gives concrete direction to these negotiations.

Ongoing Plan-Do-Review

In the real world, functional experimental assessment and associated intervention planning may not always be as neat and linear as presented in our account. In Figure 3–1 we illustrate an ongoing process of planning, doing, and reviewing that may be simultaneously at more than one point in the process, may loop back to the planning stage many times, and may be at any given stage for anywhere from a few minutes to several months. The main point is to maintain an experimental orientation to assessment and to create an institutional routine in which questions and conflicts are addressed within an experimental framework (i.e., "What should we do? I don't know. But let's see if we can figure it out experimentally!") and intervention decisions are based on the results of experimentation.

OCCHTA and Conflict Resolution

In Jim's case, a history of conflict had evolved, including disagreements among staff and between staff and family. In our experience,

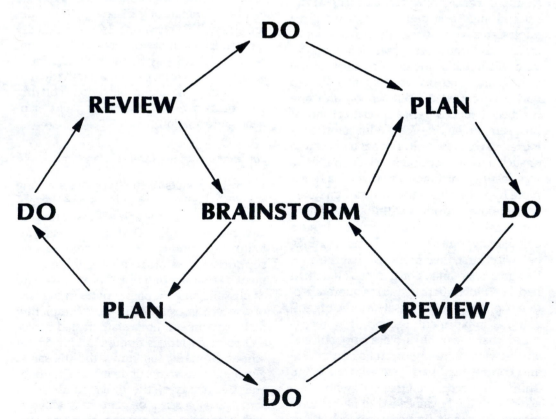

Figure 3–1. A representation of the ongoing plan-do-review process of hypothesis testing for assessment purposes.

conflicts of this sort are extremely common in the case of people with TBI and others with complex profiles of ability and troubling behavior. Rarely are such conflicts resolved through discussions that often evolve into aggravated conflicts of wills. An experimental orientation to assessment—and to conflict resolution—holds the potential to resolve differences of this sort. Within this orientation, the posture of staff is not, "I have 15 years of experience; I know I am right about this and I cannot understand why you disagree," but rather, "We seem to have different views on this important point; what do you suppose we could do to test these views and decide together how best to proceed?" To be sure, not every hypothesis is testable and not every conflict can be resolved experimentally. Furthermore, some hypotheses would simply consume too much time and money (e.g., "I feel that he needs 3 years of intensive residential behavioral programming at $1,500 per day. Could we please test my hypothesis?"). However, in our experience this open experimental and collaborative attitude goes a long way toward overcoming natural suspicions among professionals and between professionals and family members.

The same experimental attitude supports collaborative experimentation with individuals with TBI. When we worked in inpatient rehabilitation, we had countless interactions with individuals insisting that they were ready for discharge at a time when staff believed that discharge would be unconscionable. So, rather than communicating, in effect, "We know what's good for you"—a communication likely to generate alienation in adolescents and young adults with disability—we said, in effect, "OK, we seem to differ on how things will go when you leave. Let's try to think of a way for us to experiment with our conflicting views and then we might have a better basis for making a judgment about discharge."

OCCHTA: Obstacles to Implementation

The type of functional assessment described in this chapter is increasingly used by be-

havioral psychologists as an experimental approach to functional analysis of behavior (Bailey & Pyles, 1989; Carr et al., 1993, 1994; Dumas, 1986; Horner, 1994; Neef & Iwata, 1994). However, despite its solid rationale in theory and practice, the approach as a whole seems to be relatively rare in cognitive, language, and educational assessment. In our experience as consultants to varied service settings, medical rehabilitation facilities are perhaps the least likely to practice OCCHTA. We speculate that there are several possible reasons for their reluctance.

Inadequate Training in the Use of These Assessment Procedures

Most professionals who deal with the cognitive, communicative, educational, and vocational domains of rehabilitation are thoroughly trained in the administration and interpretation of standardized tests. In addition, they tend to be trained in clinical interviewing, informal observation, and possibly even experimental manipulation of assessment tasks during office-bound testing (i.e., dynamic or process assessment). However, collaboration with others in assessment and experimentation in natural environments are, in our experience, quite rare in rehabilitation facilities. Because of inadequate preprofessional training in this area, leadership in institutional program development may fall to those who appreciate the positive impact that this approach can have in developing effective rehabilitation and education plans and in creating collaborative relationships.

Administrative Requirements

In rehabilitation facilities, schools, and other settings in which rehabilitative and educational services are provided, it may be necessary to complete an assessment within a limited time period after admission or after the referral is received. Licensing and accrediting bodies may require that these assessments include a diagnosis, a prognosis, and recommendations for specific services. These administrative requirements can be met while at the same time maintaining a commitment to the process of OCCHTA. The key is to distinguish different purposes of assessment and use procedures appropriate to the purpose in question. The OCCHTA process is an ongoing component of intervention and is initiated each time an important question about the individual or the intervention program is raised, an answer to which requires organized, planned, collaborative experimentation.

Failure to Distinguish Purposes of Assessment

We frequently field objections to OCCHTA on grounds that the reliability of informants is questionable, that the tasks used in the contextualized experiments are not validated for that purpose, that without a true experimental design in place it is unacceptable to call these relatively informal explorations true experiments, and that assessment is much too important and technical a process to be turned over to untrained people. In response, we routinely remind the challenger that there are many purposes for assessment and that some of these purposes must meet exacting standards of psychometric purity and credentialing. However, for the purposes under discussion in this chapter, the functional procedures of OCCHTA are most valid, for reasons stated throughout.

Desire to Retain Special Expertise

Resistance to collaborative, contextualized assessment may be a result of general resistance to collaborating, particularly with nonprofessional people. Professionals who pride themselves in the special expertise of their discipline and the technical competence that they have acquired as a result of years of study and clinical practice may find it difficult to engage nonspecialized people as equals on the field of collaboration. Others may simply lack the confidence needed to sit at a table with several

people and brainstorm, without the support of a protective cloak of specialized, discipline-specific expertise. In Chapter 8 we address the obstacles to creating a collaborative culture in rehabilitation and offer some ways to overcome those obstacles.

ASSESSMENT CONTENT: PERFORMANCE OF REAL-WORLD TASKS

Specialists in special education (Browder, 1991; Brown & Snell, 1993) and education-related services (e.g., Nelson, 1994) increasingly recommend orienting assessments to the specific curricular needs of the student, including both academic and social curricula. That is, the goal of assessment is not simply to identify a profile of strengths and weaknesses in the abstract, but rather to identify the student's level of knowledge and skill, needs, and appropriate intervention strategies *in relation to his or her academic and social curriculum*. Similarly, functional assessment of individuals with challenging behavior requires exploration of functional relationships between behaviors and their antecedents and consequences *in the settings in which the individual must function and in the context of the people, tasks, and demands found in those settings* (Dunlap & Kern, 1993).

Curriculum-based assessment is not designed to replace but to supplement assessments with the goal of diagnosing underlying processing impairments. Translating the concept of curriculum-based assessment into rehabilitation settings, hospital staff would be expected to explore a variety of education-related skills and behaviors in preparation for a school-age patient's school reentry. We have discussed this aspect of hospital assessment in some detail elsewhere (Ylvisaker & Feeney, 1998; Ylvisaker, Hartwick, & Stevens, 1991). Similarly, hospital staff may need to be creative in exploring the effects of various types of real-world social stress on social-interactive competence. In the case of adults, assessment related to judgments about return to work and to social and family life should use tasks and contexts as closely related to the individual's work and social life as possible. Adolescents and adults with whom we have worked have experienced considerable frustration and justifiable anger when staff make judgments about their ability or inability to perform specific tasks based only on inference from performance on tasks that bear little resemblance to the "curricular" tasks to which they wish to return, that is, the important activities and settings of their lives.

ASSESSMENT CONTENT: EVERYDAY ROUTINES

The theme of this book is delivering rehabilitation to people with chronic disability after TBI through positive everyday routines. From this perspective, a critical component of assessment is exploration of those routines and of the consequences of modifying those routines.

Routines and Transitions

From the perspective of our four domains of functioning, the critical times for support and practice—and, on the negative side, for breakdowns and failure—are transitions, including large transitions (e.g., from hospital to home and community), middle-sized transitions (e.g., transitions into and out of the day; transitions from one therapy, class, or vocational activity to another), and small transitions (e.g., transitions into a therapy session, from activity to activity within the session, and out of the session).

Executive functions are most naturally exercised during transitions. Ideally, the day begins with reflection about the goals to be accomplished during the day, possible obstacles to accomplishing them (including internal states of the individual), a plan for accomplishing the goals (possibly including specific types of help from others, necessary resources, time frames, and the like), and an estimate of how successful the plan will be.

At some point toward the end of a well-designed day (from the perspective of exercising executive functions), there is a review of the day's accomplishments, including a comparison of the plan with the outcome, reflection on what worked and what did not work, and a judgment about what to try the next time. This same beginning and ending template can be applied to smaller units of time, including therapy sessions or work trials and activities within those sessions. Understood in these routine terms, important contextualized executive function practice can easily occur 10, 15, or 20 times each day.

Cognitive functions can be similarly engaged in functional ways during transitional times. Practice organizing can occur as plans are formulated. Prospective and retrospective memory, as well as compensatory strategies needed in the event of chronic impairment, are naturally engaged at the beginning of activities and during the review at the end. Reasoning and problem solving are inevitably part of planning in the face of obstacles and reviewing what works, what does not work, and what is best to try the next time.

Behavioral self-regulation is ideally addressed at the beginning and end of activities as the individual anticipates difficulties, makes decisions about what to do in the event of trouble, and subsequently reviews the effectiveness of attempts to regulate behavior. Furthermore, it is often the behavior of others during transitions that paves the way for positive behavior or, alternatively, encourages challenging behavior. For example, people with behavior problems generally do better when the transition into an activity includes clear orientation to the activity, some degree of choice, and some development of positive momentum before attacking difficult tasks. Finally, transition times are the most natural occasions for social communication and naturalistic approaches to practicing improved social skills.

With this as background, it is apparent that functional rehabilitation mandates assessment of transitions and the routines present during these transitions. Unfortunately, because people are commonly on automatic pilot during routines, it may be difficult for them to reliably describe their behavior during routine transitions or that of the person with disability. Therefore, evaluators may need to acquire information about routines in alternative ways. Direct observation has the disadvantage of interfering with the routine (i.e., people tend to behave differently while being observed) and is also logistically difficult. For this reason, we often videotape transitions and review these tapes with staff and other everyday people, using procedures described later.

Assessment of Behavior of Everyday Communication Partners

Everyday routines include settings, sequences of events and activities, and the objects needed for the activities. Importantly, routines also include language and other forms of communication, including that of the individual with disability and of his or her communication partners. We have described the importance of staff communication behavior for positive rehabilitation of people with cognitive, communication, and behavioral disability elsewhere (Ylvisaker & Feeney, 1998; Ylvisaker, Feeney, & Urbanczyk, 1993, 1993b). The language of communication partners can support all of the goal areas discussed in this book. Alternatively, that language can create learned helplessness (e.g., when the staff person takes too much responsibility for directing the person with disability), confusion (e.g., when the staff person fails to orient the individual or uses confusing language), behavior problems (e.g., when the staff person nags, talks in a disrespectful manner, rewards challenging behavior, or takes impulsive behavior personally).

Therefore, the language of communication partners is an important target for assessment and intervention. A common form of routine-based intervention, illustrated in subsequent chapters, is preparation of scripts, which are then followed by all everyday communication partners. This intervention process begins with assessment of existing communication routines, often using videos of those routines.

Videotaped Routines and Guided Video Feedback

An ideal way to gather information about everyday routines and, at the same time, to modify those routines in a positive manner is to videotape the routines and then guide staff and family members in the analysis of the video. A guide to the use of video feedback is presented in Table 3–2.

SELF-ASSESSMENT

With the goal of helping people with TBI improve executive functions, including self-awareness of strengths and weaknesses and ability to self-monitor and self-evaluate performance, there exists a strong rationale to include individuals with disability in planning, implementing, and interpreting assessment tasks. This engagement can be accomplished by using a relatively formal self-assessment instrument, by negotiating assessment tasks with the individual, and by attaching a script to everyday tasks, requesting that the person predict performance in advance, evaluate performance after completing the task, and compare predicted performance with actual performance.

Ylvisaker, Szekeres, and Feeney (1998) presented a self-assessment protocol designed for use in high school learning disability programs. It includes a detailed self-assessment rating form covering relevant domains of functioning (study skills, test taking, written expression, behavior, social and interpersonal skills, and specific academic content areas) and a protocol for using the self-assessment to collaboratively develop an individualized education plan. The form and associated process have not been subjected to psychometric investiga-

TABLE 3–2. Guidelines for video feedback for staff and others who interact with individuals with TBI.

Ground Rules for Video Feedback for Staff

➤ Videotape is not to be used for surveillance reasons or to "catch" problems.
➤ The tape will only be viewed by individuals who are approved by those being videotaped.
➤ Specialists who guide staff in video analysis of behavior should model the process by publicly analyzing their own behavior on video (including their own awkwardness and mistakes).
➤ In reviewing videos, the search is for illustrative routine events, not unusual events, however significant they may be.

Preparatory Activities

➤ Identify roles for taping and tape review (more than one can be identified for each period of taping).
  ➤ Skilled staff who will be videotaped to demonstrated skilled interaction
  ➤ Individual with brain injury who wants to demonstrate a skill or need
  ➤ Less skilled staff who are looking for feedback
  ➤ Skilled staff whose role is one of mentor or guide for actual video feedback
➤ Identify specific areas of focus as defined by the individual and by staff.
➤ Identify a specific time frame for taping.
➤ Identify an area for camera placement.
➤ Clearly articulate the existing routine and try to avoid changing the routine while videotaping.
➤ Attend to mechanical issues in advance (e.g., is the equipment working? Is there a blank tape?).

Videotaping

Let the tape run for extended periods of time. Transition times are particularly critical. There will likely be a significant amount of uninteresting, unusable tape, but that is unimportant.

Video Review

➤ Identify specific outcomes that the mentor and learner are looking for when reviewing the tape. These could include any of the following:
  ➤ Simple review of what's working and what's not working
  ➤ Hypothesis generation (functional analysis of behavior)
  ➤ Hypothesis confirmation
  ➤ Simple confirmation of skillful interaction
  ➤ Modeling of skillful interactions for others
➤ Ask the learner to:
  ➤ Describe the context prior to reviewing the tape.
  ➤ Identify specific times in which they felt successful; review successful performance first; difficulties can be reviewed later.
  ➤ Begin the discussion by describing in an objective fashion the activities and interaction illustrated on the video.
  ➤ Identify the subjective feelings that the learner experienced.
  ➤ Let the learner lead a summary discussion of what worked and what did not work.
➤ Some specific questions for guiding analysis and discussion in a nonconfrontational manner:
  ➤ What were you thinking during this activity?
  ➤ What do you think the other people were thinking during this activity?
  ➤ Why are you doing this?
  ➤ Why do you think the person with disability is doing this?

continued

TABLE 3–2. *continued*

➤ What made you decide to do that?
➤ If you could do this again, what would you do differently?
➤ What do you think worked best?
➤ OK, so now that we've reviewed the tape, what should we do now?

tion, which would not be relevant in any case. The goal of the enterprise is to provide the individual with the tools and support necessary to take a close look at his or her goals, preferences, strengths, and needs, and to generate a thoughtful intervention plan. This self-assessment and collaborative program-planning process could easily be modified to fit other settings in which people with disability are served.

Self-assessment can also be a component of everyday executive function routines, provided clinicians and everyday people encourage the individual to predict level of performance before beginning tasks, evaluate actual performance after completing the task, and explain discrepancies if they exist. With this routine in place, the individual with TBI may gain 10 to 20 or more practice sessions per day in taking an accurate measure of his or her abilities.

Finally, as we discussed earlier under the heading of resolving conflicts with OCCHTA, there is often value in negotiating assessment tasks with individuals with disability. In fact, a useful routine for professionals is to reply to clients' inflated estimates of ability with a polite invitation to the individual to prove it. Thus, a routine reply to "I am completely ready to return to my job!" should be "Great, let's think of a way for you to demonstrate your readiness" rather than, "No, I do not think you are ready. Look at your scores on the . . . ."

RECOMMENDATIONS ON VIDEO

With the goal of creating positive everyday routines as a primary context for the delivery of rehabilitation, it is important for people involved in those routines to concretely understand their role in the routines and the scripts associated with those roles. An ideal medium for communicating this information is a videotaped illustration of the routine depicted as positively as possible. All of the everyday communication partners are then asked to view the video as part of their attempt to master the script. This procedure is particularly critical for important people who may have infrequent interaction with the professional staff responsible for developing the program. This group may include night and weekend staff in hospital and residential settings as well as family members who are not readily accessible. We recommend using family members or direct care staff as actors in these model videos, as an act of respect and as a component of their training.

We have also used videos of this sort as a reminder for the individual with disability. For example, if considerable negotiation has gone into selecting an acceptable communication alternative to challenging behavior, the positive interaction using this alternative can be videotaped and repeatedly shown to the individual as a component of the reminder system needed to habituate the new manner of communicating. With some creativity, videos as self-reminders can be used in a variety of domains of functioning.

ASSESSMENT, STAFF TRAINING, AND PROGRAM MONITORING: A CHECKLIST

We close this chapter with a checklist (Table 3–3) that we have used with many staff in

TABLE 3–3. Guidelines for helping children and adults with TBI who have difficulty in the areas of behavior regulation, cognition, and communication: A program monitoring checklist.

Instructions:

Identification of gaps in the program:

1. Place an X in the right-hand box if that item is effectively addressed in the individual's program.
2. Place a line through the right-hand box if that item is only partially addressed in the individual's program..
3. Leave the right-hand box blank if that item is poorly addressed in the individual's program.

Identification of priorities:

1. Place a red P in the left-hand box if that item is insufficiently attended to and is a high priority for program development for that individual.
2. Place an X in the left-hand box if that item is insufficiently attended to.

Priority		*Meaning And Personal Engagement*
❑	❑	Does the individual have **personally meaningful goals**? Are program activities related to those goals?
❑	❑	Is the individual **as engaged as possible in making decisions** about program goals, program activities, behavior management plans, and the like?
❑	❑	Is there a process in place to ensure that the individual participates in making these decisions (including presence at meetings if appropriate)?
❑	❑	Is the individual as involved as possible in **monitoring progress** toward achievement of goals and in modifying the program when there is a need to do so?
❑	❑	Is the individual involved in **productive activity**? Paid Work? Producing products that are considered meaningful products?
❑	❑	Is the program structured as much as possible around the individual's strengths?
❑	❑	Does the individual have **meaningful roles** to play (*contributor* roles) within the program? Outside of the program?
❑	❑	Are the individuals in the program maximally engaged in **helping and supporting one another**?
❑	❑	Is the individual as involved as possible in **orienting others** to his or her strengths and needs, and to the procedures that are most effective in meeting those needs? (See Self-Advocacy Videos, Chapter 8)

Priority		*Behavior* (See Chapter 6)
❑	❑	Is there a behavior plan in place that highlights **positive interaction routines and prevention of behavioral crises** versus reaction to behavioral crises?
❑	❑	Are the behavior plan and the communication plan integrated into one plan?
❑	❑	Is there a behavior plan in place that emphasizes **antecedent management and self-management** over reactive consequent management and external control? (See Chapter 6)
❑	❑	Do written plans highlight the supports that the individual needs to succeed versus the percentage of success that is expected?
❑	❑	Are the following **antecedent management** procedures in place?
❑	❑	Whatever the individual is asked to do is **within his or her ability** to do.
❑	❑	Difficult or stressful tasks are introduced only after **positive behavioral momentum** has been built.

continued

TABLE 3–3. *continued*

❑	❑	Difficult or stressful tasks are avoided in the presence of **negative behavioral momentum.**
❑	❑	In placing demands on the individual, staff are sensitive to the total set of potential **positive and negative setting events.**
❑	❑	Every attempt is made to **increase positive setting events**. (See Chapter 6)
❑	❑	Every attempt is made to **reduce negative setting events**.
❑	❑	Every attempt is made to help the individual **manage his or her own antecedents** (as much as possible during naturally occurring stressful times). This includes facilitating:
❑	❑	Self-identification of internal states that affect behavior
❑	❑	Creation of rules to follow in the event of specific internal states
❑	❑	Identification of personal stressors and procedures to avoid those stressors
❑	❑	Creation of scripts to use during difficult times
❑	❑	Systematic efforts are made to **desensitize** the individual to stressful events.
❑	❑	Are the following **consequent management** procedures in place?
❑	❑	Are consequences (positive or negative) **logical and natural** in relation to the behavior? For example, successful behavior is followed by conversationally natural praise, sense of achievement, and, possibly, contracted payment. Successful behavior is not followed by arbitrary or unrelated "reinforcers" (e.g., points that can be traded in at the end of the day for a cigarette).
❑	❑	Is the **social environment generally positive**, that is, one in which people routinely comment on positive aspects of performance and routinely show signs of respect and affection to one another?
❑	❑	In the event of a **behavioral crisis**, do all staff know how to diffuse the crisis with minimal intervention? (See Chapter 6)

Priority		**Communication** (See Chapter 7)
❑	❑	Does the individual have a functional communication system?
❑	❑	Do all staff understand and use the individual's communication system? Do other clients understand and use the individual's communication system?
❑	❑	Do all staff use language that the individual can comprehend and interpret as respectful?
❑	❑	Do all staff interact with the individual in a way that he or she considers respectful?
❑	❑	Do all staff try to interact with adult clients more like a consultant than like a teacher teaching a young child or a trainer training an animal? Do staff avoid excessive quizzing of the individual?
❑	❑	Do staff attempt to teach the individual positive communication alternatives to negative behavior? Are the positive alternatives as effective for the individual as the negative behaviors?

Priority		**Executive Functions** (See Chapter 4)
❑	❑	Do all staff engage the individual in basic **executive function routines**: Goal-Plan-Predict-Do-Review?
❑	❑	Do all staff make a conscious effort to **avoid contributing to the individual's learned helplessness**? (See Executive System Checklist, Chapter 4.)

Priority		***Organization And Memory*** (See Chapter 5)

❏ ❏ Is there an individualized and effective system in place to ensure that the individual is **adequately oriented** (to schedule, activities, place, and people) throughout the day? Is the individual as **independent** as possible in using that system?

❏ ❏ Does the individual have **organizational support** for completing organizationally demanding tasks? Organizational supports may include advance organizers (e.g., checklists, charts, graphic organizers for specific tasks, and the like), models of completed tasks, easy-to-follow maps (for individuals with spatial orientation problems). (See Organization Checklist, Chapter 5)

❏ ❏ Is the individual's **day adequately organized**?

❏ ❏ Is the individual engaged in **meaningful projects** that by themselves contribute to organization from day to day?

❏ ❏ Do staff highlight the **usefulness and purpose** of organization and organizational supports as they relate to success in achieving goals?

❏ ❏ Is there a system in place to ensure that the individual **retains important information** (e.g., a memory book)? Is the individual as independent as possible in using that system?

❏ ❏ Are **memory cues** (e.g., Post-it notes, photograph cues) available so that the individual is as independent as possible?

Priority		***Pharmacology***

❏ ❏ Is the individual taking any **medications** that could affect cognition or behavior?

❏ ❏ Are there **multiple medications** that could interact in potentially negative ways?

❏ ❏ Is pharmacologic intervention planned and monitored by a **physician with expertise in pharmacologic management after brain injury**?

❏ ❏ Is there a system in place for **timely communication** about medication changes that may affect cognition and behavior?

Priority		***Staff Orientation And Integration*** (See Chapter 8)

❏ ❏ Are all **staff oriented** to the individual's behavioral, communication, and cognitive rehabilitation program?

❏ ❏ Are staff in **basic agreement** about the principles of the program and their implementation?

❏ ❏ Do all relevant staff **contribute to** the development of the plan?

❏ ❏ Are **family members and other everyday people oriented** to the program and its implementation?

❏ ❏ Is there a **training video** available that shows staff and other everyday people how best to interact with and support the individual? Was the individual as involved as possible in producing this training videotape? (See Chapter 8)

❏ ❏ Is there a system in place that facilitates sharing of skills and insights among staff and between staff and family members.

community-based programs as they attempt to support individuals with complex neurobehavioral disturbances after TBI as those individuals attempt to achieve a satisfying community life. The primary goal of the checklist is to ensure that staff and all relevant everyday people whose behavior has an impact on the person with disability have assumed an adequately real-world perspective in their support for the individual and that everyday routines are as positive as they can be in the domains addressed by this book. Elaboration of most of the items in the checklist can be found in Chapters 4 through 7.

A secondary goal of the checklist is to help staff gain a practical orientation to the functional approach to rehabilitation explained and illustrated in this book. To this end, we have found it helpful to assign one individual in the program to each staff person, including paraprofessional staff if managers consider that appropriate, and then ask that staff member to complete the checklist, including assignment of priorities. This may take time and many conversations with colleagues, managers, family members, and others. However, the investment yields handsome rewards as staff increasingly internalize a positive, person-centered, functional understanding of how to help other people succeed in their lives.

CHAPTER 4

Positive Everyday Executive System Routines

The primary purpose of this chapter is to describe a functional and highly contextualized approach to improving executive functions and supporting individuals with executive system impairment after TBI. We begin with a brief clarification of the concept of executive functions, an explanation of the neuropsychological basis for the importance of executive functions in brain injury rehabilitation, and a defense of a developmental, everyday approach to intervention for children and adults alike. This chapter, like all of the intervention chapters in this book, should be read together with Chapter 1, in which we present the theoretical framework that supports the clinical practices described in the intervention chapters and in which we discuss a variety of important considerations that support the approach to brain injury rehabilitation that we embrace.

THE CONCEPT OF "EXECUTIVE FUNCTIONS"

Executive functions include the self-regulatory or self-control functions that enable people to understand their own strengths and needs, formulate goals, plan ways to achieve them, and effectively execute the plans (Lezak, 1982). Discussions in cognitive psychology, developmental psychology, rehabilitation psychology, special education, and other applied fields have increasingly emphasized the role played by executive functions in academic, vocational, and social success. The general theme that emerges from these discussions is that, except in extreme cases, it is more common for people to succeed in life as a result of how effectively they *use* the capacities, knowledge, and skills they possess than as a result of their specific levels of capacity, knowledge, and skill. The concept of executive functions captures all of the mental processes needed to put capacities, knowledge, and skill to use in the pursuit of meaningful goals.

As we use the term "executive system," it refers to the control processes needed to succeed at any task that is difficult or nonroutine. These include:

➤ having a reasonable understanding of one's strengths and limitations;
➤ based on that understanding, setting reasonable goals for oneself;
➤ planning and organizing behavior designed to achieve the goals;
➤ initiating behavior (including covert cognitive behavior) included in the plan;
➤ inhibiting behavior (including covert cognitive behavior) that interferes with achieving the goals;
➤ monitoring and evaluating one's behavior (including covert cognitive behavior) to ensure successful implementation of plans and achievement of goals; and
➤ thinking strategically and flexibly, that is, trying one or more well-conceived alternative possibility in the event of failure.

Executive functions are appropriately referred to as "control" functions because they enable people to engage in controlled behavior beyond what would be done based on instinct, habit, or impulse alone. Development (and redevelopment after brain injury) of the executive system enables people to be mature, responsible, strategic, and self-controlled across a variety of domains of functioning, that is, to maintain an appropriate problem-solving set for attainment of future goals and to profit efficiently from feedback in pursuit of those goals (Luria, 1966; Welsh & Pennington, 1988).

The executive system is generally understood to be involved in the regulation of both covert cognitive behavior and overt social behavior. As such, this construct plots out territory that is intimately related to both cognitive and behavioral intervention for people with TBI. Applied to *cognition*, executive functions are involved in individuals' control of their conscious and deliberate cognitive activity (e.g., rehearsing information in preparation for an exam, preparing an outline before beginning to write an essay, considering how to succeed with any difficult task) as well as more routine cognitive activity (e.g., paying attention during a long lecture, systematically searching for a golf ball in the rough). The term "metacognitive functions" is often used to cover the territory covered by executive functions specifically in relation to cognition. This is accurate, provided metacognitive functions are understood to include both static components (i.e., knowing about one's cognitive system) and dynamic components (i.e., actively controlling cognitive behavior) (Ylvisaker & Szekeres, 1989).

Applied to *social behavior*, a mature executive system enables people to (a) inhibit socially impulsive behavior, (b) guide behavior in social context by applying learned rules of social appropriateness, (c) consider other peoples' perspectives and interests in making decisions, and (d) forego immediate gratification in the interest of long-term gain. With respect to *language*, executive functions are involved in deliberate searches of the lexicon (i.e., effortful word retrieval), comprehension of extended language requiring active organization of incoming information (both reading and listening), planned organization of extended discourse, both interactive (e.g., conversations) and noninteractive (e.g., extended narratives, descriptions, and explanations), and controlled, flexible use of abstract, ambiguous, and indirect language (e.g., irony, metaphors, puns).

The Neuropsychology of Executive Functions

From a neuropsychological perspective, these cognitive, psychosocial, and language functions are associated with prefrontal parts of the brain (Alexander, Benson, & Stuss, 1989; Stuss & Benson, 1986), which are most vulnerable in closed head injury in children and adults alike (Levin, Goldstein, Williams, & Eisenberg, 1991). In recent decades, there have been many investigations of consequences of specific prefrontal lesions, necessitating a move beyond the global notions of "a frontal lobe syndrome" or global executive system impairment (Stuss & Benson, 1986). The classical distinction is between (a) *inhibition*-related impairments (traditionally referred to as the "pseudopsychopathic personality"), associated with some degree of hyperactivity, impulsiveness, social inappropriateness, need for immediate gratification, lack of concern for others, sexual excess, and explosiveness and (b) *initiation*-related impairments (traditionally referred to as the "pseudodepressed personality"), associated with apathy, lack of drive, loss of interest, slowness, inattentiveness, and reduced emotional reactivity (Stuss & Benson, 1986). More recently, factor analyses of results of tests of executive functions, as well as specific lesion studies, have suggested the possibility of several subsyndromes associated with specific areas of prefrontal injury (Levin et al., 1996; Taylor, Schatschneider, Petrill, Barry, & Owens, 1996). Early prefrontal lesions in young children may, however, result in global executive system weakness because the injury occurs before the circuitry supporting diverse executive functions has been established.

A Developmental Perspective on Executive Functions

People with significant weakness in their executive system are often described as concrete, egocentric, impulsive, childlike, volatile, socially inappropriate, aggressive, impatient, nonreflective, nonstrategic, disorganized, inattentive, inflexible, and unlikely to direct their behavior in the pursuit of long-term goals. Of course, these descriptors also capture important characteristics of very young, normally developing children. In our opinion, there is great heuristic value in recognizing the parallels between frontal lobe injury/executive system impairment, on the one hand, and normal developmental immaturity on the other.

First, this developmental model invites application to brain injury rehabilitation of the insights and research findings from the fields of developmental cognitive psychology and educational psychology. In addition to the ever-increasing support for a vygotskyan approach to cognitive development, briefly described in Chapter 1 and applied throughout this book, recent work in developmental cognitive psychology supports an understanding of the development of executive functions as continuous rather than stagewise and as strongly influenced by experience, teaching, and expectations in the environment (Flavell, Miller, & Miller, 1993). Recent work in educational psychology supports the functional teachability of executive functions (metacognition, strategic cognitive and academic behavior), but only with long-term and highly contextualized programs of intervention (Pressley, 1995). In addition, a developmental model helps everyday people (e.g., family members, friends, coworkers, staff) appreciate the types of concrete supports that may be needed by adolescents and adults who have become vulnerable to environmental stressors because of severe frontal lobe injury and associated executive system impairment.

These everyday supports are easy to understand in the case of young children. That is, parents with no special training know that young children can behave in a way that is pleasant, productive, and socially appropriate when they are in a familiar setting, supported by familiar routines, engaged in interesting tasks (ideally self-selected and at their level of ability) and not threatened by hunger, exhaustion, or competition from others. However, in the absence of these supports, life with a young child, whose inner controls are poorly developed, can be less than pleasant—and a downward spiral of undesirable behavior followed by punishment followed by increasing deterioration in behavior becomes increasingly likely. Fortunately, effective parents understand the vulnerability of young children and put supports in place to help the child—and at the same time understand the behavioral consequences of uncontrollable environmental stressors, enabling them to respond calmly and to quickly reestablish equilibrium after the child has had difficulty with loss of control. This developmental framework yields many useful insights in assisting older individuals with serious executive system impairment after frontal lobe injury.

In addition, a developmental model for understanding executive functions helps to explain the common phenomenon of delayed developmental consequences of frontal lobe injury in children and adolescents (Benton, 1991; Eslinger, Grattan, Damasio, & Damasio, 1992; Feeney & Ylvisaker, 1995; Grattan & Eslinger, 1991, 1992; Marlowe, 1992; Mateer & Williams, 1991; Price, Doffnre, Stowe, & Mesulam, 1990; Williams & Mateer, 1992; Ylvisaker & Feeney, 1995). For example, a 3-year-old who is impulsive, egocentric, labile, episodically aggressive, disorganized, and not given to long-range planning and deferred gratification is simply an everyday 3-year-old. However, in the absence of considerable maturation of executive control functions between age 3 and age 6, that child will evidence serious disability in first grade, with the possibility of additional symptoms emerging with each subsequent developmental phase, as the demands of school and social life increasingly exceed the child's ability to perform within this domain of executive control functions. A similar phenomenon of delayed developmental consequences is often observed over the years following frontal lobe injury in early adolescence (Feeney & Ylvisaker, 1995; Ylvisaker & Feeney, 1995). To be sure, these undesirable developmental consequences are far from inevitable and the purpose of executive system supports and intervention is in part to *prevent* delayed deterioration from occurring. Nevertheless, a developmental template can be helpful in understanding the need for those supports and the potential negative long-term consequences of TBI that staff and family work to prevent.

The obvious and serious *danger* in using a developmental template is that adolescents and adults with disability are at risk for infantilization. Recognizing parallels between executive system impairment and early developmental phenomena may lead staff and families to interact with the individual in a disrespectful manner. Far from being acceptable, such interaction is the opposite of the therapeutic routines of interaction proposed in this chapter and designed to facilitate growth in this critical domain.

Populations to Which the Themes of This Chapter May Apply

This book is about people with traumatic brain injury. However, to varying degrees and in varying combinations, the attributes that characterize many people with frontal lobe injury overlap with attributes that characterize many people with other disability diagnoses, including ADHD, autism, developmental disabilities, and others—although environmental, motivational, and educational factors certainly interact with neurologic maturation and impairment to explain the behavior of specific individuals within these populations. For example, it is increasingly common for authorities in the field of ADHD to describe that disability as

an executive system impairment (Barkley, 1997; Pennington, 1991; Hallowell & Ratey, 1994). In a recent position statement that resulted from a comprehensive review of the theoretical and empirical literatures, Barkley (1997) attempted to create a coherent model of ADHD that places behavioral disinhibition at its core, with weakness in four key executive functions as the central disability. This view is consistent with most of the available behavioral and neuropsychological evidence, and identifies systematic and theoretically important relations among ADHD symptoms (e.g., disorganization, impulsiveness, inattention, concreteness, social inappropriateness) that have often been described as merely coexisting. According to Barkley, Pennington, and others, difficulty with attentional control is merely one among many symptoms of reduced central control, or impaired executive functions.

Recent investigations of adult outcomes of students with developmental disabilities and learning disabilities have highlighted the critical role played by executive functions in successful adult life, including maintaining employment, living independently, and the like (Wehmeyer & Schwartz, 1997). Intensive efforts are underway to identify effective procedures for facilitating the development of self-determination or executive functions in those populations.

More generally, the themes of this chapter apply in one specific way to virtually all children and adults with disability. Put most simply, disability is associated with difficulty performing tasks that are not difficult for people with no disability. Executive functions are called on when tasks are difficult or novel, that is, when they cannot be performed in a completely automatic, routine manner. Therefore, the development of sophisticated executive functions is an area of critical importance for most people with disability. Tragically, many children and adults with disability live and receive their services in settings where they receive a lesser rather than a greater focus on executive functions than their nondisabled peers. Reasons for this unfortunate neglect include (a) a misguided belief that executive functions are "higher order" and therefore can be deferred until basic cognitive and social processes are well developed; (b) an overriding desire to protect the individual, resulting in family members and staff assuming responsibility for all executive aspects of the individual's behavior; (c) a paradoxical decision to avoid a rehabilitation focus on executive functions because the individual is severely impaired in this area; (d) an unfortunate tendency for staff to assume that their role as helping professionals requires that they assume responsibility for executive dimensions of tasks (e.g., identifying the individuals' weaknesses, setting goals for them, planning and organizing all of their activities, helping them initiate appropriate behavior and inhibit inappropriate behavior, monitoring and evaluating their behavior, and solving their problems); and (e) professional training programs that lack a focus on this important area of intervention.

A goal of this chapter is to describe daily routines in which responsibility for executive functions is turned over to individuals with disability as quickly and effectively as possible—with whatever level of support is required. In the absence of an executive system focus, the predictable outcome for many people with disability is some combination of learned helplessness and oppositional behavior (often an appropriate response when one is stripped of meaningful decision-making power). The lessons of learned helplessness and oppositional reactions have long been available in work with other disability groups (Giangreco, Edelman, Luiselli, & MacFarland, 1997; Peterson & Seligman, 1985; Seligman, 1974).

Development of Executive Functions

Normal development of executive functions begins in infancy and continues throughout adolescence and into the young adult years (Goldman, 1971; Welsh & Pennington, 1988). This developmental fact stands in sharp contrast to the once popular notion that executive functions are at the top of a developmental hierarchy of components of cognition, a notion that supports postponing an executive system focus in habilitation and rehabilitation until other aspects of cognition and language are relatively well established. Within this traditional framework, cognitive goals for individuals who are young or early in their recovery after TBI are restricted to "basic" cognitive processes (e.g., attention, perception, memory, basic organization) and basic world knowledge (and the language associated with this knowledge).

Recent work in developmental cognitive psychology strongly suggests a developmental course for executive functions characterized by early onset of development, slow maturation of functions (continuing through the adolescent years), dynamic interaction with other aspects of development, and modifiability of development with experience and training (Bjorklund, 1990; Tranel, Anderson, & Benton, 1995; Welsh & Pennington, 1988). For example, early developments in the intelligent behavior of infant monkeys (e.g., systematic searches for hidden objects) are associated with maturation of the areas of prefrontal cortex that support behavioral inhibition (an executive control function) (Diamond & Goldman-Rakic, 1989). Human infants from the time of their first birthday have been observed to plan three-step solutions to object-acquisition problems (Willatts, 1990). Very young children can be strategic in their solutions to problems; that is, they plan solutions, remember previously successful solutions, and inhibit previously unsuccessful responses. Without being fully conscious of their cognitive activity, they engage in the kinds of important executive system routines that we advocate in this chapter.

Preschoolers increasingly attach language to their executive function behaviors, language which in turn is internalized to enable them to become increasingly deliberate and internal in their self-control behaviors. For example, 3- and 4-year-old children are quite explicit in their strategies to succeed at concrete physical tasks (e.g., "Try walking sideways on the balance beam; you won't fall down"; "hold it with both hands so it won't spill"). Four-year-old children may even formulate strategies to succeed with *cognitively* demanding tasks, provided that the task is meaningful (e.g., doing something special to remember where they left a present). Vygotsky maintained that preschoolers frequently issue controlling instructions to dolls, pets, and other children as a rehearsal for the internal self-instructions that are critical to mature executive self-control (Vygotsky, 1978). This insight has been incorporated into preschool educational programs by Bodrova and Leong (1996).

During the school years, expectations for deliberately self-regulated cognitive and social behavior are gradually increased. By the end of grade school, children are expected to be deliberate in checking their work, know how to study for tests, and understand what is particularly difficult for them so that they use appropriate strategic procedures, like requesting help as needed. These metacognitive/executive abilities continue to improve during the adolescent and young adult years, particularly in settings in which teachers emphasize these skills, and subsequent higher education and employment require increasing self-regulation of cognitive and social behavior (Flavell, Miller, & Miller, 1993; Pressley, 1995).

EXECUTIVE SYSTEM INTERVENTION: GENERAL THEMES

In Chapter 1 we listed and discussed principles that have guided our work with children and adults with TBI. From the perspective of functional intervention, we have chosen, for several compelling reasons, to operate from the premise that it is more effective to engage executive functions in an integrated and routine manner than to divide the system into components and "exercise" the components in isolation. For example, self-awareness, goal setting, planning/organizing, initiating, inhibiting, monitoring, evaluating, and strategic thinking are all targeted within the everyday goal-plan-do-review routines described in the next section. People with particular weakness in specific areas of executive functions (e.g., planning, inhibiting) can be encouraged to focus on these areas within the larger routines, while maintaining a commitment to the integrity of the interacting system of executive functions in everyday life. This approach is analogous to targeting specific linguistic targets in language intervention within the broader context of meaningful communication versus the more traditional approach of exercising specific building blocks of language divorced from meaningful interaction (Nelson et al., 1996; Fey, 1986). Just as a fragmented approach to language intervention often fails the test of generalization and functional application (Fey, 1986), similarly piecemeal, decontextualized exercising of specific cognitive and executive functions (e.g., using decontextualized exercises alone to practice set shifting, problem solving, organizing, or reasoning) runs the risk of failing to influence functional behavior in everyday life, as every teacher of undergraduate logic classes can attest (Singley & Anderson, 1989).

In this chapter we provide case illustrations under the headings general executive system routines, problem-solving routines, self-coaching routines, and flexibility routines. We then present an extended case study that is designed to show how all of the executive function themes can be integrated in a comprehensive intervention for a young adult whose needs were substantial and whose outcome was and continues to be very positive.

In presenting case material in this and the following three chapters, we identify individuals as in need of minimal, moderate, or intensive levels of support. We offer these descriptors as an alternative to the more commonly used mild, moderate, or severe injury or disability. In Table 4–1 we provide operational definitions of these levels of support, recognizing that we are dividing a continuum of possibilities in relatively arbitrary ways. We also recognize that an adult who is in need of intensive

TABLE 4–1. Levels of support: Operational definitions in three domains.

Behavioral Domain	Academic/Vocational Domain	Cognitive/Executive System Domain
Intensive Levels of Support	**Intensive Levels of Support**	**Intensive Levels of Support**
The individual's degree of impulsiveness, impaired judgment, and/or aggressive behavior creates a danger to self or others (with or without pharmacological intervention), or the individual will not engage in the most basic activities without maximal levels of external control to be safe or to minimally participate in age-appropriate activities.	The individual is not capable of participating in grade-level curriculum or work at a jobsite even with 1:1 paraprofessional or job coach support. The individual requires a fully adapted academic curriculum or segregated work setting.	Despite possibly adequate psychological test results, the individual is dependent on external supports to organize and complete tasks (relative to age expectations and life experiences), even those that are routine and occur in structured settings.
Moderate Levels of Support	**Moderate Levels of Support**	**Moderate Levels of Support**
With the flexible support of staff trained in positive behavior intervention, the individual is not a danger to self or others, but continues to be disruptive and impulsive, or nonparticipatory even with this support.	The individual can process and benefit from aspects of the grade-level curriculum or can contribute meaningfully to a work setting (either jobsite or segregated), possibly including 1:1 assistance of an aide or job coach.	The individual needs external cues and reminders to use organizing, planning, and memory supports, such as printed schedules, photo cues, graphic organizers, log books, and the like.
Minimal Levels of Support	**Minimal Levels of Support**	**Minimal Levels of Support**
The individual is not a danger to self or others and is at most minimally disruptive and impulsive, or requires minimal prompting to engage in activities, with flexible support of paraprofessional staff or in a structured or highly routinized environment. The individual continues to be disruptive, impulsive, or nonparticipatory in novel or unstructured settings.	The individual can process and benefit from substantial aspects of the grade-level curriculum, with resource room or consulting special educator support, or the individual contributes meaningfully to a job in a nonsegregated setting with the periodic support of a job coach.	The individual may require periodic prompting but is otherwise independent in using organizing, planning, and memory supports.
Periodic Supports	**Periodic Supports**	**Periodic Supports**
With no special supports, except for periodic coaching by natural support people (e.g., family members) or consultative supports by professionals, the individual's behavioral self-regulation is within acceptable levels.	With no special supports, except for periodic coaching by teachers or job supervisors, with consultative support by special educators or job coaches, the individual performs at grade level or within the expectations of a job setting and acquires new knowledge and skill at a rate the is acceptable for his or her grade level, or consistent with the expectations of his or her job.	The individual's ability to organize, plan, and remember is within normal limits for his or her age.

levels of support is likely to have a much greater impairment than a child at the same level of need.

GENERAL EXECUTIVE SYSTEM ROUTINES: GOAL-PLAN-DO-REVIEW

People who are successful in their daily lives tend to be people who set reasonable goals for themselves, formulate a plan to achieve the goals, and implement the plan. They then review their performance, determining what worked and what did not work, thereby positively influencing subsequent performance. In this section, we describe routines designed to promote this type of behavior in children and adults at a variety of ages and levels of functioning.

Individuals Who Require Intensive Levels of Support

A goal-plan-do-review routine can be implemented for preschoolers and for older children and adults with serious executive system disability. Indeed, the most popular preschool curriculum in the United States today, the High Scope Curriculum (Schweinhart & Weikart, 1993), is structured around precisely this routine. To be sure, preschoolers require that these cognitive routines be concrete and effectively supported by adults. For example, a *goal* for a 2- or 3-year-old may be to play at the water table; the *plan* may be to go to the water table with Jenny and play; *doing* is playing at the water table; and the *review* may be little more than "We played with the water and got all wet. I needed a towel. It was fun."

Clever teachers support this cognitive activity so that it is appropriately highlighted and gradually becomes more sophisticated. For example, for preschoolers there may be a large planning board with velcro pegs for photographs. To make his planning more deliberate, Johnnie may be asked to place his photo and that of his playmate Jenny on the board. Then photos of the water table and certain selected toys are placed next to

the children's photos. The review might be made more complete and interesting by having Johnnie and Jenny dictate a letter to their parents describing what they did at the water table, what problems emerged, what they did about it, and what they plan to do at the water table tomorrow. Four- and 5-year-old children are capable of specifying goals and plans at higher levels of abstractness and completeness (e.g., "We're going to make cars out of pieces of wood and glue, and then we're going to make roads and tunnels in the sand pile and drive our cars there"). Such capacities are facilitated by teachers who are good at engaging students in these relatively abstract tasks of setting goals and planning how to achieve them.

The meanings of words like *goal, plan, problem, solution, think, remember,* and *review* are learned and internalized as the children are engaged by adults in these everyday routines. Furthermore, clever teachers use these routine interactions to help children understand that some tasks are easy whereas others are difficult, but there is always something clever that can be done to succeed when tasks are difficult. Routine teacher talk at this level of executive system functioning might be something like the following:

GOAL:

Today we're going to make a big turkey out of colored paper and glue. Everybody like that idea? OK, I'm going to put a picture of what it will look like when it's done right here where it says "goal." This is our goal, this is what we are going to do—make a big turkey that looks something like this.

PLAN:

Is this going to be hard to do? Yes, I think it's going to be pretty hard. Will it take us a long time? That's right, I think it will. So we need a . . . —that's right; we need a plan. We need a plan. Let's think. A plan tells us what things we need, what we need to do, and who should do what. What do we need? That's right, colored paper, glue, and scissors. What are we going to with these things? Right, cut out the parts and glue them together. Now, let's decide who should do what.

REVIEW:

Remember, today we decided that our goal was to make a big turkey. How did we do? Does is look like the turkey I put here as our goal? It sure does—even better! So we achieved our goal! We did what we had decided to do. Great!! Now, we have to make a letter to send to your parents. So we'll say that our goal was to make this big turkey. Then we made our plan. Who remembers what problems came up? That's right. Jim got his fingers all sticky with glue. So let's write down what we had to do about that.

Very long-term follow-up of children who received their preschool education in High Scope programs (which also includes intensive efforts to help parents appreciate the importance of these aspects of development) provides striking evidence of the real-world effectiveness of the approach. For example, compared at age 15 with graduates of direct instruction preschools, the High Scope graduates had significantly fewer status offenses and reports of property damage, significantly greater sports participation and appointments to school office, and a significantly reduced likelihood that their families would report that they were generally "doing poorly" (Schweinhart & Weikart, 1986). Similarly impressive functional outcomes were reported when the experimental group reached age 27 (Schweinhart & Weikart, 1993). Our goal in reporting these findings is not to promote the use of a specific curriculum. Rather, we wish to emphasize the possibility of an early everyday focus (early in childhood and early after brain injury) on simple executive function routines and the potential for this focus to positively influence long-term outcome.

Individuals Who Require Moderate Levels of Support

An interview with a successful 10-year-old fifth grader regarding school tasks that were difficult for him revealed the following insights. He reported that Social Studies was relatively difficult because he needed to learn lots of specific information and bluffing was not possible. When asked what he did about this, he reported that he had decided that his teacher generally asked questions about the words in the text that were in italic print. So when she gave a reading assignment, he would scan the pages for italicized words. When he found one, he would look for specific information about that concept, then ask himself a question like those the teacher routinely asked, make sure he could answer it, and then proceed. By age 10, this young man had developed a habit of recognizing difficult tasks (e.g., social studies tests), setting goals for himself (e.g., I want to get an A), formulating a plan to achieve the goal, implementing the plan, and reviewing it to ensure that it was working for him. Nobody had explicitly taught him this routine; rather, he had simply internalized this way of proceeding with difficult tasks over several years and thousands of experiences in which he had goals that he wanted to achieve and was held responsible by parents, teachers, older siblings, and others for his level of success. Of course, many children require more explicit instruction and guided practice than this exceptional 10-year-old.

Educational and rehabilitation programs for grade school age children and older individuals with moderate-to-severe executive system impairment should be structured around a general *goal-plan-do-review* routine, as described above, but with the children or adults increasingly active in formulating plans and reviewing their performance. In addition to the global, daily goal-plan-do-review routine, executive system habits are more quickly understood and internalized when most activities begin with the formulation of a goal and a plan, and end with a review that includes both a general rating of success and also a listing of what worked and what didn't work—and possibly an indication of what to try next time. This routine is depicted in Figure 4–1.

GOAL

What do I want to accomplish?

PLAN

How am I going to accomplish my goal?

MATERIALS/EQUIPMENT	STEPS/ASSIGNMENTS
1.	1.
2.	2.
3.	3.
4.	4.
5.	5.

PREDICTION

How well will I do? How much will I get done?

Figure 4—1. A guide for explicitly teaching or highlighting the executive components of any task.

DO

PROBLEMS ARISE?

1.

2.

3.

FORMULATE SOLUTIONS!

1.

2.

3.

REVIEW

HOW DID I DO?

Self-rating:

1   2   3   4   5   6   7   8   9   10

Other Rating (teacher, therapist, peer, family member)

1   2   3   4   5   6   7   8   9   10

WHAT WORKED?

1.

2.

3.

WHAT DIDN'T WORK?

1.

2.

3.

WHAT WILL I TRY DIFFERENTLY NEXT TIME?

We worked with a young man with cognitive and executive system disability following treatment for a brain tumor early in his life. By the middle of fifth grade, Ben had become so inattentive in school that his teacher believed that he may have been experiencing ongoing seizures. A brief period of hypothesis testing (see Chapter 3) revealed that he was extremely disorganized, which resulted in his becoming confused when asked to do tasks with even a modest degree of organizational demands. Furthermore, he had grown dependent on his aide (i.e., learned helplessness unconsciously fostered by the aide), so that when he became confused, he simply "spaced out" until his aide stepped in to show him how to proceed.

Ben quickly learned how to use an executive system routine, which was then implemented for all of his academic tasks. It began with a written statement of his goal, followed by an extremely concrete checklist of all of the steps needed to complete the task. The form, which he referred to as a "task sheet," then directed him to rate his performance on a 10-point scale. His work was also rated by a teacher or his aide, with discrepancies in ratings necessitating discussion. Finally, the form included parallel columns for analysis of what worked and what did not work for him. These guides were collected in a large notebook that Ben referred to as his "Independence Book," which not only helped him work more independently, but also showed his aide how to reduce her unnecessary levels of support.

With this system of executive function supports in place, global ratings in areas of executive system functioning, given by Ben's regular education teacher, special educator, and mother, increased from kindergarten-to-second grade levels (preintervention) to third-to-fifth grade levels (end of fifth grade). This system of supports did not reduce Ben's executive system impairment (i.e., "cure" him), which was demonstrated by near total regression in sixth grade when the supports were inappropriately removed. However, the executive sys-

tem routine did substantially reduce Ben's educational disability and handicap while it was in place, and had the same positive effect when a modified system of supports was reimplemented in seventh grade.

Positive, Everyday Problem-Solving Routines

Some people greet problems in their daily lives positively and thoughtfully, knowing that their success ultimately depends on their choices and efforts, and that there is usually something that can be done to create a relatively positive outcome. It is likely that these people have a long history of accepting responsibility for solving their own problems and engaging in successful solutions, derived and implemented with whatever help may have been necessary. Other people, including some with disability, react to problems passively, expecting somebody to step in and solve the problem for them, or fearfully, because they have no confidence that a solution will be found, an attitude possibly encouraged by overprotective service providers. It is a goal of this section to describe everyday routines designed to increase the likelihood that people with TBI will fall into the category of resilient, effective, and autonomous problem solvers. Based on the principles described in Chapter 1, this positive outcome is largely dependent on the daily problem-solving routines that are put in place for individuals with disability.

Individuals Who Require Intensive Levels of Support

In staff training sessions, we frequently show a videotape of a father interacting with his 15-month-old son. The father hands his son an interesting, mechanical windup toy duck and says, "That's a funny thing. I wonder how it goes." The toddler takes the toy and tries to wind it up. He is unable to do this, so he tries a few alternatives, such as pushing down on the duck's legs, twisting it, and throwing it on the table. The father then says, "Boy, that's hard to do. I wonder what else you could do." The toddler tries the windup key again, pushes down on the duck's head, drops it, and finally hands it to his father with a vocalization meaning, "You do it." The father praises his efforts and then collaborates with his son, "You tried lots of things. That's great! But it's still not working, is it? This is hard to do! Here, let me show you." After he models the correct way to wind up the toy, the toddler tries again, fails, and again asks his father for help. The father winds the toy again, saying, "Boy, that's a hard thing to do, isn't it? You tried real hard; that's great. But it didn't work. Here, let me do it for you. Dad can always help."

At age 17, at the time of this writing, this toddler is a National Merit Scholarship finalist and is on his way to the National Science Bowl competition. We mention this because of our conviction, supported by the developmental framework of Vygotsky (see Chapter 1) and data from a variety of fields of inquiry, that his success as a critical thinker and problem-solver at age 17 is in part a result of the thousands of mediated problem-solving experiences he has enjoyed over his 17 years of life, experiences similar to the mediated problem solving with the mechanical toy at 15 months, but at increasing levels of complexity and abstractness as he matured. The general structure of these everyday problem-solving routines is as follows:

Facilitator:	Engages the apprentice in an interesting task, somewhat beyond the apprentice's ability to succeed independently.
Apprentice:	Attempts to complete the task, possibly working collaboratively with the facilitator.
Facilitator:	Encourages a variety of solutions; highlights the difficulty of the task, the characteristics of the task that make it difficult, and the strengths and limitations of the apprentice.
Apprentice:	Indicates frustration or perseverates with one unsuccessful solution.
Facilitator:	Again highlights the difficulty of the task and the reason for the difficulty; models one or two successful solutions; works with the apprentice to get the job done; communicates that there is always something clever to do to get the job done.
Both:	Enjoy the fruits of their collaborative labor.

Staff and parents who have made these teaching interactions routines in their lives are typically able to create many such interactions every day. Some of the interactions may be planned. For example, snack time for children yields many opportunities for solving problems, including one too few necessary items (e.g., chair, spoon, glass, cookie), difficulty distributing the items, spills, and the like. Alternatively, many of the teaching interactions may be unplanned. Any nonroutine event requiring a thoughtful solution can be turned into a brief exercise in problem solving with the appropriate adult routine: "Woops; we've got a problem. What's wrong here? Can anybody think of a smart thing to do about this? Do you think that will work? Why? Why not? Can you think of anything else? Who thinks this solution would be the best one to try? Did it work? Why? Great! That was a smart thing to do, wasn't it? We'll have to remember to do that again!" Some of the language and associated thought processes in these exchanges may be somewhat beyond the level of some preschoolers. However, it is precisely these verbally mediated adult-child daily interactions that are the source of abstract meanings and the basis for what gradually become internal thought processes.

Unfortunately, many children and adults with disability live and receive their rehabilitation, education, and training in environments characterized by unhelpful routines like the following, observed during an assessment of a 4-year-old's problem-solving ability.

Adult:	Gives the child a pill jar with a secure lid. The jar is filled with candy.

Child:	Turns the lid several times and complains that it won't come off. Continues trying to turn the lid.
Adult:	After a minute or two, takes the jar from the child, says "Good job!" opens the jar and gives the child a piece of candy.

The problem with this adult routine is that it involves unhelpful feedback (i.e., the child had not done a very good job) and fails to highlight for the child the nature of the problem, the possibility of varied solutions, the reason for the child's failure, the appropriate solution, and the general principle that there is usually a clever, strategic solution to daily problems. In this case, a positive, appropriately mediated problem-solving routine would have the adult say something like the following: "That's not working, is it? You're trying as hard as you can, but just turning the lid isn't working. I wonder what the problem is here, anyway. Oh, look! It says here that you have to push down while you turn the lid. That was hard for you to figure out because you can't read yet. I guess they don't want kids to open these jars. Here, now we know what to do; let's do it together. There's always some way to get the job done, isn't there?"

Positive and negative illustrations of everyday problem-solving routines with adults with TBI are presented in the following two sequences, both of which were observed during an hour-long team meeting about an adult client, Steve, who was present at the meeting. Steve, who had significant physical disability (e.g., he walked slowly with a walker) and cognitive disability (e.g., he had weak planning and problem-solving skills, as well as impaired spatial orientation), had only visited the office twice before the meeting in question. What follows is a positive interactive routine (private exchange with a familiar staff person).

Steve:	"I need to go to the bathroom." (He begins to leave the room.)

Staff 1:	"Do you know how to get to the bathroom and back?"
Steve:	"Yes." (He proceeds to turn the wrong way down the hall.)
Staff 1:	(As Steve returns past the door of the office, appearing frustrated) "Steve, you finding things OK or do you need some help?"
Steve:	"I'm not sure where to go."
Staff 1:	"Need a plan, huh? Let me show you how to get there and back. And what would be best if you get lost?"
Steve:	"Ask somebody how to get to this office."
Staff 1:	"Great; maybe it would be good to carry the number of this office; what do you think? Here. I think these are probably useful plans."
Steve:	(Finds the bathroom and returns.)

This is a positive routine in a variety of ways. Steve was allowed to attempt an unassisted solution first and, in effect, predicted that he would succeed. In a positive, nonthreatening way, the staff person helped Steve realize that his first plan was weak, helped him create a better plan, and provided no more assistance than necessary. The following unhelpful problem-solving routine (unfortunately typical of negative interactions Steve had with some staff) occurred later during the same meeting.

Steve:	"I'll be right back. I gotta go again." (Turns the wrong way again.)
Staff 2:	"Steve, that's the wrong way. Here, I'll take you there." (Accompanies Steve to the bathroom.)

This is an unhelpful routine because it lacks all of the positive elements of the first routine and because it continues the pattern of staff assuming responsibility for the executive function dimensions of most tasks. In this case, there is nothing to help Steve learn from his mistakes, nor is there practice of any of the executive functions as Steve struggles with a difficult everyday task. Routines of this sort begin the slippery slope toward learned helplessness. As a result of his brain injury, Steve needs many more experiences like the first routine than does a person with no disability. In an environment characterized by routines like the second illustration, he will tragically receive fewer rather than more needed learning trials.

Individuals Who Require Moderate Levels of Support

During a visit to a special education classroom for children in the 5- to 7-year-old range, we observed the following exchange between Dave, a 7-year-old with a history of TBI, and his teacher. They were preparing the script for a transition video designed to orient Dave's new staff at his next level of education in the fall.

Teacher: "OK, Dave. We need to show how you use this window that covers the page except for the line you're reading."

Dave: "No, I don't think I need that any more."

Teacher: "But don't you remember? We decided that it's easier for you to keep your place when you only have to look at one line?"

Dave: "But I don't need it any more."

Teacher: "Well, I don't know. Maybe you're right. Let's try an experiment." (They try one page with the window and one page without.) "Well look at that! You were right and I was wrong. You don't need this window any more. It used to be helpful, but now your reading has improved and you don't need it! That's great! And I'm very happy that you got us to do this little experiment. I guess this is how we find out what you need and what you don't need, right?"

In this case, the teacher capitalized on a very meaningful issue to engage the child in important problem solving that influenced his educational program. Many adults are disinclined to collaborate in this way with children or older individuals with disability, because they do not see the individual as a potential contributor to problem solving and decision making, or because of

a misguided sense of professional status that requires that the professional must always remain in authority and appear to have all the answers. In either case, the child or adult with disability is denied important mediated learning experiences, with learned helplessness or oppositionality or both as the likely consequences.

With grade school level children who are very impulsive and disorganized in their problem solving, we have used graphic organizers for problem solving—again in a routine, everyday manner. A simple example of such an organizer is presented in Figure 4–2. This organizer can be available for unplanned, ad hoc problem-solving exercises or for planned exercises, for example, during reading class when comprehension requires discussion of problems that arise in the readings. The goal with this and other graphic advance organizers is to highlight the components and the organization of the thought process and then practice using the organizer so that the components and their organization become internalized as routines of thought.

Individuals Who Require Minimal Levels of Support or Periodic Consultative Supports

The types of mediated problem-solving experiences described in the previous sections can be used across the age span, with appropriate changes in content, complexity, and interactive style. With some adults with ongoing problem-solving difficulty after TBI, we have encouraged the use of somewhat more complicated advance organizers. However, it must be made clear that complicated and time-consuming problem solving is required only in the event of serious problems that arise when there is time to devote to serious reflection. Nobody devotes large quantities of time and intellectual energy to minor, everyday problems. Asking this of individuals with disability may induce a generally negative attitude to the enterprise of thoughtful, deliberate problem solving and decision making. That is, the internal scales of costs and benefits that everybody carries unconsciously through life must tip on the benefits side or cost-intensive procedures will be quickly discarded.

A problem-solving guide that is more complete than that presented in Figure 4–2 may include the following components:

1a. Specify the problem (e.g., conflict with staff over . . .).
1b. Indicate the personal goal that the problem is related to (e.g., greater autonomy).
1c. Specify the general nature of the problem (e.g., this has to do with getting

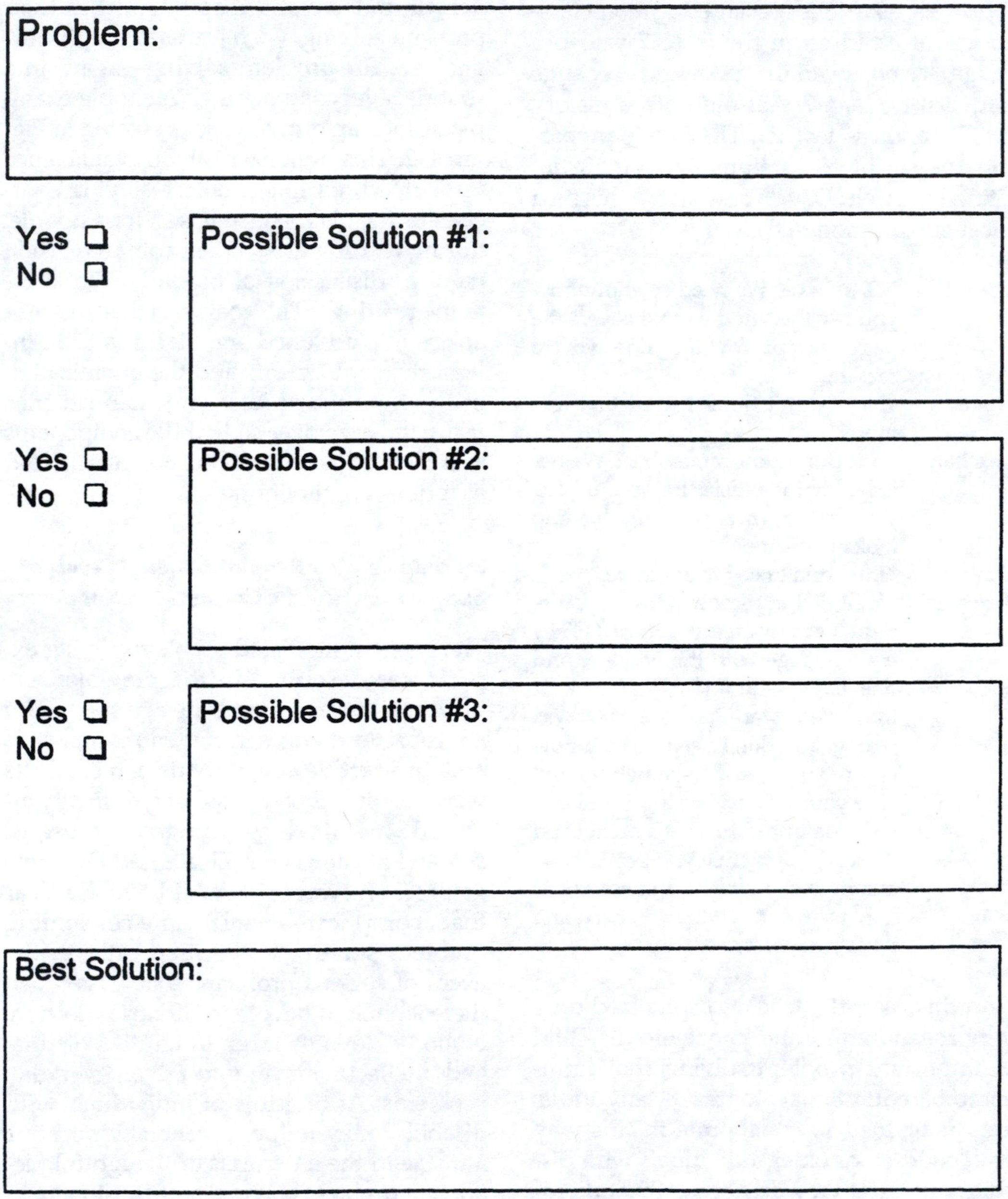

Problem:

	Possible Solution #1:
Yes ☐ No ☐	

	Possible Solution #2:
Yes ☐ No ☐	

	Possible Solution #3:
Yes ☐ No ☐	

Best Solution:

Figure 4–2. A simple graphic organizer for problem solving.

along with others; this has to do with following others' instructions; this has to do with managing my time effectively).

2a. Indicate information that is relevant to a solution to this problem (e.g., history with this staff person, level of success of previous efforts).

2b. Identify information that needs to be gathered before a solution can be selected (e.g., staff person's perspective).

3a. List possible solutions.

3b. List pros and cons associated with each possible solution (e.g., predicted effectiveness in relation to goals, time, and other resources required, difficulty of implementing the solution, potential for other problems being created by the solution).

4. Select the most attractive solution.

5. Act on the solution.

6. Monitor the results: What worked? What did not work? What will I do the next time?

Teachers and therapists will recognize that this organized problem-solving process is very much like the process used by professionals to identify issues of concern in their students or clients, to select goals, to complete a functional evaluation, to choose a course of treatment or instructional program, to monitor its effectiveness, and to make modifications if necessary. There is a great irony and tragedy implicit in the reality that people who are weak in the important area of strategic thinking and problem solving are often served by professionals who hoard all of these "executive" activities for themselves, denying their students or clients the practice they need to improve in meaningful, functional ways. The predictable result is, once again, learned helplessness or oppositional behavior.

Therefore, in our practice with adolescents and adults, we work hard to turn over to them responsibility for this problem-solving activity. In many cases, we have a problem-solving routine visible on the wall of the classroom or intervention

setting. Individuals know that they are responsible for selecting the areas of concern to work on, for identifying their goal, for discussing relevant issues, for selecting solutions/strategic procedures based on solid reasoning, for monitoring their progress, and for making judgments about where to go next. In group sessions, all of the group members can participate in the organized, deliberate problem solving. As always, sufficient support is provided so that this process is efficient and successful, but not so much that the individual grows unnecessarily dependent on it.

This process is illustrated by an episode that occurred during an adult TBI group session. Members of the group had gathered to discuss their plans for the day and the week ahead, and to review important events of the previous few days. Bob, who was 6 years postinjury at the time, was able to manage his daily routine adequately, but had significant difficulty with novel events.

Bob: (Enters the meeting late, visibly upset.) "Somebody wrote some stuff on the wall about me, and it's not nice. I want to know who did it. I want to get my hands on him."

Staff: (Turning to the group.) "This is tough. Bob needs help. What do you think?"

Group: (Make a variety of suggestions. Help Bob think through the pros and cons of each as he tries to select the best solution following a script similar to that presented above.)

Bob: "OK, thanks. What I'll do is find out who wrote the graffiti, tell him I'm real upset about this, and that we won't be able to do anything together until he apologizes."

Later, the staff person reviewed Bob's plan and asked him what he would do if he became upset during the confrontation with the person who wrote the graffiti. Together, they considered options to ensure that this would not happen. Bob elected to practice his confrontation with a peer using video feedback. In addition, he decided in advance that he would have to practice until he could role play the confrontation with a peer without becoming upset. He did this and ultimately confronted the guilty party in a way that turned out to be successful for him. Later, the staff member reviewed the episode with Bob, systematically listing the components of the process that contributed to its success.

We highlight this as a positive routine because (a) it occurred in a meaningful, everyday context; (b) the problem to be solved was a genuinely important problem that needed to be solved (versus an artificial exercise); (c) members of a support group all obtained practice in meaningful problem solving; (d) because a group was involved, there was a rich array of possible solutions that emerged along with several considerations associated with each; (e) the group proceeded systematically through the problem-solving process; (f) Bob ultimately accepted responsibility for making his decisions based on group and staff suggestions; rather than acting impulsively, he chose a deliberate plan; (g) the outcome was positive; and (h) a review of the process highlighted for Bob the components and value of this deliberate, supported problem-solving process. After this and other positive experiences using peer support to formulate a solution to personal problems, Bob acknowledged that his own judgment and problem-solving abilities were weak and therefore was willing to work at routinizing his use of staff and peer problem-solving support.

Positive, Everyday Self-Coaching Routines

In our discussion of the highest level problem-solving routines, we highlighted the analogy between controlled, deliberate, personal problem solving and the planning activity of teachers and therapists. This is also like the strategic planning activity of corporate executives, which explains the origin of the metaphor "executive functions." For obvious reasons, this metaphor fails to resonate with most children and young adults with TBI. An alternative metaphor that

has meaning for many adolescents and young adults—and even many younger children—is that of a coach. Individuals with executive system weakness can then be equipped with everyday routines that exploit the features of coaching and the status associated with coaching.

Individuals Who Require Intensive Levels of Support

As a result of her TBI at age 10, Jan had a significant initiation impairment as well as hemiplegia necessitating daily physical therapy and occupational therapy exercises. She received therapy twice each week in school and was expected to do her exercises at home the other 5 days. Because of her initiation impairment, she routinely neglected her exercises, which resulted in her mother having to remind her—an activity naturally perceived by Jan as nagging. Working with the physical therapist, we helped Jan to produce an "exercise video"—complete with art work and background music of her choice—in which she gave herself instructions and modeled the exercises that she was to do at home. With the introduction of this home video, Jan's mother reported that she improved from reluctantly doing her exercises one to two times per week at home to four to five times without resistance. In addition, her education staff reported that the introduction of this self-coaching program with her exercise video was associated with a noticeable increase in social initiation in school.

We have used these "self-coaching" video routines with children as young as 6 years old. In addition to helping individuals accept responsibility for their improvement and engaging them in personal problem solving, the videos also help children internalize a positive self-concept as competent helpers and coaches, as opposed to the generally negative self-concept of "person with a disability always needing help from others." This potentially positive contribution of carefully designed video self-observation has been explored in a series of studies by Dowrick (Dowrick, 1979; Dowrick & Raeburn, 1995).

Individuals Who Require Moderate Levels of Support

Jim was severely injured in a motor vehicle accident during his senior year of high school. After extended hospitalization and inpatient rehabilitation, he returned home and began an extended period of outpatient rehabilitation and tutoring. Motor problems included dysarthric speech, a labored gait, and generally slow motor responses. Academically, Jim tested in the late grade school range on basic academic tests. His goal was to pass the graduate equivalency exams, thereby securing a high school diploma, and proceed on to a private, liberal arts college, which was his preinjury goal.

At 1 year postinjury, Jim's perception of his academic abilities was strikingly inconsistent with his progress. Confrontation designed to help him understand the severity of his deficits was greeted with anger and accusations that staff were insufficiently competent to enable him to achieve his lofty goals. Although his brain injury was widespread and his disability generalized across all functional domains, his most debilitating disability was in the area of executive functions. His awareness of his profile of strengths and weaknesses was limited. He had difficulty setting realistic goals and he consistently relied on others to plan activities that were related to his achieving his goals, to initiate his activity, to monitor and evaluate his performance, to think strategically for him, and to solve his problems. In summary, despite his ambitions, hard work, and spirited engagement with many tasks, he was becoming increasingly dependent on others and increasingly angry about his situation—all of this in a rehabilitation setting dedicated to helping people achieve independence and create a positive life for themselves! The irony was that by accepting responsibility for planning Jim's rehabilitation and making his decisions for him, rehabilitation staff were actively contributing to his growing helplessness and resistance to accepting responsibility for himself.

Recognizing the dangers in this dynamic and knowing that Jim had been a star athlete before his injury, staff worked with Jim to create a format for "self-coaching" that was then implemented in all of his therapy and tutoring sessions. It was his choice to proceed through every session by (a) identifying the problem that he wished to focus on; (b) identifying the goal that he set for himself related to that problem; (c) making a "game plan" for achieving the goal (combining a practice activity with a strategic maneuver to use during that practice activity); (d) giving himself specific instructions based on this plan; (e) practicing the skill using those instructions; (f) monitoring his performance (i.e., reviewing the "game films"); (g) identifying what worked and what did not work; and (h) making a decision about what he would try the next time or what other type of help he might need in order to achieve his goals. He referred explicitly to this routine as "self-coaching" and he knew that it was a general goal for him to internalize this self-coach so that he would routinely approach every difficult task as both "athlete" and "self-coach." We frequently talked about "the coach in his head" and what that coach was telling him.

With this routine in place, it was no longer necessary to use confrontational procedures with Jim—when necessary, he confronted himself. Furthermore, his accusations of staff incompetence were quickly eliminated once he became an active collaborator with staff and came to consider himself his own coach. With increasing patience and fewer signs of anger and frustration, Jim ultimately passed all of the GED exams and began college as a part-time student. Because there was no experimental design in place, it is unclear if his physical and academic success increased as a result of these self-coaching routines. There is no question, however, that his sense of personal responsibility and general executive functioning improved in important ways.

Positive, Everyday Routines for Dealing with Changes in Routines: Cognitive and Behavioral Flexibility

Cognitive and behavioral inflexibility are among the most salient symptoms for many people with frontal lobe injury (or immaturity). Many people with executive system impairment become disorganized and upset when established routines change. Their response patterns tend to be inflexible, they have difficulty shifting cognitive and behavioral sets, and they often perseverate on single solutions to problems, even if that solution is inadequate. In this section we present simple "flexibility routines" for people whose concreteness in thinking, inflexibility, and need for routine is problematic after TBI.

Individuals Who Require Intensive Levels of Support

Dave (described earlier) had a severe TBI at age 2. At age 6, when we first met him, his parents' primary concern was his rigidity and the serious tantrums that were associated with changes in routine (e.g., a new bus driver) or with his expectations not being met (e.g., canceling an expected visit of a friend). The parents described themselves as, to some degree, hostages of Dave's need for routine. That is, they worked very hard to ensure that his life was predictable and that there were no surprises.

When we described Dave's need as a need for "a routine to deal with changes in routine," his parents quickly designed an experiment that proved to be successful. They placed a small blackboard in their family room and negotiated with Dave a list of favored activities. Subsequently, each time they had to tell him that there would be a difficult change in routine or disappointing change in plans, they did it at this choice board and invited him to select an alternative activity. After several weeks of this new routine—or "meta-routine"—tantrums had been eliminated and were re-

placed by, at most, a brief expression of disappointment. Dave continued to use this system, with decreasing dependence, for about 1 year. He continued to need predictability and routine, but he and his parents had a system in place that created much greater flexibility in their home, reversed Dave's downward behavioral spiral, and served as a model for the parents in creating other positive routines to deal with chronic difficulties.

About 18 months after initiating this routine to deal with changes in routine (6 months after he had stopped using the system), Dave looked at the board and commented, "I used to need that when I didn't know what to do. But now I know, so I don't need it any more." Just as Vygotsky described normal development 70 years ago, Dave's parents supported performance in a demanding area of development with adequate scaffolding and subsequently dismantled the scaffolding as Dave internalized procedures to manage his own reactions and behavior.

Individuals Who Require Minimal-to-Moderate Levels of Support

Jerry incurred bilateral frontal lobe injury associated with closed head injury at age 27. Prior to his injury, he had a checkered employment history (e.g., he lost several jobs because of oppositional behavior) and there had been considerable conflict with his family. After the injury, he experienced excellent physical and general intellectual recovery (e.g., WAIS Full Scale IQ: 110). However, neuropsychological tests sensitive to prefrontal injury (e.g., Wisconsin Card Sorting Test) suggested ongoing executive system weakness, particularly in the area of cognitive and behavioral inflexibility. This inflexibility manifested itself in Jerry's becoming seriously upset when staff were late or even when the subway was late. When we first met him, Jerry was living in a supervised apartment with 24-hour 1:1 staffing. The service provider responsible for his care maintained that his judgment was so weak and his organizational functioning so impaired that he required around-the-clock supervision for his own safety.

The concreteness of Jerry's thinking and his need for routine resulted in his becoming agitated when staff behaved in ways that deviated from his expectations, for example, in their manner of interaction with him and in their level of expectations and support. Because of normal staff turnover, these deviations were quite common Therefore, Jerry's negative reactions were quite frequent, including escaping from staff supervision and visiting places that were explicitly against the rules imposed by staff.

Intervention for this major difficulty proved to be quite simple. Jerry learned to ask a scripted question ("This is not part of the plan. Is there a new plan?") every time he sensed a deviation from routine. This question was a cue for staff to negotiate a new plan with Jerry. In addition to the concrete reorientation that this afforded Jerry, it also took him out of an oppositional mode (because of the respect implicit in the negotiation process) and helped staff to organize themselves in a usefully concrete way around an explicit plan. Over the 6 months since the introduction of this "routine for dealing with changes in routine," Jerry has not attempted to escape from supervision and the program has been able to reduce supervision from 24 to 8 hours per day.

CASE ILLUSTRATION OF AN EVERYDAY, ROUTINE-BASED APPROACH TO EXECUTIVE SYSTEM REHABILITATION

Jason's injury occurred at age 24 as a result of an automobile-motorcycle accident. Widespread injury gradually evolved into primarily prefrontal symptoms. Although he had been a good student in his university program before the injury, Jason had a history of oppositional behavior, which was exacerbated by the injury. Following his acute rehabilitation, he underwent two involuntarily placements in neurobehavioral TBI rehabilitation programs and four involuntary psychiatric hospitalizations, all associated with episodes of uncontrolled behavior. On several occasions, his poorly controlled behavior brought him into conflict with the law, and he had spent time in several jails.

In his epilogue to this book, Jason describes the downward spiral of his life over the first few years after his injury and explains why the interventions attempted in the neurobehavioral rehabilitation programs, psychiatric hospitals, and jails did not work for him. The theme that runs through those explanations is *control*. Jason demanded a reasonable amount of control over his life. Service providers either judged him to be incapable of exercising good judgment or simply demanded that he fit into their predesigned system of services. Unfortunately, with each successive crisis in Jason's life, medical professionals and authorities in the criminal justice system were accumulating evidence that increasingly convinced them that he was incapable of making good decisions, particularly when he was under stress.

We met Jason 4 years ago as he was preparing for discharge from his last psychiatric hospitalization and resumption of community living. We have worked with and collaborated with Jason since that time. During these 4 years, we have come to respect him as solid contributor to our support programs in New York state for adults with neurobehavioral problems after TBI. For 2 years, Jason has joined us in conducting 1- and 2-day training sessions for community-based providers of services. He also serves as a peer counselor for adults receiving services in a TBI-substance abuse rehabilitation program. Four years ago, few people who knew Jason would have predicted this positive outcome.

In his epilogue, Jason groups the interventions that worked for him under six headings: choice and control, networks of support, prevention and scripting, reality checks, responsibility and personally meaningful activities, and being in charge. His discussion is an excellent description of critical aspects of executive function intervention. Our current goal is to present aspects of Jason's successful rehabilitation as illustrations of contextualized, person-centered, routine-based intervention for individuals with executive system impairment.

General Executive System Routines

Because of Jason's history of crises resulting in part from inadequate anticipation and planning on his part, we proposed to him that he adopt a daily goal-plan-do-review routine, using a simple executive system advance organizer. Jason predictably rejected the proposal, in large part because of his habit of opposing all "therapy-like" proposals from rehabilitation professionals, particularly if the proposal appeared to him to be designed to impose external control over his behavior. Subsequent discussions emphasized the opposite goal—namely, that he would acquire the tools needed to set his own goals and control his own behavior, thereby eliminating the need and provocation for external control. He then designed his own form that for 3 years of successful independent living has served as his daily goal-plan-do-review routine (see Figure 4–3). Every day begins with Jason listing his priority goals for the day and his schedule of activities (a routine similar to that recommended by time management experts). Over the course of the day, he records his accomplishments and other noteworthy events. In addition to this daily planner, Jason has a system for weekly, monthly, and yearly planning to ensure that he attends to major needs, such as paying his rent.

Self-Awareness and Self-Advocacy

Jason's many hospitalizations, his bewildering variety of psychiatric diagnoses, and his growing pattern of oppositional behavior had combined with the normal consequences of severe prefrontal injury to create confusion in his mind about his identity. When our intervention began, Jason's primary sense of himself seemed to be that he was a person who hated the system within which he was forced to operate and who fought against anybody who chose to try to control him. This sense of self is clearly presented in the first part of Jason's epilogue, in which he describes the downward spiral of the early years after his injury. Recognizing that pure oppositionality is hardly a sense of self upon which to re-establish a meaningful life and that endless recitations of brain injury related deficits would not help him, we engaged Jason in the production of an autobiographical video tape. This project was subsequently expanded to include two videos designed to serve different purposes.

Jason made the first video as he was beginning community living after his last psychiatric hospitalization. The primary purpose of the video was for Jason to introduce himself to potential support staff and to give them important guidance in how to help him. Giving this responsibility to Jason was consistent with the general executive system themes driving the intervention. Jason also participated in interviewing and hiring his support staff.

In addition to serving its stated purpose, the production of an autobiographical video gave Jason a natural and meaningful context for serious reflection about himself, his life, and his new life story. Throughout his previous hospitalizations, therapists told Jason that he needed to acquire a realistic understanding of himself and his limitations after the injury, because it is clinically important to do so. Predictably, Jason angrily rejected these earlier proposals. However, because he now saw this self-reflection as part of a concrete and obviously important project to screen, orient, and train potential staff—and because he was told that it was his project—Jason worked hard at writing lengthy scripts about himself and his history.

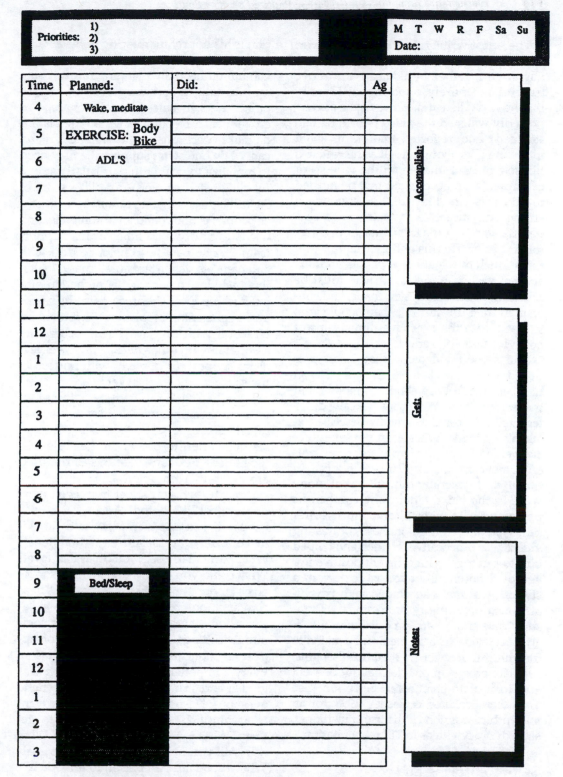

Figure 4–3. A self-designed system for daily planning of activities and self-monitoring of agitation (Ag = agitation). (Reprinted with permission from "Executive Functions: Supported Cognition and Self-Advocacy After Traumatic Brain Injury," by M. Ylvisaker and T. Feeney. *Seminars in Speech and Language, 17,* 217–232.)

The script writing itself played a powerful role in helping Jason to put his personal narrative together in his head and move beyond the purely oppositional identity that he had fallen into. However, he also repeatedly watched the video (which he had scripted) and reported that he received many insights about himself as he watched himself present himself on the video. For example, Jason once noted that he needed to live his life like Clint Eastwood—a strong and attractive character, but also a person who is at the same time both director and actor. This insightful metaphor captures much of the effort of people with executive system impairment who must be much more deliberate, systematic, and concrete in their director role than people who succeed with the executive dimensions of behavior with little effort.

The second videotape that Jason produced was a video letter to his mother. Jason had positive feelings about his mother, but their face-to-face interactions typically disintegrated into conflicts, vividly described in Jason's epilogue. Whereas in the self-advocacy video for professionals, Jason presented himself as abrasive, irascible, oppositional, and generally difficult to get along with, in the video letter to his mother, he presented a thoughtful and much softer self. Watching himself on these contrasting videos was provocative for Jason and helped him to put together a coherent positive image of a potentially successful person, a clinical goal that had eluded both psychiatric and brain injury professionals. In Jason's case and others, production of a self-advocacy video is a concrete and personally meaningful occasion to organize thoughts, evaluate others' impressions about oneself, and formulate changes in behavior. (See Ylvisaker, Szekeres, & Feeney, 1998, for an in-depth discussion of the use transitional, self-advocacy videos in TBI rehabilitation.)

Self-Monitoring and Self-Regulation

A critical component of Jason's concrete, externally supported system of self-regula-tion is his hourly monitoring of his level of anxiety or agitation (recorded in the "ag" column on his daily planning form). Using an internalized *agitation barometer*—a 100-point scale with rules for behavior associated with each 10-point range on the scale—he makes decisions about what he can and cannot do and what supports he may need to mobilize to deal with particularly stressful circumstances. For example, a score of 90 to 100 means that he cannot be with other people, cannot be in an automobile, and needs to notify a member of his support team that he may need help. To deal with emergencies, Jason formulated a 911 plan that includes contacting his probation officer and the local sheriff to gain their support in managing problems with limited interaction with the law. Lower scores are associated with other rules, with lower levels of support, or possibly with no restrictions on activity whatsoever.

Jason had little difficulty learning to attach numbers in a reliable way to his level of agitation or anxiety. Associating rules of self-regulation to points on the scale was facilitated by conversations structured around rather common sense questions, such as "When you are at that level, what do you feel like doing? And what would happen if you did that? How difficult is it to control your impulses at that level? What particularly sets you off at that level? What could you do to avoid an undesirable crisis under those circumstances?" These conversations primarily took place in Jason's home and in various relevant community settings, making the interaction appear as "nonclinical" as possible to Jason. Every component of the intervention was guided and structured by the more general questions: "Jason, what do you really want to accomplish? What can you do to get there? What is standing in your way? What help will you need to accomplish the goal? Who will be the best person to provide it?" It was clear to Jason that the goal was to enable him to take control of his own life. As these conversations crystallized important themes and lessons that Jason had learned through bitter experience, barometer-related rules of self-regulation emerged and were adopted.

Over the course of the following weeks, Jason created the habit of recording a barometer reading on his daily planning sheet every hour and following the behavioral rules associated with that reading. Because effort is required to create new habits, Jason needed the encouragement of support staff and family members to use this system when he was calm and under control. Furthermore, guided observation of his life increasingly convinced him that he needed to be relaxed, and that, after the injury, great effort was required to maintain acceptable levels of relaxation. Jason new that he did not want to resume his out-of-control life, with its associated serious restrictions on his freedom. Therefore, he worked hard to create a positive everyday routine of self-monitoring and self-instruction using a concrete set of rules of self-management.

Scripting

By his own admission, Jason's difficulties with others were largely a result of his being unprepared for stressful interaction and unable to control his anger in a crisis. He elaborates on this theme in his epilogue. With this as background, we worked with Jason to anticipate difficult interactions and prevent crises by preparing advance scripts to guide his behavior. For example, Jason knew that his mother would be upset when he told her that he planned to share an apartment with his girlfriend. In preparation for this interaction, Jason prepared a script with our assistance. The following conversation took place at a restaurant and illustrates this script-writing intervention.

Jason:	"You know my levels are high. I gotta tell my mother that I'm moving and I know she's gonna go nuts. I'm sure she's gonna make me crazy. I don't know what to do!"
Staff:	"OK, so you're saying that you're sure that she's gonna give you a hard time, right?"

Jason:	"Guaranteed."
Staff:	"Well, what do you expect her to say or do?"
Jason:	(Gives a number of possibilities, including, crying, yelling, making him feel guilty.)
Staff:	"OK, we've got 7 or 8 things that she might do. If you had to predict which ones are more likely and which ones are less likely, what would that list look like?"
Jason:	(Makes a list based on ranking of priorities.)
Staff:	"OK, we've got 4 or 5 likely scenarios, and maybe some other things that she might do that you don't expect. Do you have an idea how you'll deal with them?"
Jason:	"Well, no. I don't know what to do."
Staff:	"OK, lets try to script it out—you know, anticipate what your mom will likely say and then develop your best responses to those possibilities."
Jason:	(Makes scripts with staff for the likely scenarios.)
Staff:	"OK, now do you feel ready to deal with these if they happen?"
Jason:	"Yeh, sure."
Staff:	"OK, do you have a plan for things that she might say that are unexpected?"
Jason:	"No, but I don't think I've got to worry about that really."
Staff:	"So there's absolutely no way that she'll do or say something that you would not expect?"
Jason:	"Well, yeh, I guess she might, but there's no way I could tell all of the possibilities."
Staff:	"So if you can't be specific, what do you think you can come up with?"
Jason:	"How's about a 'punt' plan? You know, I can't deal with this ma, I'm outta here for a while."
Staff:	"Sounds like a plan to me!"

Soon thereafter, Jason told his mother his plans. She responded in ways that he felt were designed to make him feel guilty. He had anticipated this as one of the possibilities and therefore was prepared with a script. He successfully negotiated the potentially stressful conversation, maintaining low agitation levels. He commented later that he felt good about himself for doing as well as he did, and added that he continues to develop and use scripts for many potentially difficult scenarios (e.g., "OK, I hear you. What can I do to help you? You're upset, but I can't deal with it when you become so emotional. Can you please tell me when you're calm enough to talk about this in a more controlled way?"). He also routinely creates a respectful "bail out" plan to implement if the interaction becomes too painful for him. This plan includes a place to which he can retreat. In his role as peer counselor, Jason has coached others in the use of advance scripting.

With some assistance, Jason has also oriented his family and friends to scripts that they need to use in their interaction with him. For example, when his mother calls him on the phone, the script requires that she ask what his level of agitation is, identify what she would like to talk about, and specify how long she would like to talk. These scripts have been very useful for Jason, who has been more effective in using them than a number of support people in his life!

Managing a System of Supports

Jason's system of support people has evolved over the last 4 years of successful community living. Family members, close friends, and his fiancé are critical members of his support team. During his first year out of the hospital, he also had access to a community support staff person several hours each day. Jason helped to hire this person and decided when that support was no longer necessary. The consulting psychologist, Jason's probation officer, and his attorney have also served as supports for some aspects of his life. Our job was to help Jason learn how to use and manage his supports in an efficient and effective way, without alienating any of them. We spent time with Jason and people in his support system, helping him to orient them to his goals and plans. We also provided contextualized coaching to Jason and members of

his support team in positive ways to interact, particularly during tough times.

An ongoing goal was to help support people learn how to assist Jason in a way that did not create learned helplessness or elicit Jason's oppositional reactions. It was particularly important for Jason's mother to learn how she could support her son without treating him like an adolescent (a natural maternal reaction in light of Jason's history of self-destructive behavior). All of the brainstorming and planning meetings took place in community settings, such as restaurants or homes, to underscore the reality that we were not delivering a medical intervention analogous to an antibiotic for pneumonia. Rather, we were facilitating the development of positive routines of life—positive executive function routines—designed to help Jason manage his life despite ongoing disability associated with executive system impairment.

Creating Meaning

In his epilogue, Jason highlights the importance for him of playing positive roles in which he is a contributor, not just a person who receives services and complies with others' plans for him. In addition to the increasingly positive roles he plays in his family and circle of friends, he has a successful history as a presenter at head injury workshops, he has designed illustrations for several projects (including the cover design for this book), and he is a peer counselor in a TBI-substance abuse rehabilitation program. In his peer counselor role, he is seen as a powerful role model by individuals in the program and has had an undeniably positive impact on many lives. In our list of intervention premises in Chapter 1, we included the fundamental premise, "In the absence of meaningful engagement in chosen life activities, all interventions will ultimately fail." In executive system intervention, this theme cries out for special attention. In the absence of genuine goals, there is no true executive functioning. In the absence of meaningful activities with important goals, there is no executive function rehabilitation. Executive functions exist to enable people to achieve their goals in the presence of obstacles. Rehabilitation of people with impairment in this domain of functioning must, therefore, take place within the context of their pursuit of genuine goals.

Following TBI, many people have difficulty identifying goals for themselves that are at the same time personally compelling and also consistent with their new profile of abilities. The creativity of staff and family members is often stretched as they join the individual with disability in searching for this often illusive territory. However, the overriding importance of meaningful goals in the lives of people like Jason creates a mandate. The success of intervention for people with executive system impairment is contingent on attaching intervention activities to the pursuit of meaningful goals.

Jason's Story: Summary

Using these self-managed executive system supports along with a steadily decreasing level of community supports, Jason has maintained successful independent living for 3 years, has managed to reduce the costs associated with his post-TBI services from over $100,000 per year to around $2,500 per year, and has played an instrumental role in orienting community providers in the state of New York to behavioral issues associated with TBI. In addition, Jason has completed his undergraduate degree and is now formulating plans for advanced studies. Over the past 4 years, there have been no incidents of physical aggression, a remarkable accomplishment in light of their frequency and intensity over the previous 4 years (see Jason's Epilogue).

Because of his frontal lobe injury, Jason remains vulnerable to external stressors and may need to use some form of self-managed external executive system support and other types of assistance indefinitely. However, he agrees that the effort needed to maintain his current system of daily planning, advance scripting, reality checks, and self-imposed antecedent controls over his behavior is clearly preferable to facing the negative consequences of inadequately planned and poorly controlled behavior. The general theme illustrated by Jason and many people like him is that if a type of cognitive activity—in this case planning and self-regulating behavior—does not efficiently and effectively take place *in* the individual, then it often becomes necessary to implement a structured routine with customized supports. These routines, which may change frequently over time, should involve only as much support from other people as is absolutely necessary.

In Chapter 1 we described an approach to rehabilitation that essentially reverses the traditional hierarchy of impairment-, disability-, and handicap-oriented interventions. In Jason's case, external systems of support, including people and procedures like his daily planner and mediated scripting, were first put in place to reduce his social handicap and keep him out of jails and psychiatric hospitals. As he habituated his compensatory procedures, his reliance on external supports decreased, thereby reducing his disability. However, his impairment remained, necessitating frequent deliberate use of compensatory procedures. He now reports that many of his compensatory procedures, including advance planning and scripts for stressful interaction, have become internalized and automatic, thereby reducing, at least to some degree, his executive system impairment. We present Jason as an illustration of the vygotskyan approach to executive system rehabilitation described in Chapter 1. That is, mediated and externally supported executive system interaction, with thousands of appropriately scaffolded learning opportunities in the context of important everyday routines, was gradually transformed into internal and at times automatic cognitive activity.

SUMMARY

In this chapter, we have described and illustrated with case material a variety of positive everyday routines for people with executive system weakness after TBI. These routines can be implemented in very simple, concrete, and highly supported ways for young people or older people with severe impairment, or in ways that are appropriate for more mature and better recovered individuals. We hope that the illustrations presented in this chapter will serve a heuristic purpose for professionals or family members needing to create positive executive system routines for people with varied needs and at varied developmental levels and varied levels of recovery after TBI. The general ideas are simple and straightforward: As much as possible, people need to be supported in pursuing meaningful goals. When achieving success is difficult, there needs to be a system in place so that the individual considers, at some level of deliberateness, "What am I trying to accomplish? What's my plan? How's it going? Do I need to do something different? Is my plan working?" In contrast, when the routine is, "You're not good at that. You need help. Let me do that for you or let me tell you what to do," the predictable result is some combination of learned helplessness and resentment. Without a great deal of effort, well oriented staff and family members can typically implement at least 10 meaningful positive executive function routines daily. At this rate, the individual annually receives at least 3,650 meaningful learning trials and 36,500 over the course of 10 years, numbers sufficiently large to make a difference in the person's life.

We understand fully that a few case illustrations are insufficient to validate an approach to rehabilitation. Additional theoretical and empirical considerations are presented in Chapter 1. Our own commitment to this positive, everyday, highly contextualized approach to rehabilitation is based largely on our work with several hundred individuals with executive system impairment after TBI, including children and adults of all ages and levels of recovery, and in settings that include hospitals, rehabilitation centers, schools, work places, family homes, group homes, and other community settings.

A chapter on executive functions represents an interesting intersection of cognitive and behavioral themes. Most of the individuals described in this chapter were considered to have "behavior problems" after their injury. Indeed, in some cases their early intervention was traditional behavior management which, rather than helping, was a contributor to growing behavior problems. We hope that this chapter convinces its readers to at least consider the types of everyday routines described here for people diagnosed with behavior problems after TBI.

We could easily have added other important executive system routines to this chapter. For example, the discussion of self-assessment in Chapter 3 fits the theme of the current chapter. Inadequate support for people with executive system impairment easily leads to failure, frustration, and behavioral maladjustment; too much support or the wrong kind of support easily leads to learned helplessness, resentment, and failure to mature as a person capable of using strategies to overcome the obstacles created by disability. In Table 4–2, we present a checklist that we hope will help staff and family members create an appropriate executive system focus for individuals with TBI and create supports that are at an appropriate level to ensure active engagement, success, and ongoing progress toward meeting their goals in life.

TABLE 4–2. Intervention for individuals with executive system impairment: A checklist.

General Considerations

❑ Is intervention in the areas that fall under the heading "executive functions" structured around the individual's own **meaningful goals**?

❑ Is intervention infused into **everyday activities**? Are all **everyday people** oriented to how they can facilitate improved executive functions? Are all everyday people aware of the dangers of **learned helplessness**?

❑ Are everyday people aware of the strategies that the individual is being taught or is expected to use?

❑ Is successful performance in the areas grouped under this heading richly and naturally **rewarded**? Is the individual held **responsible** for effective strategic performance?

❑ Is the individual given **ample opportunity** to identify and solve his or her own problems (with guidance if necessary)?

❑ For individuals who are young or very concrete, are executive function tasks structured around **concrete physical activities** (versus **abstract or cognitive activities**)?

❑ Do everyday people in the environment routinely **model** expert use of executive functions?

❑ Is the individual given sufficient **practice** so that strategic behavior becomes **automatic**?

❑ Are everyday people in the environment **supportive** of strategic or compensatory ways to accomplish tasks?

❑ Does the individual **respect** a strategic or compensatory approach to everyday problems? If not, have reasons for this been explored? Have varied approaches to motivation been attempted?

❑ Are everyday people in the individual's environment fully **aware of possible limitations** in the individual's executive functions (especially initiation and inhibition) so that they do not misinterpret behavior?

Age and Level of Development

❑ **Preschoolers:** Are preschoolers introduced to relevant vocabulary, including "hard/easy to do"; "plan"; "do something special"; "review"; "what works? what doesn't work?" Are they actively engaged in identifying what is hard and easy for them (especially physical activities)? Are they actively engaged in identifying clever ways to accomplish difficult tasks? Are they richly and naturally rewarded for clever solutions to difficult everyday problems?

❑ **Grade school age:** Are grade school age children actively engaged in identifying what is hard and easy for them (including cognitive/academic activities)? Are they actively engaged in identifying clever ways to accomplish difficult tasks? Are they actively encouraged to seek help on their own when tasks are hard? Are they richly and naturally rewarded for clever solutions to difficult everyday problems? Are they encouraged to help each other solve problems?

❑ **Older students and adults:** See entire checklist. Is interaction related to the development of strategies respectful of age and self-concept?

Level of Recovery

❑ **People who are minimally responsive:** Is the individual prompted (physically, if necessary) to engage in familiar activities (e.g., activities of daily living), so that he or she is **acting**, not just being acted upon? Has every attempt been made (e.g., remote switch control) to enable the individual to **control** meaningful events? Do everyday people in the environment **respond** to the individual as an agent—a person who acts and is not only acted upon?

❑ **People who are alert but confused:** Is the individual given **choices** whenever possible (short of increasing confusion)? Is the individual thoroughly **oriented to the purposes** of intervention activities? Do staff **negotiate** activities with the individual? Does the individual have opportunities to experience **natural and logical consequences** of choices?

❑ **People who are no longer seriously confused:** See entire checklist.

continued

TABLE 4–2. *continued*

Self-Awareness of Strengths and Needs

❑ Is the individual maximally engaged in **identifying what is easy and hard to do**, and what makes activities easy or hard?

❑ Is the individual given opportunities to **compare performance** when an activity is completed in a usual way versus when it is completed with special strategic procedures?

❑ Does the individual keep a **journal** in which strengths and needs are recorded?

❑ Is the individual given opportunity to **identify strengths and needs in others** and **strategic procedures** that others may use (e.g., peer teaching)?

❑ Is the individual given appropriate informative **feedback** (e.g., peer feedback, video feedback, confrontational feedback, if appropriate)?

Goal-Setting

❑ Is the individual routinely asked to **predict** how well he or she will do on activities?

❑ Are predictions recorded in journals and **compared with actual performance**?

❑ Does the individual maximally participate in rehabilitation/special education **goal-setting**? Is adequate support provided if this is difficult?

❑ Are intervention activities structured around **the individual's personal goals**?

Planning

❑ Does the individual participate maximally in **planning his or her intervention activities**?

❑ Is a **planning guide** available, if needed?

❑ Does the individual begin the day by **preparing a plan** on a planning board or in a journal? Does the individual begin each activity by preparing a plan?

❑ Do therapy activities include attempts to plan meaningful complex events (e.g., parties, outings, etc.)?

❑ Does the individual participate maximally in **long-term future planning**? rehabilitation planning? IEP development?

Organizing: See Organization Checklist, Chapter 5

Self-Initiating

❑ Do everyday people give the individual **opportunities to initiate** and wait an appropriate length of time? Are **signals** available to remind the individual to initiate activities?

❑ Do the activities that the individual engages in make **appropriate demands** on the individual's ability to initiate (e.g., board games may require little initiation; conversations may require much initiation)?

❑ Are all forms of institutional **"learned helplessness"** avoided?

❑ Are **prosthetic initiators** available if needed (e.g., alarm watch, NeuroPage)?

❑ If initiation cues are necessary, are they provided as much as possible by peers versus staff? Is nagging avoided?

Self-Inhibiting

❑ Do everyday people give the individual **opportunities to inhibit** that are realistic in their demands?

❑ Do the activities that the individual engages in make **appropriate demands** on the individual's ability to inhibit (e.g., unstructured and unfamiliar activities in a distracting environment require considerable inhibition)?

❑ If inhibition cues are necessary, are they as subtle as possible and provided as much as possible by peers versus staff? Is nagging avoided?

Self-Monitoring/Evaluating

❑ Do everyday people give the individual **opportunities to self-monitor and evaluate** performance? If cues are necessary, are they subtle? Is nagging avoided?

❑ Is the individual maximally involved in **charting** his or her own performance? Keeping a **journal** in which performance is recorded? Graphing performance?

❑ Is the individual routinely asked to fill in a form regarding his or her own performance: **What Works?** and **What Doesn't Work?**

Problem Solving/Strategic Thinking

❑ Is the individual maximally involved in **solving everyday problems** as they arise? Are **everyday people** thoroughly oriented to the importance of problem solving?

❑ Is the individual maximally engaged in **selecting strategies** to overcome obstacles and achieve important goals?

❑ Is there an appropriate amount of **external support for strategic thinking**?

    ❑ Does the individual have a **form** that cues the appropriate kind of strategic thinking?

    ❑ Do everyday people in the environment **expect and cue strategic performance**?

    ❑ Do everyday people in the environment avoid **learned helplessness**, that is, do they resist solving all of the individual's problems?

❑ Is there consistency among staff and family members in how problem-solving tasks are presented and in the kinds of external problem-solving support that are provided? Is there consistency in **reducing external support** as the individual becomes increasingly independent in problem solving?

Source: Reprinted with permission from "Cognitive Rehabilitation: Executive Functions" by M. Ylvisaker, S. Szekeres, and T. Feeney, 1998, pp. 260–262. In M. Ylvisaker (Ed.), *Traumatic Brain Injury Rehabilitation: Children and Adolescents* (2nd Ed.). Boston: Butterworth-Heinemann.

CHAPTER 5

Positive Everyday Cognitive Routines

Our primary purpose in this chapter, as in the other intervention chapters, is to describe a functional and highly contextualized approach to helping people with types of disability commonly observed after TBI. It is certainly not our view that the effort, illustrated in this chapter, to positively influence everyday routines of life exhausts what can be done for individuals with cognitive impairment after brain injury. However, our work with large numbers of children and adults with chronic impairment suggests that this effort is among the most important contributions of specialists in rehabilitation and has been undervalued in the intervention and research literatures. In our experience, the themes illustrated in this chapter apply not only to many individuals with TBI, but also to people with cognitive impairment associated with other diagnoses, such as ADHD, learning disability, and developmental disability.

After a brief general discussion of cognition, we suggest a framework of categories for thinking about cognition and cognitive impairment, outline the types of cognitive impairment most commonly observed after TBI, and review intervention premises. The bulk of the chapter is devoted to case material that we hope will illustrate this approach to intervention and stimulate its creative application to unique individuals. This chapter should be read along with Chapter 1, which presents the theoretical framework that underlies this everyday approach to rehabilitation and the rationale for working within this framework, Chapter 2, in which we describe mechanisms of injury and common features of outcome, and Chapter 3, in which we discuss functional assessment procedures, which are an aspect of intervention.

Our goal is to illustrate a functional approach to cognitive rehabilitation by describing specific interventions that were successful for individuals widely ranging in age and level of disability. Our focus is on chronic disability associated with impaired organization and memory, types of cognitive impairment common in TBI. In Chapter 4, we address executive control over cognitive functions, problem solving, and cognitive flexibility, areas of intervention that could easily have been included in this chapter on cognitive rehabilitation. Similarly, the case illustrations presented in Chapters 6 and 7 could equally appear in the current chapter—and, conversely, the individuals described in this chapter could easily serve as illustrations in Chapters 4, 6, and 7—underscoring the inseparability of executive functions, cognition, behavior, and communication after TBI. We conclude with a brief indication of implications of this approach for types of disability and types of intervention that we have not selected for special attention.

COGNITION AND COGNITIVE DEVELOPMENT

A Framework of Categories for Describing Cognitive Functioning

As we use the term here, cognition includes all of the mental systems and processes that are postulated to explain the acquisition and use of knowledge. Within the tradition of information processing theory, cognition has come to be understood as "encompassing the processing of information, which occurs within certain mental systems or structures and for purposes of achieving meaningful goals in natural contexts" (Ylvisaker & Szekeres, 1998, p. 126). Table 2–1 outlines one among many ways of analyzing cognition into components. Discussion of this classification system, with special application to cognitive disability after TBI, can be found in Szekeres, Ylvisaker, and Cohen (1987) and Ylvisaker and Szekeres (1998).

As with all attempts to classify aspects of cognition, there is some arbitrariness in this scheme. Category schemes inevitabley suggest clear separation of processes and systems which, in reality, may be inseparable or alternative ways of describing the same realities. More importantly, there are critical relationships among components of cognition and between these components and other domains of human function (Flavell, Miller, & Miller, 1993; Graham & Harris, 1996; McClelland et al., 1995; Posner, 1992; Pribram, 1997). For example, attentional processes, organizational processes, working memory, the knowledge base, and the executive system all interact to enable a person to focus on and make sense of complex and novel experiences (Dennett & Kinsbourne, 1992; Luria, 1973a; Newman & Baars, 1993; Posner & Dehaene, 1994; Posner & Peterson, 1990; Stuss & Benson, 1986). It is hard to identify any human behavior that does not engage a variety of interacting cognitive processes and systems, a fact that we emphasized in Chapter 3 because of its importance for dynamic assessment. Similarly, it is critical to understand that cognition does not operate in a motivational and emotional vacuum. That is, cognitive behavior is driven in part by goals, by the individual's history of reinforcement, and by current emotional states (Flavell et al., 1993; Kantor, 1959; Michael, 1982, 1989). Furthermore, cognitive and motor functioning interact. For example, if conscious effort is required to remain upright or maintain balance, then effectiveness of performance of other tasks from a cognitive perspective will likely diminish. These complex relationships underscore the importance of a collaborative approach to assessment and intervention.

It is equally important to be sensitive to the domain specificity of cognitive processes. Common sense, studies of transfer of cognitive skill (Singley & Anderson, 1989), and the history of cognitive training and retraining (Mann, 1979) all point to the conclusion that people can improve their cognitive abilities in specific domains of content and task without affecting their ability to perform tasks in other domains that apparently involve the same aspects of cognition. For example, college students are famous for their ability to improve deductive reasoning skills in logic class without transferring those skills to other academic domains. Similarly, athletes might be great strategic thinkers on the playing field, but fail to apply the same strategies to academic or social tasks. Adolescents with attention deficits might evidence admirable control over attentional processes at the video arcade without improving their ability to focus and maintain attention in class. This domain specificity of cognitive skill serves as one of the primary theoretical supports for a richly contextualized approach to intervention.

Developmental Acquisitions: Linguistics, Academic, Vocational, and Social Knowledge and Skill

The category scheme presented in Table 2–1 does not explicitly list developmental acquisitions like language and academic, vocational, and social knowledge and skill. As aspects of the knowledge base, they would most naturally be included under long-term memory. One could also highlight content-specific aspects of cognitive processing, such as social perception and problem solving, verbal organizing, job-related judgment, and the like. The important points are that these domains of content and processing efficiency are important components of cognition and, therefore, facilitating their reacquisition and ongoing development is part of cognitive rehabilitation.

Patterns of Cognitive Development: Implications for Rehabilitation

In serving *young* children with TBI, it is obviously important to understand principles of normal cognitive development and ways to facilitate ongoing development after the injury. For reasons discussed in Chapter 1, we believe that these principles also yield important guidelines for serving *older* children and adults, particularly in the case of frontal lobe injury. Our heuristic principle is that, in cognitive rehabilitation, *there must be a good reason to deviate in substantial ways from what are known to be important general principles of normal cognitive development.* This developmental heuristic carries the authority of Luria, who commented toward the end of his career that the primary sources of insight for his work in neuropsychology were the clinic and the kindergarten (Luria, 1979).

We have selected the following three general developmental principles because they yield useful implications for the conduct of cognitive rehabilitation:

Cognitive Development Progresses from Concrete and Context Dependent to Abstract and Decontextualized

This general progression takes many forms (Flavell et al., 1993): (1) The content of early concepts includes concrete things, people, and actions (e.g., mommy, doggy, truck,

cookie, eat, hug), whereas only later do children develop more abstract concepts of attributes, space and time, relationships, numbers, and the like. This progression toward increasingly abstract thinking continues into adulthood. (2) Preferred ways of organizing things and people progress from concrete, everyday routines and activities to more general scripts and more abstract, hierarchically organized categories. (3) Whereas young children focus only on the concrete here and now, older children can increasingly reflect abstractly on the distant past and future. (4) The behavior and learning of young children are highly dependent on context. More mature children and adults are increasingly able to transfer learning from one context to another. (5) Young children tend to solve problems by manipulation of objects in a concrete trial-and-error manner; older children and adults are increasingly able to use hypothetico-deductive reasoning to solve problems, although trial and error tends to persist into adulthood in areas of minimal expertise. (6) Whereas young children have difficulty seeing the world from another's perspective, older children and adults are better equipped to assume a nonegocentric perspective, although cognitive egocentrism is routinely observed when people of any age are under stress.

The everyday cognitive routines described later in this chapter are designed to be at an appropriate level of concreteness and context sensitivity for the individual, with the expectation that ongoing neurologic recovery, combined with coached practice and planned generalization, will facilitate positive movement along all of these concrete-to-abstract dimensions of development. Unfortunately, many commercially available cognitive rehabilitation materials (e.g., workbooks, computer programs) initially target processing at a high level of abstractness, and only later inject concreteness into the program (Butler & Namerow, 1988; Craine, 1982; Harrell, Parente, Bellingrath, & Lisicia, 1992; Levin, 1991). For example, many programs attempt to exercise attention, perception, memory, or other functions with tasks that are relatively "contentless" and in contexts unrelated to application contexts (Craine, 1982). Alternatively, the "content" of exercises may be concepts that are not concretely meaningful, the exercises may be unrelated to relevant action contexts, organizing schemes used in cognitive exercises are often at a level of abstractness that does not fit the head of the learner, and problem-solving exercises are often based exclusively on discussion of hypothetical situations. In each case, "cognition" is initially targeted in the abstract, a progression that is the reverse of normal cognitive development. In contrast, our goal is to facilitate maximum abstractness, independence of context, and flexibility, but starting at the individual's current level of concreteness and systematically progressing upward and outward.

In highlighting sensitivity to meaningful context in serving individuals with brain injury, we do not wish to suggest that there is no value in intervention provided in clinical settings. Controlled tasks in controlled environments can serve a variety of purposes. For example, they are important in practicing skills that can be improved with decontextualized remedial exercises, highlighting for individuals their strengths and needs, exploring procedures for compensating for deficits, and negotiating how best to practice skills in more natural contexts. Furthermore, individuals who are extremely distractible may accomplish very little in natural environments. Similarly, those who are self-conscious may be willing to practice new skills only under controlled circumstances. Controlled small group interaction may be the best context for emotional support and adjustment counseling. Having recognized the value of controlled clinical interactions, we repeat our call to be sensitive to the importance of natural contexts in rehabilitation, a call that is justified in part by the many forces at work in medical rehabilitation that would keep rehabilitation out of natural settings and divorced from natural activities.

Cognitive Development Progresses From Involuntary to Deliberate, Strategic Processing and Learning

Young children learn efficiently when they have a concrete goal and the information to be learned must be processed to achieve that goal (Schneider & Pressley, 1989). Conversely, the learning of young children can be rendered inefficient if the teacher orients the child to the specific goal of learning and tries to teach outside of the context of meaningful activity. For example, color words might be effectively taught in a preschool classroom by engaging the children in fingerpainting, with relevant color words processed correctly *in order to* get the desired paint to make the painting. Involuntary (or "incidental") learning under these learning conditions tends to be more efficient for young, concrete, relatively nonstrategic children than deliberate (effortful, strategic) learning, which resembles more traditional pedagogy (e.g., "Today we are going to learn red—and remember, there will be a test on Friday. This is red; please say that after me—red; good; is this red or yellow?").

The gradual progression from nonstrategic to controlled, strategic learning is often discussed under the heading "metacognitive development." Deliberate learning tasks are useful only if the learners can orient themselves to the abstract goal of learning, have procedures to achieve that goal (i.e., learning strategies), know that they must use those procedures when oriented to the goal of learning or remembering, and do so. Many children and adults after brain injury are relatively concrete and nonstrategic, therefore requiring teaching within an involuntary or incidental learning paradigm, at least during the initial stages of their cognitive improvement. Often deliberate learning tasks (e.g., "You must remember to bring your memory book to memory group") are introduced too early, generating frustration for the individual and staff alike.

Cognitive Development Progresses From Dependent or Supported Thinking to Independent and Unsupported Thinking

Vygotsky's developmental theory portrays young children as "apprentices in thinking" (see Chapter 1). That is, at any developmental stage, they are able to perceive, think, solve problems, and make decisions independently at a certain developmental level, but can also engage in those cognitive activities at a higher level with the support of an adult or more mature peer. It is this support, often taking the form of social interaction during cognitively demanding tasks, that is the driving force behind cognitive development. In this sense, higher cognitive processes are internalizations of repeated social interaction with a mentor or facilitator (i.e., cognitive mediation). Well-conceived supports and contextualized coaching in strategic thinking teach the child the next level of thinking, organizing, or problem solving. When the next level is mastered, the supports can be systematically withdrawn or the level of difficulty increased or both.

In this model of teaching and cognitive rehabilitation, dangers lurk on either side of ideal levels of support. If supports are not withdrawn as appropriate, the result may be a combination of general learned helplessness and specific dependence on context cues. Persisting intensive use of classroom aides for students with TBI, beyond their legitimate need, illustrates this danger. At the other extreme, if intelligent supports are not provided when they are needed, the individual can experience an intolerable frequency of failure and not learn the strategies, organizing schemes, or skills that are most useful in successfully completing difficult tasks and acquiring higher levels of cognitive processing. We have observed many children return to school and adults return to work without needed supports, with teachers and supervisors assuming a "let's see if he can make it" attitude. Subsequent efforts to reverse a downward spiral of failure are often too little and too late.

Dangers in an Inflexible Use of a Developmental Template in Brain Injury Rehabilitation

An understanding of normal development yields important insights for rehabilitation.

However, we caution against applying a developmental template rigidly. Our recommendation in Chapter 3 for flexibility in the generation of hypotheses and application of hypothesis-driven intervention applies to cognitive rehabilitation. Furthermore, there are other genuine dangers associated with applying a developmental template to the cognitive rehabilitation of older children and adults, including the following:

➤ It is never acceptable to interact with older children, adolescents, or adults in an infantilizing manner or to present tasks that may be interpreted as infantilizing.

➤ Following TBI, careful analysis and structuring of tasks may need to be much more intense than that needed by normally developing children.

➤ Because of processing weakness, the tasks used for teaching may need to be artificially simplified, targeted, supported, and intensified relative to what is needed by normally developing children.

➤ Because of the potential for chronic disability and the consequent need for strategic compensations, it may be important to focus on metacognition and strategic behavior at a younger age and more intensively than with normally developing children.

➤ Unlike young children, older children and adults bring a world of acquired content knowledge to the task of rehabilitation.

➤ Following TBI, it is critical to be sensitive to the possibility of "gappy" profiles of ability and disability quite unlike those of normally developing children or of individuals with disability from birth.

➤ Specific types of injury, for example, severe hippocampal damage associated with anterograde amnesia, may create cognitive profiles and needs completely unlike those of typical children at any developmental age.

➤ Motivated by the goal of placing helpful supports in place for people with cognitive disability, it is easy to provide too many supports or leave them in place too long, thereby flirting with learned helplessness and the maintenance of childlike behavior when the goal is the opposite.

COGNITIVE IMPAIRMENT ASSOCIATED WITH TBI

Virtually any combination of strengths and needs is possible after brain injury. In the case of closed head injury, the most common type of TBI, commonalities in cognitive profiles—and associated themes in cognitive rehabilitation—result from the vulnerability of prefrontal and limbic regions of the brain (see Chapter 2) (Bigler, 1990; Levin et al., 1991, 1993; Pang, 1985). In individual cases, cognitive impairment following injury to these regions may be combined with preinjury learning disability and specific damage to posterior regions of the brain, thereby affecting specific domains of processing (e.g., specific difficulty with linguistic processing, including reading; loss of stored knowledge, including academic, social, and general world knowledge) (Benton, 1991; Mateer & Williams, 1991, 1992). Furthermore, young children may evidence growing disability over the years after their injury in part because of their greater vulnerability to new learning impairment (Dalby & Obrzut, 1991). That is, adults who recover much of their preinjury knowledge and skill but who have significant new learning disability after TBI may have little difficulty succeeding in social and vocational contexts that place minimal demands on new learning (Grattan & Eslinger, 1991). Young children, on the other hand, look forward to a world of learning, with each element of knowledge contributing to the acquisition of subsequent elements. Therefore, new learning impairment may take a greater cumulative toll in their lives than in the lives of comparably injured adults (Asarnow et al., 1991; Eslinger et al., 1992; Grattan & Eslinger, 1991).

As discussed in Chapter 4, prefrontal regions of the brain are associated with executive or control functions. Therefore, the manifest cognitive problem is typically not a deficit in processing under ideal conditions, but rather difficulty controlling cognitive processes under less than ideal conditions (Damasio et al., 1990, 1991; Stuss & Benson, 1986). For example, working memory impairment may only be obvious when the individual must process more than one stimulus or simultaneously consider a variety of issues in solving a novel problem. Similarly, people with prefrontal injury may be able to attend to relevant stimuli for adequate periods of time, but not when there is competition for their focus of attention or when they are expected to flexibly shift their focus or attend to more than one stimulus at the same time. They may have little difficulty perceiving and making sense of visual and auditory stimuli under ideal conditions, but experience surprising breakdowns when the task becomes complex, requiring controlled perceptual processing. They may reveal age-appropriate knowledge of organizing schemes (e.g., organization of concepts and event schemata), but fail to guide their behavior and their discourse with those organizing schemes (i.e., frontal apraxia). They may be able to learn new information under ideal conditions, but fail to appropriately direct their encoding of new information or their searches of memory when stressed (i.e., ineffective deliberate or strategic learning and memory). They may solve problems effectively when the requisite thinking is relatively automatic for them, but have great difficulty with novel problem-solving tasks and problem solving under stressful circumstances.

Language and communication disability associated with cognitive impairment due to prefrontal injury may include any of the following, consistent with apparently well recovered language and speech (Biddle, McCabe, & Bliss, 1996; Campbell & Dollaghan, 1990; Chapman, 1997; Chapman et al., 1992, 1995, 1997; Dennis, 1992; Dennis & Barnes, 1990; Dennis & Lovett, 1990; Ehrlich, 1988; Ewing-Cobbs et al., 1987, 1989; Hagen,

1981; Hartley, 1995; Hartley & Jensen, 1991; Jordan, Murdoch, & Buttsworth, 1991; Knights et al., 1991; Liles, Coelho, Duffy, & Zalagens, 1989; Luria, 1970; McDonald, 1992a, 1992b, 1993; Mentis & Prutting, 1987, 1991; Petterson, 1991; Prigatano, Roueche, & Fordyce, 1985; Rutter, Chadwick, & Shaffer, 1983; Sarno, 1980, 1984; Sarno, Buonaguro, & Levita, 1986; Turkstra & Holland, 1998; Ylvisaker, 1986, 1989, 1992, 1993; Ylvisaker & Feeney, 1995):

1. difficulty controlling and organizing discourse, including conversation and noninteractive discourse (e.g., narratives, explanations, descriptions); extended discourse may be rambling, copious, and tangential; alternatively, the individual may produce little connected language because the organizational task is too difficult or because of initiation impairment; receptively, organizational impairment expresses itself as difficulty comprehending extended spoken or written language, despite little difficulty comprehending language that does not go beyond a few sentences;
2. difficulty searching for words in an organized manner, resulting in word-retrieval problems and possibly disfluent speech;
3. difficulty with demands for linguistic flexibility (e.g., processing ambiguous words and expressions with multiple meanings) and abstractness (e.g., comprehending metaphors and figures of speech); and
4. difficulty interacting with others in a socially appropriate manner; effectiveness of social interaction may be reduced by verbal disinhibition, lack of initiation, and failure to perceive and act on social cues.

Just as tests of intelligence typically fail to uncover cognitive weakness associated with prefrontal injury, so also commonly used tests of aphasia and language development in children often fail to identify these common language and communication weaknesses.

The most common site of limbic region impairment after TBI is the hippocampus, which is particularly vulnerable to secondary hypoxic injury (see Chapter 2). The classic presentation of individuals with selective hippocampal damage includes anterograde amnesia—specifically difficulty with declarative and explicit memory—despite an adequately preserved preinjury knowledge base and possibly relatively preserved procedural and implicit memory systems (Squire, 1992; Tranel & Damasio, 1995). Rehabilitation of individuals with severe memory impairment is often based on the relatively intact procedural and implicit memory systems (Diller & Gordon, 1981; Schacter & Church, 1992; Schacter & Glisky, 1986). Because of the complexity of human memory systems (see Table 2–1), it is critical to explore all types of memory processes, memoria (e.g., verbal versus nonverbal information, auditory versus visual information, facts versus episodes versus rules and procedures), and learning tasks to ensure a complete and useful understanding of the individual's memory and learning potential. Ylvisaker and colleagues (1990) presented an organized list of probe tasks that can be used to explore these and other aspects of cognitive functioning.

Earlier we highlighted the difficulty in isolating specific components of cognition and precisely determining which component or combination of components is responsible for success or failure on a specific task. For example, it is unfortunately easy to misdiagnose a memory impairment when the basis of the problem is actually weak attentional or organizational skills. Similarly, individuals are often identified with an attention deficit when their real problem is difficulty organizing behavior or incoming stimuli. Comparable misdiagnoses can occur across broader domains of functioning. We have worked with many individuals like Doug, described later in this chapter, who were diagnosed with a primary behavior problem that was clearly secondary to improperly diagnosed cognitive weakness (see Feeney & Ylvisaker, 1995). In Chapter 3, we describe a contextualized, hypothesis-testing process designed to sort out these potentially confusing realities, a process described in greater depth by Ylvisaker and Gioia (1998).

FRAMEWORK FOR INTERVENTION

We invite readers to review the intervention premises that were described in Chapter 1, including those that apply across domains of functioning after brain injury, as well as those that apply specifically to cognitive rehabilitation. In that chapter, we isolated four traditional types of approaches to helping people with cognitive impairment after TBI improve their performance of important real-world tasks: (1) a process-specific, hierarchically organized restorative approach that attempts to improve underlying cognitive processes and systems with relatively "contentless" cognitive exercises (e.g., Sohlberg & Mateer, 1989); (2) a task-specific, skills-based approach that attempts to improve performance of important real-world tasks by practicing those tasks, without necessarily expecting cognitive functioning to improve in a generalized way (e.g., Butler & Namerow, 1988; Mayer et al., 1986); (3) a compensatory approach that attempts to improve performance by equipping individuals with strategic procedures designed to compensate for ongoing cognitive impairment (e.g., Parenté & Anderson-Parenté, 1991); and (4) a compensatory approach that attempts to improve performance by modifying the individual's tasks or environment, or by providing other external supports (e.g., Ylvisaker, Szekeres, & Haarbauer-Krupa, 1998). Pharmacological treatment is a possible adjunct to any of the other types of cognitive intervention (Lombardi & Weingartner, 1995).

The "tradition" that emerged in the field of cognitive rehabilitation during the 1970s and 1980s was one in which initial emphasis was placed on restoration of function

with process-specific exercises (Ben-Yishay, Piasetsky, & Rattok, 1987). In the event of residual disability following intensive exercises, compensatory procedures were taught. Finally, if functional disability persisted, then functional task-specific training, combined with possible task and environmental modifications, was highlighted. Our suggestion is that all four of these goals can and should be simultaneously addressed within a vygotskyan approach to intervention. That is, by engaging people in real-world tasks with sufficient "scaffolding" or external supports to ensure success, by encouraging the use of helpful strategic behavior during performance of these tasks, by practicing these tasks to mastery, by highlighting specific components of cognitive processing while practicing the tasks, and by systematically withdrawing the supports and expanding the tasks and environments in which the individual can be successful, all four approaches can be integrated into one functional approach to rehabilitation.

This framework is one in which the fundamental role of strategic cognitive behavior in *normal* cognitive functioning is highlighted; that is, strategic behavior is not considered second best and therefore targeted only after "restorative" approaches have either failed or achieved their maximum benefit. Improving strategic behavior *is* restorative. Furthermore, supporting performance with various types of external scaffolds is an important component of normal cognitive growth, not only in childhood, but into adulthood as well (e.g., internships and other vocational apprenticeship programs for adults).

Our perception of the natural history of program development in cognitive rehabilitation after brain injury—from (1) a primary focus on decontextualized, process-specific exercises designed to remediate the cognitive deficit to (2) a focus on acquisition of discrete compensatory strategies in clinical training tasks to (3) a richly contextualized approach to improving cognitive functioning by practicing skills, practicing specific tasks, using strategic behavior, and employing supports and modifications—appears to mirror earlier histories of cognitive intervention for individuals with developmental disabilities and congenital learning disabilities (Mann, 1979). That is, early reliance on remedial exercises was enriched by recognition of the need for compensatory strategies, and both were enriched by recognition of the value of contextualizing the intervention (cf. supported employment programs, inclusionary education programs, "push-in" therapy programs).

Controversy persists about the value of process-specific, remedial, cognitive retraining exercises (Mateer & Mapou, 1996; Ponsford, 1990; Sohlberg & Raskin, 1996). What is undeniable, however, is that many people with severe TBI have residual and possibly debilitating cognitive impairment after intensive exercises have achieved their maximum benefit. The everyday, contextualized, multifaceted approach to intervention described in this chapter is, at the very least, relevant for this group of people, along with many groups of people with congenital disability, including mental retardation, learning disability, ADHD, and others.

Cognitive Rehabilitation, Cognitive Development, and Generalization

It is sometimes argued that training that begins—or is largely provided—in real-world contexts using real-world content is doomed to fail. That is, the individual may learn specific behaviors and apply them in those training contexts, but requires targeted cognitive exercises that are free of specific context and content in order to improve functioning in a generalizable way (Sohlberg & Raskin, 1996). In our view, cognitive development sheds light on this important issue. Young children acquire many important behaviors (e.g., avoiding the hot stove in their kitchen) and routines (e.g., a rigid bedtime routine) in highly specific real-world contexts without being consigned

to those limited contexts, behaviors, and routines for life. Normal child development, which begins with contextualized acquisitions, includes stimulus and response generalization, to use behavioral terms, or development in abstractness from concrete routines to flexible scripts and schemas, to use cognitive terms. An analogous process of generalization is always a focus of intervention following brain injury whether the clinician chooses to start with contextualized or decontextualized practice. However, if the individual remains extremely compromised cognitively and is therefore capable of minimal generalization, it is better that the training results in functional, albeit limited, contextualized improvement than in improved performance of decontextualized training tasks that are of no value in the real world. (See Chapter 1.)

EVERYDAY COGNITIVE ROUTINES: ORGANIZATION, MEMORY, AND LANGUAGE

In Chapter 1 and earlier in this chapter, we described some of the many ways in which apparently discrete components of cognition are highly interrelated. For example, the ability to organize perceptions, thoughts, and behavior clearly depends on the ability to focus and maintain attention. Conversely, the ability to focus and maintain attention depends in part on the ability to impose organization on incoming stimuli. Similarly, the ability to learn and remember is dependent on many cognitive factors beyond specific memory processes, including attention, organization, and, at least for older children and adults, executive direction of the learning process.

We have chosen to focus on organization and memory because impairments in these areas are among the most common and disabling after closed head injury. We have chosen to connect organization and memory in this discussion because of the overwhelming evidence of their intimate connection in both normal and memory-impaired populations. This connection was a major theme in the study of memory in the 1960s and 1970s (e.g., Mandler, 1967). The fundamental reality is that information that is organized effectively and in a way that fits the organizational schemes of the learner is easier to attend to, comprehend, encode in memory, store over time, and retrieve when desired. This theme, initially explored and elaborated by cognitive scientists, has been preserved in recent neuropsychological accounts of memory. According to Baddeley (1995), information that is encoded in an organized way leads to "a well-integrated trace that stores the information in more than one dimension, hence making it resistant to forgetting. Furthermore, the presence of several dimensions will increase the number of retrieval routes" (p. 9). Furthermore, intervention focused on organizational strategies has been found to be useful in working with various populations of children with developmental learning and memory problems (Pressley & Associates, 1990; Deshler & Schumaker, 1988), adults with memory problems associated with TBI (Levin & Goldstein, 1986), and adults with age-related memory problems (West, 1995). Szekeres (1992) summarized the literature that connects organization and memory impairment and intervention for individuals with TBI.

Language appears in the heading of this section for two reasons. First, within a vygotskyan cognitive framework, cognitive organization is largely the internalization of language.

> The acquisition of language can provide a paradigm for the entire problem of the relation between learning and development. Language arises initially as a means of communication between the child and the people in his environment. Only subsequently, upon conversion to internal speech, does it come to organize the child's thought, that is, becomes an internal mental function. (Vygotsky, 1978, p. 89)

This hypothesis motivates the use of everyday interactive language routines, described later in this chapter, with the goal of improving cognitive organization and memory. In addition, even if the goal for the individual is not an internalization of a form of language, the language of intervention and scripts associated with task demonstration and clarification are still critical components of cognitive intervention.

Organization, Memory, and Language: Individuals Who Require Intensive Levels of Support

Research in developmental cognitive psychology has emphasized the role of parent-child conversations about the past in facilitating the child's development of thought organization and autobiographical memory (Fivush, 1991; Fivush & Fromhoff, 1988; Fivush & Reese, 1992; Hudson, 1990; McCabe & Peterson, 1991; Nelson, 1992; Reese & Fivush, 1993; Reese, Haden, & Fivush, 1993). The evolving view is that parents who frequently interact with their preschool children in a collaborative, elaborative, and socially enjoyable way have children who develop internal organization and autobiographical memory more effectively than comparable children whose parents interact with them less frequently or in a way that is not supportive. Although these interactions can focus on a variety of topics, developmental investigations in this area have largely targeted parent-child interaction while jointly talking about events that they have experienced together, that is, socially co-constructed narratives about the past.

The positive and facilitative parental style of jointly constructing narratives with children is characterized in several overlapping ways in the experimental literature, for example, as an elaborative style (Fivush & Fromhoff, 1988), and a positive cognitive style (Nelson, 1973). In Table 5–1, we attempt to capture the competencies associated with this positive style under two general headings: collaboration and elaboration. That is, these parents tend to *participate with* their children rather than *demand perform-*

TABLE 5–1. Collaborative and elaborative competencies in socially co-constructing narratives about the past with young children and older individuals with cognitive disability.

Competencies Associated With a Collaborative Style

Collaborative intent

1. Partner shares information; does not just demand it.
2. Partner uses collaborative talk (e.g., "Let's try to remember the day we ..."; "I enjoy thinking about these things with you.").
3. Partner confirms partner's contributions (e.g., "That's right, that was next.").

Cognitive support

1. Partner gives information when needed (within either statements or questions).
2. Partner makes memory/organization supports available (e.g., photos, memory book, gestures).
3. Partner gives cues in a conversational manner.
4. Partner responds to errors by giving correct information in a nonthreatening, nonpunitive manner.

Emotional support

1. Partner respects other's concerns.
2. Partner explicitly recognizes difficulty of task.

Questions: positive style

1. When questions are used, they are used in a nondemanding and supportive manner.
2. If needed, partner uses specific questions that include cues.

Competencies Associated With an Elaborative Style

Topics

1. Partner introduces topics of interest and with potential for elaboration.
2. Partner maintains topic for many turns (e.g., repeats partner; affirms partner's contribution; adds information; asks open questions; reviews topic; expresses interest; if necessary, corrects partner in nonthreatening manner).
3. Partner contributes many pieces of information per topic.
4. Partner invites elaboration (e.g., "I wonder what happened ...").

Organization

1. Partner tries to organize information as clearly as possible.

   ➤ sequential order of events (e.g., "First, we ..., then we ...")
   ➤ physical causality (e.g., "It broke because you dropped it.")
   ➤ psychological causality (e.g., "You ran because you were scared.")
   ➤ similarity/difference (e.g., "Yes, they are similar because ...")
   ➤ analogy/association (e.g., "That reminds me of ..., because ...")

2. Partner reviews organization of information.
3. Partner makes connections when topics change.

1. Partner adds explanations for events.
2. Partner addresses problems and solutions (e.g., "I wonder if we can think of a better way to handle this if it comes up again.").

Explanation

---

ance from them; in addition, they use these conversations to help their child understand how things, people, and events in the world are organized, that is, they gradually clarify for their children the many ways in which things in the world go together. In effect, parents, as well as teachers, therapists, and others, are able to teach children how to think and how to organize their thoughts while at the same time enjoying pleasant conversations about topics of mutual interest. Within a vygotskyan framework (see Chapter 1), the processes of organizing information and remembering events first exist as part of the interaction between child and parent (i.e., *interpsychic* cognition) and are over time internalized to become the child's subjective cognitive processes (i.e., *intrapsychic* cognition). This supportive style of interaction and its rationale parallel the style and corresponding rationale associated with reciprocal teaching of reading comprehension, applicable to older children and discussed later in this chapter (Brown & Palinscar, 1989; Palinscar & Brown, 1984, 1989).

It is ironic and unfortunate that many professionals and family members alike switch to an unhelpful, performance-oriented manner of interacting when talking to a child or adult who is disorganized and has difficulty remembering as a result of brain injury (or developmental disability). That is, interaction comes to be characterized by interrogation, more like a teacher quizzing a student than a parent conversing with a child. Many adults justify the string of performance-oriented questions they ask on grounds that they are trying to help the person remember more effectively (e.g., "I'm trying to jog his memory"), despite solid evidence that this type of interaction actually interferes with rather than facilitates the development of cognitive organization and autobiographical memory.

Case Illustration: Child Who Required Intensive Levels of Cognitive Supports

Dave, described briefly in Chapter 4 in the section on cognitive and behavioral flexibility, was injured in a motor vehicle accident at age 2. Neuropsychological testing at age 5 revealed significant disinhibition, distractibility, and impulsiveness. Receptive and expressive language were delayed, motor strength and coordination were weakened, and visual-spatial and visual-motor deficits were documented. At age 7, a verbal IQ of 91 and a performance IQ of 70 were derived using the Wechsler Intelligence Scale for Children—III. Performance IQ was reduced by specific visual-perceptual deficits and generalized slowness. Interestingly, at the time of this testing, Dave's classroom teacher asserted unequivocally that his chief difficulties in the classroom were related to language—in contrast to what would be predicted by the results of intelligence testing—and included word-retrieval problems and general expressive organizational weakness as well as difficulty with verbal problem solving and reading. This pattern of relatively superior verbal functioning on testing but serious language-related disability in the real world is common in both children and adults with TBI (Alexander et al., 1989; Ylvisaker, 1992, 1993).

We met Dave when he was 5. In addition to his cognitive and behavioral rigidity, described in Chapter 4, Dave's parents and teachers were concerned about his difficulty verbally expressing himself, his resistance to even modestly complex discourse tasks, and his relatively weak memory. Parents and teachers asked Dave many questions over the course of the day (to "exercise his memory"), to which he frequently replied "You say it!" or some such rejection of the performance demand. That is, Dave knew that these tasks were difficult for him and that adults were in the habit of asking him questions to which they knew the answers. It was, therefore, natural for him to suggest that they answer their own questions. The following conversation, which served as a baseline for the parent training program, is an illustration of the short and unsatisfying conversations that occurred at this time:

Mom: Dave, you want to tell Dad about Matthew's game?

Dad: You guys go to the game?

Dave: No, Mom, you tell him.

Dad: You tell me; how did Matthew do today?

Dave: Ah . . .
Dad: C'mon.
Dave: Ah . . . good.
Mom: How many points?
Dad: How many points did he have?
Dave: Mom, you tell him.
Mom: Matthew had six points.
Dad: Did they end up winning the game?
Dave: Yeh.
Mom: Ok.

As this "conversation" illustrates, most of the language directed at Dave, both at school and at home, was a demand for his performance, which he knew would be difficult and therefore something to avoid. Under these circumstances, conversations are not a context for expanding and organizing Dave's framework of concepts and understanding of relations in the world.

To address these problems with cognitive and linguistic organization and memory, we implemented a parent training program, designed to increase their use of the positive interactive competencies listed in Table 5–1, thereby positively modifying their everyday interaction with Dave. The training program began with coached observation of a videotaped conversation between a father and his normally developing preschool son. This model conversation was about a trip that the two had recently taken to an amusement park and included excellent examples of all of the interactive competencies listed in Table 5–1.

Following this general orientation, the parents tried to find at least three times a day (usually after school, over dinner, and before bed) during which they could practice their competencies in collaborative and elaborative conversations with Dave. Over the course of the next 3 months, we made monthly visits to the home to review with the parents tape-recorded conversations between Dave and his mother or father and to provide them with additional coaching and cheerleading in this collaborative, conversational approach to teaching Dave how to organize his thoughts, more effectively remember, and express himself in a more fluid and organized manner. During that

time, the parents dramatically reduced their proportion of performance-oriented questions, increased the typical number of turns per topic of conversation from 1 or 2 to 10 or more (thereby facilitating Dave's development of thought organization), learned how to use concrete organizational and memory supports (e.g., photographs, graphic organizers), and in general became more elaborative and collaborative in their interaction with Dave.

Four months after the parent training program began, an outcome conversation between Dave and his mother was videotaped, illustrating the extent to which she had evolved a collaborative and elaborative style and the increased willingness and ability of Dave to maintain and contribute to the construction of narrative descriptions. The conversation took place at home and was about Dave's day at school. The cognitive supports for this conversation included a letter home from school listing all of the day's activities and a set of photographs that depicted most of the activities that could take place at Dave's school. The conversation continued for about 15 minutes and included segments during which the two maintained a specific topic for several minutes. One segment of this conversation was a discussion of a game Dave had played in school that day, and involved 13 turns per partner. During her 13 turns on this topic, Dave's mother used a variety of elaboration procedures (e.g., introducing a rich topic, inviting elaboration [2 turns], explaining events [2 turns], suggesting analogies or similarities [2 turns], requesting needed information [3 turns], highlighting important information, constructing a relevant plan) as well as a variety of collaboration procedures (e.g., expressing enthusiasm for the topic, giving necessary information [2 turns], expressing her reactions, responding to Dave's contributions with obvious interest, requesting clarification [2 turns], and offering useful memory supports [photographs]).

At the same time, staff at school reported that, despite ongoing organizational and word-retrieval problems, Dave increasingly volunteered to answer questions in class and to report about events that had occurred in school (e.g., describe art or music class activities to the regular classroom teacher). Observation of Dave in his classroom 1 year later revealed a student with confidence in his ability to express himself and the ability to organize several thoughts in his answers. For example, during a half-hour full-class discussion, Dave raised his hand to answer questions or contribute information more than 10 times. When called on, he expressed his thoughts clearly, although with obvious effort. Teaching staff indicated that this was typical of his classroom performance. That is, despite Dave's ongoing organizational impairment, which interferes with efficient word retrieval and fluid organized expression of ideas, his positive, collaborative, and elaborative everyday interaction with his parents has contributed both to his confidence that he can express himself and to the efficiency and organization of this expression.

In addition, Dave's parents reported that their interaction with him at home was profoundly more pleasant than when they felt that it was their job to routinely test their son, thereby making his job that of escaping these tests. In a videotaped message designed to support Dave's transition to another classroom, his mother observed,

> We've seen a lot of progress in his ability to tell stories and communicate longer versions of things to us. When we first started working with Dave to try to get him to be more verbal, we did a lot a quizzing. He got a little sick of that constant questioning and put us off because he always felt he was being put on the spot. We then learned a few techniques to get him to elaborate more on his stories and to collaborate with us in a conversation. So the quizzing has stopped. We encourage him to participate with us in the storytelling rather than perform for us. And we've seen a huge improvement in that area—and I think he also has enjoyed it so much more.

Older Adults With Severe Organization and Memory Problems

There is a growing literature on memory intervention and supports for adults with neurogenic memory disorders, stimulated in part by the growing population of older adults with Alzheimer's disease. Options include buddy systems (i.e., another person who serves as prosthetic memory), memory books, posted reminders, electronic reminder systems (briefly discussed below), and internal memory strategies (reviewed in Parenté & Anderson-Parenté, 1994), as well as daily repetition of critical information and pharmacologic intervention (reviewed by Lombardi & Weingartner, 1995), among others. In addition to exploring combinations of these approaches when serving adults with memory impairment, we have found it useful to review the competencies associated with an elaborative and collaborative interactive style with their everyday conversation partners. Although conversing about the past in a supportive way (versus demanding performance from adults with memory impairment) may not have the effect of improving memory and thought organization, as it does with normally developing children and apparently did with Dave, it does serve to reduce some of the stress, frustration, and discomfort that both parties experience when the conversation is performance oriented (i.e., largely a series of quizzes) and unsupported.

With this as background, we have coached spouses, nursing home staff, and others in the use of the competencies listed in Table 5–1. In addition, we have encouraged them to make use of photographs and other memory cues as they converse and to try to organize their own contributions to descriptions or narratives using advance organizers like those depicted in Figures 5–1 and 5–2 as guides. The typical report from adults with memory impairment is that, when their partners shift from an inquisitorial to a collaborative and elaborative style of interaction, the conversations are more satisfying for both. Furthermore, individuals with memory impairment can often contribute more information when they are not forced by their partner's conversational style to feel like an incompetent child.

Implicit Memory, Errorless Learning, and Scaffolding

In a series of studies, Wilson and her colleagues have introduced the traditional developmental disabilities concept of error-less learning into brain injury rehabilitation (Wilson, 1995; Wilson et al., 1994; Wilson & Evans, 1996). Their conclusion from these studies is that, at least in some situations, people with *severe* memory impairment learn better if they do not make mistakes in the early stages of their learning. Because individuals with severe amnesia often have relatively preserved *implicit* memory despite severely impaired *explicit* memory, their performance on tasks may be influ-

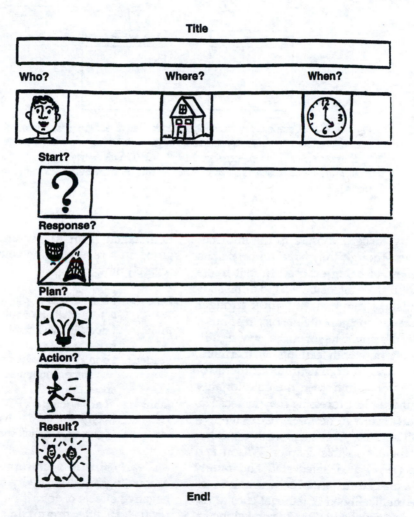

Figure 5–1. A simple graphic organizer for narrative information. (Reprinted with permission from "Cognitive Rehabilitation: Organization, Memory, and Language," by M. Ylvisaker, S. Szekeres, & J. Haarbauer-Krupa, 1998, p. 206. In M. Ylvisaker [Ed.], *Traumatic Brain Injury Rehabilitation: Children and Adolescents.* Boston: Butterworth-Heinemann.)

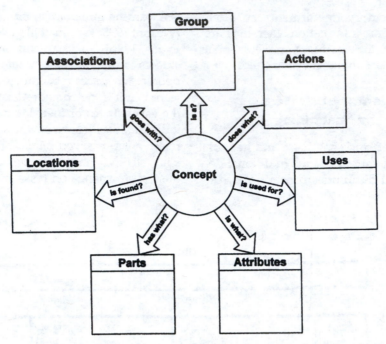

Figure 5–2. A graphic organizer for semantic feature analysis. (Reprinted with permission from "Cognitive Rehabilitation: Organization, Memory, and Language," by S. Szekeres, and J. Haarbauer-Krupa, 1998, p. 210. In M. Ylvisaker [Ed.], *Traumatic Brain Injury Rehabilitation: Children and Adolescents.* Boston: Butterworth-Heinemann.)

enced by earlier exposure to the information even though they have no conscious awareness of being exposed to that information. If their exposure was to a mistake, that mistake may persist with a stronger representation than the correct response. That is, the practicing of errors may significantly interfere with learning. Furthermore, if there was an argument about the erroneous information, then the emotionality surrounding its processing may increase its strength of storage, despite no explicit memory of learning. Consistent with the other main themes in this chapter, Wilson and Evans (1996) also urged staff and family members (1) to *contextualize* teaching to increase the likelihood of retrieval cues at the time of retrieval and (2) to maximize the individual's engagement in learning tasks, in part by making them personally *meaningful*.

The importance of these themes is illustrated by the following misguided interac-

tion, taken from a morning orientation group in a rehabilitation center. John was severely amnesic.

Leader: John, Let's start with you. Could you tell me what you do after group today?
John: I don't know; I think I go to PT; I go to PT.
Leader: I don't think so; let's check the schedule; Nope, you have a break and then speech.
John: That's wrong; it's PT I told you.
Leader: Maybe you used to have PT; but now it's break and then speech.

Clearly this is a performance-oriented routine, with no sensitivity to the possibly negative effects of John's rehearsing an error (i.e., PT after group). In addition to the serious interpersonal problems associated with beginning the day with a failed test followed by an argument, John's repetition of "PT after group" is likely to be retained as an implicit memory, thereby contributing to disorientation and agitation over the course of the day—the opposite of the goal of the Orientation Group. In contrast, the following alternative interaction includes sufficient scaffolding to ensure that John does not rehearse errors.

Leader: John, let's try to get clear about what your day looks like.
John: I don't need your help.
Leader: Well, you might be right about that; but let's double check your schedule. We're starting with group, then— take a look here—it's break time then . . . aha, speech.
John: No, I don't think so; it's . . .
Leader: Hold on. It's silly to argue, isn't it? The minute we're done here, we'll double check with Lorie in speech; she'll know for sure, right? I think it's speech after group—you see, here is Lorie's picture, your speech therapist. We know how to find out; we'll check with Lorie.

This interactive routine has several important characteristics. It involves no performance demands, it provides sufficient support for the individual to process correct information, the information (speech next) is meaningfully processed four times, the learning is errorless, and disagreements are dealt with in a respectful, experimental manner (i.e., we will check with Lorie), thereby avoiding pointless arguments. As in so many cases, it is critical that everyday communication partners learn their scripts well; only then will the cognitive routines for individuals with cognitive impairment be positive and potentially helpful in relation to cognitive improvement.

The more severe the memory impairment, the more important it is that errors are not practiced. This principle may seem contrary to an intuitive understanding of amnesia. That is, when people cannot explicitly recall information, it would seem benign to practice errors because they will be quickly lost with no harm done. Indeed,

it is common to hear staff and others say, "Don't worry about what you say to John; he won't remember it anyway!" However, the increasing evidence of relatively preserved implicit memory in even severe cases of amnesia argues for intense efforts to prevent these individuals from practicing errors or in other ways processing misinformation. This goal dovetails nicely with the Vygotskyan goal of errorless teaching through appropriate scaffolding. Errorless learning is also a component of the scripted teaching routines associated with Direct Instruction, an approach to teaching academic content that has been found useful for many students with TBI (Glang, Singer, Cooley, & Tisch, 1992; Madigan, Hall, & Glang, 1997). The relative preservation of implicit memory and procedural learning in TBI also argues for careful attention to supported behavioral routines, thereby avoiding the possibility that the individual "practices" negative behaviors (e.g., acting out to avoid difficult tasks) that may inadvertently become lodged in memory (see Chapter 6).

In highlighting the value of errorless learning for individuals with severe memory impairment, we do not wish to suggest that mistakes cannot be useful for other individuals in rehabilitation. For many people, including professionals, mistakes followed by meaningful, natural feedback can be a rich source of learning and insight. Indeed, it is not uncommon for people with brain injury to believe that they have no problems associated with the injury until they begin to make serious mistakes and experience unexpected failure. As in so many cases, good clinical judgment is required.

Organization and Memory: Individuals Who Require Moderate Levels of Support

The two individuals chosen for illustrative purposes in this section, an adolescent and a young adult with moderate cognitive impairment after severe TBI, demonstrated an ability to succeed in school and at work, but only with the support of well rehearsed routines that included advance organizers. Without these supports, they were both on the road to failure. With the supports, they succeeded—and gradually internalized the external supports so that they became progressively less reliant on external cues.

Case Illustration: Adolescent Who Required Moderate Levels of Cognitive Supports

At age 13, Doug was struck by a car while riding his bike on the side of the road. He was the only son in a deeply religious family that lived in a rural setting. He was described as a bright student before his injury, who succeeded in school and helped his father at work. Following his injury, he was hospitalized for approximately 3 weeks, followed by 2.5 months of inpatient rehabilitation. His brain injury included bilateral damage, but was localized primarily in his left hemisphere, specifically frontotemporal and dorsoparietal regions.

With intensive rehabilitation, Doug's physical recovery was relatively rapid. However, he was extremely disoriented and disorganized, could not remember locations and routes in the center, had difficulty following simple directions, and was unable to remember recent events, despite adequate recall for events that occurred prior to his injury. While in rehabilitation, Doug carried a memory and orientation book with him at all times, writing down daily events and referring to the orientation cues (e.g., schedules, maps, photos of staff, assignments) as needed to remain oriented. He continued to be dependent on this system when he was discharged. At that time, he received a Verbal IQ of 94 and a Performance IQ of 101 on the WISC-III.

After 3 months of summer home tutoring, Doug returned to school in a small, religious school in which there was heavy reliance on independent work. The students were expected to ask the head teacher or assistant for assignments and for quizzes, to complete work at their own pace, and then ask for feedback from the teaching staff when the assignments were completed. In addition, students had homework every night for each class.

Doug experienced relatively complete recovery of academic skills mastered before the injury and evidenced an adequate learning rate for new material. One-and-a-half years after the injury, he was still scoring at grade level on basic academic measures and reported that he still liked school work. However, he continued to be disorganized in his thinking and behavior, with ongoing episodic memory problems. Academic learning tended to be much more efficient than day-to-day recall of events and assignments. Doug resisted help for these problems, saying that if parents and staff would leave him alone, he would be fine. Because of his weak awareness of his ongoing disability, he became progressively more angry about others' concerns and their attempts to help him. Ultimately, reduced initiation, combined with impaired organization, emerged as his most salient disability in school. Doug often sat at his cubicle in school doing nothing, despite repeated reminders that he was supposed to be working.

The teachers were understandably frustrated with his failure to initiate work and to stay focused on and complete his assignments. In addition, they were increasingly offended by his negative attitude toward their attempts to help. Doug frequently "talked back" to the head teacher following prompts to work or offers of help. Doug's parents were increasingly upset about his apparent lack of concern for and failure to complete school work. Their impression was that he primarily needed to exert greater effort, but was refusing to do so. Doug characteristically responded to his parents' admonitions by going for a walk or taking a nap, which often resulted in grounding or other punishment.

In summary, neither parents nor school staff recognized the contribution of organically based initiation and organizational impairment to his problematic behavior. In both locations, he was urged to work harder. The following is an illustration of a typical negative communication routine based on this misdiagnosis, a routine similar to those that occurred repeatedly at home:

Doug: (sits at his desk; not working)
Teacher: "Doug, what's the matter?"
Doug: "Nothing, I'm fine."
Teacher: (walks away)
Doug: (still doing nothing)
Teacher: "Doug, there is something the matter; what is it?"
Doug: "Nothing; just leave me alone; I'm working"
Teacher: "How come there is nothing done?"
Doug: "I'm thinking."
Teacher: (punishing tone) "Whatever you don't get done now, you'll have for homework!" (walks away frustrated)
Doug: (Remains angry; does not complete his work)

At this time (1.5 years postinjury) we were invited to work with Doug, his school staff, and family. The problem was initially framed by staff and family as a behavior problem, highlighting Doug's "laziness" and "oppositionality." After some discussion, we convinced staff and family to test an alternative hypothesis, namely that the difficulty was largely a consequence of organizational and initiation impairment. To test this hypothesis, staff, family, and consultant negotiated with Doug a daily planning routine that included the following elements:

➤ Upon entering school in the morning, Doug and his teacher created a Daily Plan. Doug's contribution to the creation of the plan systematically increased.

➤ This plan included specific academic content to be covered, and specific time tables for the completion of the activities. In addition, following completion of each activity, the plan called for Doug to seek out a teacher for immediate review of the work, with feedback and corrections if necessary.

➤ In the event that he became "stuck" (i.e., confused), Doug proceeded through a set of questions that were listed in his plan:

What's the problem?

Can I figure this out myself?

Who can help me?

Did I ask for help?

These self-queries were laminated and placed in his cubicle as concrete cues.

➤ The plan also included a self-evaluation of academic work (i.e., on a scale of 1–10 how did I do in completing the assigned activities, and on the same scale, how much do I understand?). This allowed for interaction with the head teacher that was positive, self-initiated, concrete, and easy for Doug to understand.

➤ Finally, at the end of the day, Doug and the head teacher reviewed the daily activities, reviewed the homework assignments, making sure that Doug had the materials that he needed, and set some priorities for the next day.

➤ At home, Doug followed the same general Goal-Plan-Do-Review routine with his mother and tutor.

Three weeks after implementing this routine, the head teacher reported a reduction of problem behaviors to zero. Doug no longer talked back, and, although he continued to have memory and organizational impairments, he completed his work in a timely manner, and was generally able take correction with little difficulty. At home, Doug's mother reported that he continued to demonstrate limited interest in completing his homework assignments (not uncommon among adolescents), but that he routinely created a plan at home similar to the plan negotiated each morning at school. Doug's mother regretted that he did not demand more of himself, but she recognized great value in his structuring his work around self-generated plans and organizational routines.

For the following 4 months, Doug was not grounded or sent to his room. Two years later, he was still performing at grade level in all academic areas, with ongoing tutorial support. The tutor helped Doug with his school work, ensured that he continue to formulate written plans, and brainstormed with him about organizational strategies for large tasks (e.g., term papers). As Doug improved in planning and organizing, the tutor and school staff provided systematically less external support for these activities. Doug graduated from high school with his age peers and, as this book went to print, was planning to attend college. He may need help indefinitely with organization and initiation, a service we have referred to elsewhere as "supported cognition" (Ylvisaker & Feeney, 1996). This need may increase or decrease, depending on the demands that Doug faces. For example, he may require more support on the job than is customarily given to new employees until vocational routines are mastered. At least the contextualized cognitive intervention provided in high school showed Doug and subsequent professionals what positive, productive routines look like for him and what supports enable him to be successful and as independent as possible. Furthermore, Doug's insight into his needs gradually grew as he habituated his planning and organizing routine, without the confrontations and behavioral outbursts that had characterized earlier attempts to call his attention to these needs.

Concrete Advance Organizers

Doug was successful using an advance organizational system that mainly consisted of written cues and reminders within a general Goal-Plan-Do-Review format, with specific checklists embedded as needed. Similar supports were needed for specific assignments, such as papers that he wrote for school (organizers at a somewhat more abstract level than those depicted in Figures 5–1 and 5–2). This system of advance supports increased his success at school and, perhaps more important, undercut the increasingly self-fulfilling prophecy that his problem was a "behavior problem."

Many people, children and adults alike, benefit from advance organizers that are more concrete than those used by Doug.

For example, preschoolers and older individuals who are concrete in their thinking, effectively use physical containers (e.g., toy boxes, "cubbies" in school) to remain organized. At a slightly higher level of abstractness, sequences of photographs are often used by preschoolers to remain organized over time. A similar form of organizational support may be used by older children and adolescents with chronic organizational impairment. Graphic advance organizers often take the form of flow charts or sequences of boxes connected by arrows. The purpose of all such cognitive "maps," which can be used by individuals ranging in age from preschoolers to adults and representing a wide range of cognitive ability levels, is to guide people through unfamiliar or potentially confusing tasks so that they can be successful without relying on reminders or "nagging" from others. With repeated use, graphic organizers may be internalized as cognitive structures, releasing the individual from dependence on the concrete support. If this goal of internalization is not achieved, at least the person has the supports necessary to successfully complete important tasks of daily life without having to rely on other people (Ylvisaker, Szekeres, & Haarbauer-Krupa, 1998).

In Chapter 6, we present an illustration of an adolescent with organizational impairment and associated severe aggressive behavior whose intervention began with a photograph routine as an advance organizational system. Eventually, the photographs gave way to a written routine. We are frequently asked why we would suggest photographs or drawings to guide a disorganized person through a complex task if that person can read. The answer to this question is no further than the nearest product bearing the ominous phrase, "some assembly required," which invariably includes a sequence of pictures to guide the purchaser—in most cases a competent reader—through the novel or organizationally complex task. As we have said earlier, in the case of organizational impairment following brain injury, the initial goal is to identify the supports that enable the individual to complete the task as independently as possible and then reduce those supports, increase the difficulty of the task, or both.

Case Illustration: Adult Who Required Moderate Levels of Cognitive Supports

Bill incurred a severe traumatic brain injury at age 24 attempting suicide by jumping out a fifth floor window. He reported that he had been on a "partying binge for a whole bunch of days" and was "miserable with [his] life" and "couldn't deal with it no more." Prior to his injury, he had lived on city streets for several years where he sold and used drugs, and was arrested on several occasions on drug-related charges.

Bill was in coma for 3 weeks and hospitalized for a total of 6 weeks, after which he received approximately 13 months of inpatient rehabilitation. His brain injury included severe bilateral frontal lobe injury with additional primary impact damage to the temporal and occipital regions. A subsequent MRI scan revealed diffuse bilateral degeneration of the dorsal and medial frontal regions and the dorsooccipital regions, with significant ventricular enlargement. Despite relatively rapid physical recovery, Bill remained disoriented and disorganized during the first several months of his rehabilitation program. He had difficulty learning routes, following simple instructions, and remembering information from day to day. In addition, he frequently resisted his therapies, choosing to sleep instead.

The initial focus in Bill's rehabilitation was on motivating him to participate in all aspects of the program. He typically went only to those therapies that he believed were integral to his physical recovery (OT and PT), although it was evident to members of the rehabilitation team that he also had significant cognitive impairment, particularly in the areas of memory and organization. However, Bill was unaware of these problems and angrily resisted all efforts to have him use compensatory procedures (e.g., memory books, schedules, and the like). With concerted efforts to make prosthetic memory and organizational systems functional for him, Bill began to use a memory book that included written schedules and appointments, with which he could decrease his dependence on others. Using advance organizers, he was able to follow most of his daily routine. At the time of discharge from inpatient rehabilitation, he obtained a Full Scale IQ of 80 on the Wechsler Adult Intelligence Scale (Verbal IQ: 84; Performance IQ: 79).

Upon discharge, he moved into an apartment with no support or follow-up services. Predictably, he resumed his preinjury life of alcohol and drug abuse, and was arrested for disorderly conduct. In lieu of incarceration, he agreed to participate in a recently implemented dual diagnosis brain injury and substance abuse residential rehabilitation program. He was initially belligerent, refused to participate in scheduled activities, and spent most of his day in his room complaining about the program and insisting that he was ready to leave. He rejected the notion that he had functional cognitive problems that would interfere with daily life in the real world, even in the face of concrete evidence.

During these early weeks in the program, everyday communication routines with staff often had the following snowballing negative characteristics:

Bill: (in bed)

Staff: "Time to get up."

Bill: "[curse]; get out of my face!"

Staff: "Bill, you know it's time for you to get going."

Bill: (curse)

Staff: "That's inappropriate; you can't talk to me like that."

Bill: (more cursing)

Staff: "You know it's important to work your program; you know you have a brain injury; we're here to help you."

Bill: (escalates; more cursing)

Staff: "You know you have a lot to do; you need to practice using memory aids; you have some vocational activities that will help you get a job; you have group today—that will help you understand your drug problem."

Bill: (more cursing)
Staff: (becoming agitated) "You know, if you don't work your program, you can't be here; we're here to help you." (leaves)

Far from helping, these confrontational communication routines created a negative setting event that affected the rest of the day (see Chapter 6) and, despite Bill's difficulty explicitly remembering morning interactions later in the day, created an implicit memory of conflict and negative feelings about specific staff. At about this time, we were engaged by the program to help staff create daily routines that would be helpful for the dual diagnosis group. A first step in this process was to engage the residents in a process of identifying their strengths, their goals, the obstacles to achieving their goals, and the most effective ways that the program could help them achieve their goals. In many cases, the residents worked with each other in this exploratory process, which was intended in part to replace a process that the residents perceived as essentially designed to coerce them into compliance with program goals.

Bill identified as strengths his unshakable desire to return to "the good life," defined as his job, his woman, and his place to live. He also correctly identified his endearing personality (under ideal conditions) and sense of humor as strengths. Within this framework of personal goals and strengths, he became willing to accept help from others, but only when they negotiated the assistance with him, whether it was general supports or specific ad hoc advice. His injury-related needs were identified as ongoing disorganization in thinking and acting, significant recent memory impairment, and a short temper when challenged by staff. Bill, staff, and the consultant then negotiated a daily planning routine with the following elements:

➤ He got up, dressed, ate breakfast, and found a staff person to review his goals for the day and his plan for accomplishing the goals.

➤ The plan was based on specific time frames (e.g., clean group room between 2:00 and 3:00 P.M.). Bill requested this type of schedule because he had difficulty with temporal awareness, which he knew would be an obstacle to maintaining a job.

➤ The morning planning session included identification of activities that would be difficult for him to complete independently. He then negotiated a plan for asking for help (e.g., "When should I ask for help? Who will be the best help to me?"). Because Bill could accept help and discuss the need for help only when in a positive frame of mind, it was critical that this be negotiated and written into his plan at the beginning of the day.

➤ Bill's daily routine also included the use of other individuals for feedback. He negotiated a script that he practiced and eventually followed: "Before I make a decision, check it out with someone I know." The goal was to make this script a routine part of Bill's interaction with others. Following contextualized modeling and coaching from the consultant, other staff, and peers in the program, he increasingly asked trusted peers and staff for feedback. For example, he frequently asked peers if they heard the same thing that he heard after conversing with others. Following several weeks of coached practice and his gradual acceptance of this script as a "smart move" and not a sign of weakness, he had largely internalized this self-instruction: "Check it out, man." That is, his learned response to internal confusion or agitation was "Check it out, man," as opposed to his previously habituated acts of verbal aggression.

➤ Bill also engaged in periodic (approximately once a month) video reviews of himself planning and reviewing in everyday contexts (see Chapter 3). One of the results of this video feedback was an increase in Bill's acceptance of everyday feedback from others, especially in areas that he had reviewed on the videotape. In Bill's words, if he sees it, he can believe it—"it's not BS."

It took only one afternoon to negotiate this positive daily routine, which included rich opportunities to practice planning and organizing, monitoring the need for help and acquiring needed help, and requesting and accepting feedback from others. Several months were devoted to making the routine operate smoothly. During that time, the program was relocated and there were many staff changes, which predictably interfered with the smooth operation of the routine.

Two years after implementation of his new routine, Bill continued to have chronic memory, organizational, and general executive system impairment. However, he had a part-time job as a mover, shared an apartment with a roommate, and participated in several community-based activities (e.g., a local church group, Narcotics Anonymous and Alcoholics Anonymous groups). His boss indicated that he routinely completed his work with little need for monitoring and that he was a reliable employee. For more than a year he had worked with no job coach support. He continued to use his "I gotta check this out" routine at work, typically when angry at his boss because of a misunderstanding. In his residential setting and at work, Bill generally met scheduled obligations in a timely manner and was able take correction with less difficulty than before the intervention began. He reported that he found the daily routine and associated scripts helpful: "It reminds me to do what I gotta do without no hassles from the staff." He reported that he felt that his life was "going in the right direction, for once."

Organization and Memory: Advance Organizers

Advance organizers, including graphic advance organizers, continue to be helpful throughout life when tasks are complex and nonroutine. For example, virtually every purchase bearing the ominous phrase, "some assembly required," includes a graphic organizer to help the purchaser succeed with the assembly. Even a task as apparently simple as slipping a new ink cartridge into a laser printer is typically supported by a series of pictures because the manufacturer knows that, no matter how many Ph.D.s the individual may have, the task is probably not routine and therefore requires concrete organizational support. Even very high level tasks, like writing a Ph.D. dissertation or a book, are characteristically supported by detailed outlines, time lines, and other organizational supports. Furthermore, at all levels of education, including the highest levels, educators know that their students process information more efficiently and therefore remember more and remember longer if they are alerted in advance to what is critical for them to learn.

Because people with TBI often have ongoing difficulty with organization and memory, in many cases subtle difficulties that do not meet the eye, supports of this sort continue to be useful. The goal for cognitive specialists, functioning as consultants, is to customize these organizational supports to meet the individual's specific needs and then help the person to habituate the use of such supports in everyday routines. In many cases, these external supports come over time to be internalized and can therefore be faded. In other cases, they may be needed indefinitely.

Case Illustration: Adolescent/Adult Who Required Varying Levels of Cognitive Supports

Jane represents that group of people whose need for concrete organizational support continued indefinitely. She was severely injured in an automobile accident at age 14 in the spring of ninth grade. Prior to the injury, she had been a solid student (mainly As and Bs), with a measured IQ of 120. Her injury included a right frontal hematoma and bifrontal hygromas. She was deeply comatose for several days, and evidenced minimal intellectual interaction with her environment for another 4 to 6 weeks. Six months postinjury, she received a Verbal IQ of 88 and a Performance IQ of 74 (relatively depressed by slowed processing and motor impairment) on the WISC-R. As with Dave (described earlier), this suggestion of relatively preserved language functioning was an artifact of the limited language processing demands on the IQ test, which did not sample the types of language tasks that were difficult for Jane. Subsequent neuropsychological evaluations performed 2 years postinjury and again 9 years postinjury revealed initial improvement in global intellectual functioning (i.e., IQ scores came to be within normal limits and then remained essentially unchanged from 2 to 9 years post), but with clear signs of a "frontal behavioral syndrome," that is, executive system impairment, along with generalized slowing of cognitive and psychomotor processing. Executive system impairment was evidenced by disinhibited social interaction, cognitive and behavioral rigidity, concrete thinking, weakness in strategic learning (particularly verbal information), and limited self-monitoring.

During the last 2 months of her 7-month inpatient rehabilitation program, Jane was involved in an intensive effort to improve her reading comprehension and memory for text. Like many students with TBI, her reading/decoding skills returned quickly (e.g., at 6 months postinjury, she obtained a grade equivalent that exceeded the twelfth grade on the Reading subtest of the Wide Range Achievement Test), but at the same time she performed at a second grade level in comprehending a lengthy paragraph. This difficulty was believed to reflect a general difficulty organizing significant amounts of information and processing abstract information, an interpretation supported by her Listening Comprehension grade level score of 3.5 (Spache Diagnostic Reading Scales). Extremely depressed scores on two verbal learning tests, the Auditory-Visual Learning Subtest of the Woodcock-Johnson Psychoeducational Battery and the Consistent Long Term Retrieval measure of the Selective Reminding Test, confirmed the severity of her verbal learning impairment when this functional intervention began 5½ months post onset. (See Figure 5–3.)

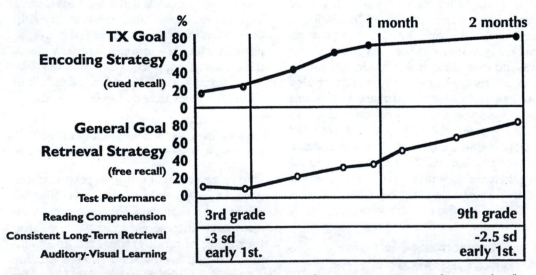

Figure 5–3. Results of a 2-month training program in the use of a compensatory strategy for comprehending and remembering narrative text. Pre- and posttesting with the Consistent Long-Term Retrieval (CLTR) measure of the Selective Reminding Test and the Auditory-Verbal Learning subtest of the Woodcock-Johnson Psychoeducational Battery suggested little change in the underlying verbal memory impairment. However, disability was substantially lessened, as evidence by improvement in cued recall and subsequently free recall performance on functional reading tasks, and by improved performance on a reading comprehension test.

Because she was concrete in her thinking and processing of language, the intervention began by helping her understand the concept of organization (e.g., how clothes are organized in a room) and the importance of organization for remembering (e.g., we would have great difficulty retrieving clothes if there were no organization to their storage in our bedrooms). This was followed by clinician-coached experiments to determine if special organizing procedures and advance organizers would help her understand and remember reading material and, if so, what types of organizers would be most effective (see the discussion of hypothesis-testing assessment in Chapter 3). Visually complex graphic organizers were not helpful because of her visual perceptual problems at that time. However, a simple, vertical outlining advance organizer, accompanied by conversational exploration of the organization of the information, proved to be extremely helpful.

The conversational exploration of the organization of textual information was similar to the procedures associated with "reciprocal teaching," a method developed by Brown and her colleagues (Palinscar & Brown, 1989), based on Vygotsky's principle that strategic and organized thinking begins as well planned social dialogue between children and adults. That is, in the early stages of intervention, Jane and the clinician read together, with the clinician leading a discussion that included identification of main ideas, prediction of consequences, and descriptions of relationships, as well as more specific clarification of facts and sequences. There was little performance-oriented questioning, and Jane contributed what she could to the discussions and to the written outlines and summaries. Gradually more and more was turned over to her, and she made outlines (using a standardized advance organizer) and wrote summaries on her own.

Jane's mother attended some of these sessions and continued the conversational support for comprehension with Jane as they read fiction together on the weekends.

With these supported everyday routines in place, Jane's comprehension and memory for text improved over the course of the 2 months prior to discharge from inpatient rehabilitation. Improvement was first noted on cued recall tasks and subsequently on free recall, suggesting that she quickly began to use the organizational cues to encode information into long-term storage, but needed special training to use the same cues to retrieve the information on free recall tasks. Figure 5–3 shows Jane's marked progress in text processing and memory, combined with severe ongoing impairment in verbal learning and memory. That is, she continued to have significant, neurologically based difficulty processing and remembering complex language, but effectively used organizational strategies when reminded to do so.

Unfortunately, Jane continued to be relatively dependent on others to remind her to use the organizational strategies and supports that she needed to succeed academically. When she left the rehabilitation hospital, insights about her need for concrete organizational support for reading comprehension (and other cognitive activities) were passed on to her high school teachers who continued these supports, with gradual paring back over the course of her final 3 years of high school. Jane then entered college, where she had the support of special tutors within a learning disabilities support program. Six years later, after she had graduated from college (2 years behind her entering class), Jane maintained that the college tutors were less effective than they could have been because they expected her to be able to organize larger amounts of information than she was capable of organizing, thereby causing some confusion and frustration. When she returned home after college, she gave up reading for several months because it was more frustrating than it was enjoyable for her.

Jane's 9 years following her severe brain injury illustrate a theme that, in our experience, is important for many people with brain injury. Because of her organizational supports and ongoing reminders from educators to use the supports, she was able to succeed at levels that far exceeded early predictions for her after the injury. However, throughout high school and college, she remained somewhat dependent on others to ensure that her daily reading, writing, and study routines were well designed to meet her learning needs. Presumably because of the severity of injury to that part of her brain associated with strategic thinking and initiation, she needed, and may indefinitely continue to need, external support to ensure that organizational strategies are a part of her life. Elsewhere we have presented this aspect of cognitive rehabilitation under the heading *supported cognition* (Ylvisaker & Feeney, 1996).

Organization and Memory: Compensatory Strategies and Prosthetics

In this chapter we have described a variety of strategic procedures that can be used by some individuals to compensate for chronic organization and memory disability. However, none of the people we chose for illustrative purposes used electronic prostheses. With rapid developments in computer technology have come applications for individuals with disorders of organization and memory. Several useful reviews of rehabilitation technology in cognitive rehabilitation are available (Chester, Henry, & Tarquino, 1998; Harrell et al., 1992; Kapur, 1995; Parenté & Anderson-Parenté, 1991). With rapid advances in the field of rehabilitation technology, lists of available products are virtually obsolete the minute they are published. For this reason, clinicians are well advised to make effective use of vendors or specialists in the field so that consideration of technological supports is as current as possible.

Rather than describe products, we have chosen to highlight six clinical principles that are unfortunately easy to neglect in prescribing compensatory strategies and devices for people with disorders of organization and memory. Decision making in the area of rehabilitation technology is more than diagnosing a cognitive deficit and prescribing a strategy or device that holds the potential to compensate for that deficit. When this is the process, the all-too-common outcome is a product that gathers dust in a closet or a compensatory behavior that is never used in the real world.

Negotiation and Experimentation

There are several important reasons to base strategy and equipment decisions on negotiation and experimentation. Even in cases in which a clinician is convinced that a product is ideally suited to meet an individual's functional needs, it is wise to present the decision making as an experimental process, in which the person with TBI, family members, and possibly other significant everyday people are involved. Decisions based on negotiation and experimentation have a greater likelihood of winning compliance with the decision. Furthermore, it is difficult to foresee all of the potential obstacles to functional integration of a device or strategy into the individual's everyday routines. Experimentation is designed in part to reveal these obstacles and develop plans to overcome them.

Having a Strategy Versus Being Strategic

The process of deciding on a compensatory strategy or device is also an ideal context within which to engage the individual in functional strategic thinking. As discussed in Chapter 4, the ultimate goal of strategy intervention is to help the individual become increasingly strategic, that is, become a flexible and creative problem solver. When clinicians do all of the strategic thinking, solve all of the problems, and make all of the decisions, they are in effect denying the individual prime opportunities for practice in this critical domain of cognitive functioning (Ylvisaker, Szekeres, & Feeney, 1998).

Integration Among Settings and Among Components of Technology

We have frequently observed strategies (e.g., use of a memory book or schedule cards) and products (e.g., computerized day planner, pager, alarm watch) used in a rehabilitation setting, but discontinued when the individual reentered home, school, or the workplace. Similarly, we have seen therapists, working in isolation, prescribe products that meet a specific need in their area of concern, but that do not constitute an integrated system when brought together. For example, the individual may use separate products to communicate, control environmental events, and operate a wheelchair. Integration across settings and across functional needs must be considered a clinical priority, requiring cross-disciplinary collaboration among clinicians in each setting as well as integration of technological support and compensatory strategies across settings.

Among other things, this principle of integration implies that reports from rehabilitation facilities or clinics to schools or workplaces should not include recommendations for equipment and strategies unless the equipment and strategies have been successfully explored under conditions similar to the school or work conditions, and staff in the school or work setting have indicated that there are no major obstacles to use of the equipment and strategies. Achieving support for technology or other compensatory behaviors in work, school, and home settings may require effort and salesmanship from rehabilitation specialists. Without this effort, environmental support may be lost and the equipment and procedures abandoned.

Sensitivity to the Individual's Entire Cognitive Profile of Abilities and Disabilities

With an exclusive focus on single cognitive impairments, it is possible to make decisions about compensations that prove to be failures because of the impact of other cognitive impairment. The classic example of this principle is the apparently sound prescription of memory aids or organization aids for individuals who not only have organizational and memory problems, but initiation impairment as well. In this case, the predictable and common outcome is a well-designed product or strategy that is rarely used. Similarly, an individual who is short tempered and disinhibited may quickly destroy an expensive memory aid because of frustration experienced in attempting to use the product.

Sensitivity to Aesthetics and Life Style

Equipment and compensatory behaviors can be rejected for a variety of reasons, including failure to meet the individual's aesthetic standards or general life style sensitivities. For example, we have worked with older adults with serious problems with organization, memory, and orientation who have shown under clinical conditions that they profit from compensations such as large schedule boards in their immediate environment, labels on locations and storage areas in their living environment, and the like. However, in some cases they refuse to allow their home and natural routines to be altered in a way that seems clinically appropriate to professionals. In such cases, there is no substitute for flexible experimentation with a variety of procedures and products, with the goal of identifying the best compromise between facilitation of cognitive functioning and personal satisfaction of the individual. Staff and family must also be alert to the possibility of change. For example, it is common for individuals to reject a device or compensatory behavior during the first year after the injury, but later come to recognize its value.

Sensitivity to Costs and Benefits: Practice and Automaticity

Everybody operates with an internal scale of costs and benefits. When the costs of an effort outweigh its benefits, then that effort is abandoned. Considerable effort goes into using new procedures and devices to achieve goals (like remembering and organizing) that were once achieved with minimal effort. Skilled clinicians respect cost-benefit considerations by ensuring that there is a considerable payoff for using a new device, particularly in the early stages, and that the individual practices using the device or behavior enough that it becomes as automatic as possible. For individuals who are embarrassed using a new device or procedure, extensive practice may need to occur outside the context of social interaction so that the individual is as adept as possible before introducing the device or strategy into everyday routines. If embarrassment is not a concern, contextualized practice has the advantages listed earlier in this chapter. In either case, practice to the point of automaticity helps tip the internal cost-benefit analysis in the direction of benefits.

SUMMARY

In this chapter, we have presented and illustrated an approach to cognitive rehabilitation that highlights the importance of positive everyday routines and the interaction of everyday people within those routines. We focused on disorders of organization and memory, which are commonly

debilitating after severe TBI. We invite readers to consider the discussions of planning, problem solving, flexibility, self-coaching, and attention in Chapters 4, 6, and 7 as also falling within the domain of cognitive rehabilitation. The difficulty we experienced in deciding where to place specific content and associated case illustrations underscores the arbitrariness in separating cognition, executive functions, behavior, and communication.

Our focus was on individuals with chronic disability. The everyday interventions that we described had the effect in some cases of reducing the impairment and thereby improving functioning in varied contexts (e.g., Dave). In other cases (e.g., Jane), improvements in everyday functioning (i.e., reduction in disability) were not effectively generalized or maintained without significant support. However, even in the latter cases, improvements were substantial and enabled the individual to succeed beyond expectations created by the severity of the brain injury.

We close this chapter with a checklist (Table 5–2) designed to help staff maintain an appropriate focus on organizational abilities and on consistent application of compensatory procedures in the event of ongoing impairment. As always, staff must reduce the intensity of cognitive supports as the individual's functioning improves. In this way, learned helplessness is avoided and reduction in disability is facilitated.

TABLE 5–2. A checklist for intervention for individuals with organizational impairment.

❑ Are the individual's *life experiences adequately organized?*

   ❑ Is there thematic or other organization *within* therapeutic or instructional sessions? Is the organization of the session obvious to the individual?

   ❑ Is there thematic or other organization *across* therapeutic or instructional sessions? For example, are the activities in speech therapy or occupational therapy related in a clear way to activities in academic instruction or vocational intervention?

   ❑ Is there thematic or other organization *from day to day?* Is the individual involved in activities or projects that require integrating information over several days or weeks?

   ❑ Is the individual's life organized around well-understood routines?

❑ Is the *content* that is used for organizational tasks personally meaningful or directly related to social, academic, or vocational success?

- ❑ Are organizing tasks correctly placed on the *continuum of involuntary (incidental) to deliberate (strategic) learning tasks!*
  - ❑ For the concretely thinking person. is there a concrete. meaningful goal that he or she wishes to accomplish and that requires organizational thinking?
  - ❑ If appropriate, is the individual engaged in trying to understand the concept of organization and what he or she can do to organize more effectively?
- ❑ Is there an appropriate amount of *external organizational support* for individuals who have difficulty organizing?
  - ❑ Are advance graphic organizers available for complex tasks? That is, is the task mapped out in a way that makes it easy to follow (e.g., sequence of photographs or drawings; written outline: flowchart or checklist)?
  - ❑ Does the organization of the advance organizers correctly capture the way in which the information should be organized in the head of the learner?
  - ❑ Is a log book, day planner, or memory book available that contains schedules, maps, photographs of critical people, assignments, and other important information needed to stay organized?
  - ❑ Are plans illustrated in appropriately concrete ways (e.g., photographs)?
  - ❑ If organizational reminders must be provided by other people, are they presented in a way that is not perceived as nagging?
  - ❑ If the individual is confused about his or her past life, is a visually clear *life line* available, representing important events in that person's life?
- ❑ Is there *consistency* among staff and family members in how tasks and information are presented and in the kinds of external organizational support that are provided?
  - ❑ Do *all everyday people* understand how to use everyday activities to facilitate improvement in organizational functioning?
  - ❑ Is there consistency in *reducing external organizational support* as the individual becomes increasingly organized?
- ❑ Is the individual as engaged as possible in:
  - ❑ Determining the *goal* of activities?
  - ❑ Creating a *plan* to achieve the goal?
  - ❑ *Monitoring* performance during the activity?
  - ❑ *Evaluating* success of the activity?
  - ❑ *Determining what worked and what did not work* in the plan?

Source: Reproduced with permission from Ylvisaker, M., Szekeres, S., & Haarbauer-Krupa, J. (1998). "Cognitive Rehabilitation: Organization, Memory, and Language." In M. Ylvisaker (Ed.), *Traumatic Brain Injury Rehabilitation: Children and Adolescents* (p. 217). Boston: Butterworth-Heinemann.

CHAPTER 6

Positive Everyday Behavioral Routines

Our primary purpose in this chapter, as in the other intervention chapters, is to describe a functional and contextualized approach to helping people with chronic disability after TBI. This approach has evolved primarily out of our work with several hundred children and adults with challenging behavior associated with acquired brain injury. Components of the approach also have a pathophysiologic rationale (see Chapter 2) as well as empirical support from studies of individuals with TBI as well as a variety of other etiologies (see Chapter 1).

After a brief discussion of behavioral outcome after TBI, we present a positive, antecedent-focused approach to behavior management, which is followed by several case illustrations. Most of these cases could equally have been presented in Chapters 4, 5, or 7, because the individuals had injury-related challenges in the areas of cognition, executive function, and communication, all of which contributed to their total package of behavioral difficulties. The chapter should be read with Chapters 1 and 2, which present theoretical and physiologic information relevant to supporting our approach. In Chapter 3, we describe the type of assessment most relevant to formulating an intervention plan and achieving compliance in its implementation.

The individuals we describe in this chapter exhibited a variety of behavioral challenges, some based on patterns of behavior established before the injury, others related quite directly to the injury, others related indirectly to the injury (e.g., associated with cognitive or communication disability secondary to the injury and associated academic, vocational, and social failure), and, finally, others associated with psychological adjustment to the injury or with reactions to changes in life circumstances and possibly inappropriate interventions.

The creation of positive everyday routines, illustrated in this and other chapters of this book, does not exhaust the domain of interventions that may be appropriate for people with challenging behavior after TBI. In many cases, behavioral interventions are effectively complemented by pharmacologic management and possibly also counseling. Psychopharmacologic approaches for individuals with challenging behavior after brain injury are summarized by O'Shanick (1990, 1998) and Silver and Yudofsky (1994). Methods of counseling for individuals with brain injury are described by Sherwin and O'Shanick (1998) and Prigatano (1991).

BEHAVIOR PROBLEMS AFTER TBI

The ways people behave and adjust to their circumstances in life are dynamic, responsive to many influences, determined by many causes, and subject to change over time. This complexity is at least as true of people with brain injury as it is of people who are neurologically intact. In the section that follows, we list a variety of possible contributors to social maladjustment and challenging behavior after TBI, including (1) preinjury behavior problems, (2) direct behavioral consequences of the injury, (3) cognitive impairment that affects behavior, (4) communication impairment that affects behavior, (5) emotional reactions to changes in life after the injury, (6) overly restrictive interventions in inappropriate settings, and (7) delayed consequences as a young person fails to mature in certain domains of functioning because of earlier injury.

In most cases, a thorough explanation of the individual's behavior would include a unique blend of several of these contributors. The importance of maintaining keen awareness of the multitude of factors that influence behavior lies in the flexibility and creativity of behavioral hypothesis testing that it supports as we search for effective ways to help people create satisfying lives for themselves (see Chapter 3).

Preinjury Behavior Problems

TBI does not randomly select its victims. The high-risk group for TBI includes children, adolescents, and young adults who were risk takers before the injury, who had frank learning and behavior problems, or who lived in poverty or other challenging circumstances associated with behavioral difficulties. Epidemiologic studies suggest that 30 to 50% of young people with TBI have some combination of these risk factors in their preinjury history (Alberts & Binder, 1991; Asarnow et al., 1991; Fletcher et al., 1990; Greenspan & MacKenzie, 1994; Hart & Jacobs, 1993; Pelco et al., 1992). We estimate that at least half of the individuals we have worked with who demonstrated chronic behavior problems after the injury had preexisting behavior problems, in most cases exaggerated by the injury.

Knowledge of a person's behavioral history and associated intervention serves several purposes. If the individual and significant others were locked in a vicious cycle of negative interaction before the injury, clinicians should be alert to the first signs of re-sumption of this interaction so that they can help break the cycle before it is again entrenched. Second, if staff know that specific behavioral interventions were particularly successful or unsuccessful before the injury, they have guidance in developing behavior plans, should they be necessary after the injury. We have worked with adolescents whose behavior management system in their schools had included a token economy component for several years before the injury. After the injury, we reinstituted the familiar system, not because we judged it to be the most effective intervention, but rather because the student demanded it. We then worked hard to eliminate the student's dependence on extrinsic reinforcers, using a combination of the proactive procedures described below.

Knowledge of preinjury behavioral difficulties is *misused* if it discourages clinicians or agencies from providing intensive intervention or if it creates self-fulfilling prophecies of behavior problems after the injury. We have worked with several individuals whose serious preinjury behavioral impairment combined with severe TBI to create a most pessimistic prognosis. In many cases, however, intensive intervention yielded a behavioral outcome superior to preinjury functioning. Therefore, clinicians are well advised to be realistic about the people with whom they work, but at the same time remain optimistic about the potential impact of their efforts.

Pathophysiology and Behavioral Outcome

In Chapter 2, we discuss the pathophysiology of behavioral impairment after TBI in some detail. Our goal in this section is simply to highlight the main points of that discussion. Frontal lobe lesions have classically been associated with two general behavioral syndromes, (1) the so-called pseudopsychopathic personality, associated with orbito-frontal lesions and characterized by some combination of disinhibition, impulsiveness, restlessness, hyperactivity, euphoria, facetiousness, social inappropriateness, need for immediate gratification, lack of concern for others, sexual excess, crude humor, explosiveness, fearfulness, withdrawal, and lability and (2) the so-called pseudodepressed personality, associated with dorsolateral or dorsomesial prefrontal lesions and characterized by some combination of reduced initiation, apathy, lack of drive, loss of interest, lethargy, slowness, inattentiveness, reduced spontaneity, unconcern, lack of emotional reactivity, dullness, poor grooming, and perseveration (Stuss & Benson, 1986). People with widespread frontal lobe injury may appear to lack initiation under some conditions (e.g., in low stimulation environments with few demands), but to be disinhibited and explosive under others (e.g., high stimulation, demanding conditions).

Subsequent investigations of behavior problems after brain injury have demonstrated that lesions elsewhere (e.g., in the limbic regions) can create profiles similar to classic prefrontal syndromes (Adolphs et al., 1994; Aggleton, 1992; Bechara et al., 1995; Izard, 1992; LeDoux, 1995, 1996). Furthermore, greater prefrontal differentiation has been revealed than is suggested by the two syndromes described in the last paragraph (Goldman-Rakic, 1993; Pribram, 1987; Rezai et al., 1993).

The value of a correct diagnosis of organic pathology underlying problem behavior is that it may lead to potentially helpful interventions (Bachman, 1992; Jacobs, 1990; Wood, 1990). For example, under the hypothesis that a problem behavior is related to brain injury and is not primarily a learned behavior, a medication may be tried or forms of support may be offered that prove to be useful. The point of an organic hypothesis is not to excuse the behavior. Seriously aggressive and disruptive behavior is not excusable. However, the first step in managing behavior is to understand it. If there is an organic component, it must be understood and considered in designing effective interventions. Finally, identification of a problem behavior as based in part

on organic pathology is most certainly not a call to give up hope that intervention will be effective. All of the individuals described in this and other chapters of this book had severe TBI. In each case, the behavior problems were related in some way to the injury. However, in each case, intervention had a positive effect.

Cognition and Behavior

Beyond the early stages of recovery after brain injury and in the absence of ongoing active neuropathology (e.g., seizures), problem behavior is most often intimately associated with other aspects of impairment. Cognitive impairment, often undiagnosed in those whose recovery seems generally good (see Chapter 3), is a frequent contributor to behavior problems (Asarnow et al., 1991; Eames, 1988, 1990; Feeney & Ylvisaker, 1997; Gaultieri & Cox, 1991). For example, acting out may be related to general confusion and disorientation, which may heighten anxiety and result in disorganized, acting-out behavior. Alternatively, the individual may have difficulty attending to or interpreting others' language, resulting in noncompliance and associated conflicts. People with difficulty planning and organizing their behavior, or remembering what to do, may fail to complete assigned tasks, which, if followed by reprimands or excessive nagging, may lead to aggressive outbursts. In other cases, cognitive impairment takes the form of cognitive and behavioral rigidity, creating anxiety and possible acting-out behavior when the demands for flexibility exceed the individual's neurological capacity. Individuals who are concrete in their thinking and acting may acquire acceptable behaviors in a training setting, but fail to apply them in functional, real-world interaction, frustrating staff who fail to appreciate the severity of the cognitive impairment.

Furthermore, the memory and learning profile commonly associated with TBI in school-age children and adolescents—namely, adequate recovery of knowledge and skills acquired before the injury combined with significant difficulty learning new information and skills—predictably results in adequate academic performance when the student returns to school, but steadily increasing difficulties as the consequences of impaired new learning snowball. As failure and frustration in school increase, negative behavior tends to increase. These observations about the potential cognitive basis for behavior problems after TBI mandate collaboration between professionals who specialize in behavior management and those who specialize in cognitive aspects of rehabilitation and education (Ylvisaker & Feeney, 1996).

Communication and Behavior

The intimate relations between communication and behavior are discussed in Chapter 7. Here we wish to highlight only one of these relations after brain injury, namely the evolution of challenging behavior out of early reflexive behavior or early attempts to communicate in the presence of significant speech and language impairment. As they emerge from coma, individuals with severe TBI often engage in problem behaviors that have no communicative intent (e.g., yelling, pulling at tubes, randomly hitting out). If this phase of recovery is protracted and staff and family inadvertently reward these behaviors (e.g., by allowing the person to escape painful or difficult treatments or by giving the person attention only after such behavior), there is every likelihood that the behavior will gradually become a component of the individual's deliberate communication system. That is, if communication partners respond to yelling and hitting as though the communicative intent were "I want to escape this" and release the individual contingent on those behaviors, it is only reasonable for that person to subsequently choose those behaviors when sufficient cognitive recovery has occurred to allow the person to deliberately select means of communication. These observations about the potential com-

munication basis for behavior problems after TBI mandate collaboration between professionals who specialize in behavior management and those who specialize in communication disorders (Ylvisaker & Feeney, 1994).

Psychoreactive Consequences and Behavior

We have observed many patterns of psychological reaction to acquired brain injury-related disability, ranging from serious emotional breakdown to extraordinary resilience, determination, optimism, and generally effective adjustment. We have found it helpful to look for individuals to progress slowly from (a) complete unawareness of disability to (b) a focus on what they were to (c) a focus on what they are not now to (d) a focus on what they will never be to (e) reasonable adjustment, including reasonable plans for the future. We do not propose this as an invariant stage-wise progression, nor do we suggest that every person with severe TBI experiences phases of psychological response adequately captured by any of these descriptions.

People in the "I was" phase dwell on their life before the injury, possibly exaggerating their successes, and refuse to entertain the possibility that the future will be substantially altered by the injury. Associated with this focus may be anger directed at those who challenge their self-perception and judgments about personal goals. It is tempting to understand this psychological state as psychoreactive denial. However, in many cases organically based unawareness of deficits is a likely contributor (see Chapter 2).

People in the "I'm not" phase recognize that they are unable to do many of the things that they did before the injury and entertain the possibility that their previous goals may be unattainable. In many cases, this phase is characterized by perplexity (Lezak, 1982, 1987b) about abilities and disabilities and their implications for the future. This perplexity is often associated with anxiety and anger directed at those who try to impose labels, such as "disabled." Many adolescents and young adults in this phase of reaction strongly resist association with other people with a history of TBI or other disabling condition.

People in the "I'll never be" phase recognize that they have persisting problems that block the achievement of cherished goals that they had tried hard to maintain. This recognition may be associated with depression, which in many cases includes withdrawal from social interaction and possibly suicidal thoughts. We often hear adolescents and young adults in this phase say, "I just wish the crash had finished it off." One expects people in this phase to resist discussion of alternative careers, peers, and social activities. Adequate recognition of ongoing disability and active engagement in efforts to achieve a satisfying educational, vocational, and social life within limits imposed by the disability—that is, adjustment—is ideally achieved, but typically not until after 2 or more years of effort to reestablish critical aspects of preinjury life.

Creative counseling, peer support, and carefully monitored attempts to achieve preinjury goals may help facilitate movement toward productive adjustment to life with chronic disability (Becker & Vakil, 1993; Pollack, 1994a, 1994b; Prigatano, 1986, 1991). Our current point is simply that the individual's psychological reaction to the injury and associated disability may contribute to challenging behavior and problematic social interaction.

Restrictive Treatments and Behavior

Hart and Jacobs (1993) highlighted the frequency with which individuals with brain injury receive the diagnosis of behavior disorder because of their responses to settings and interventions that they consider inappropriate, infantilizing, overly restrictive, or meaningless for them. Behaviors that they consider reasonable under the circumstances—including angry outbursts, noncompliance with program demands, and attempts to manipulate the system to achieve their goals—are predictably considered inappropriate by staff, leading in many cases to power struggles and escalation of negative behavior on the side of the individual, and intensification of restrictions on the side of staff. To the extent that these behaviors can be labeled problem behaviors, their origin is iatrogenic, that is, a placement or intervention that is intended to be therapeutic is the cause of or a contributor to the disorder.

We have worked with many adolescents and young adults who wore a diagnosis of severe behavior disorder but who, following discharge from a highly restrictive setting (that they protested) and resumption of personally meaningful activities, had little difficulty behaving in ways that others found easy to live with. The pervasiveness of this phenomenon is unknown to us. Furthermore, in most cases, the problem behavior results from a combination of ill-conceived interventions, a reduced threshold of tolerance for frustration, and impaired cognition. Although difficult to identify in individual cases, iatrogenic behavior problems are sufficiently widespread to justify serious consideration of the hypothesis that troubling behaviors may not be entirely or even partially a sign of a disorder internal to the individual. In these cases, experimentation with decreased restrictions, increased client choice, and possibly a change in setting is warranted.

A second form of iatrogenic behavior problems is that which occurs when challenging behavior (e.g., yelling, physical aggression) is negatively reinforced (e.g., followed by release from an aversive task or situation). For example, a therapist may end a difficult therapy session or a teacher may discontinue math exercises following the individual's disruptive behavior. This is analogous to the classic situation in poorly managed school programs when disruptive students are removed from class and taken to an in-school suspension room where they chat with their friends. The predictable consequence of this type of intervention, assuming that the individual has minimally adequate learning mechanisms, is an increase in the behavior that resulted in release from an aversive situation. Ylvisaker, Feeney, and Szekeres (1998) described the evolution of serious self-injurious behavior in a young adolescent, a process that began with reflexive, neurologically driven behavior and ended with frequent episodes of self-injury as a means of communicating escape. In this case and in many others, well-intentioned staff inadvertently teach negative behavior.

Influences of the Natural Environment on Behavior

Just as inappropriate treatment settings and professional interventions can affect behavior negatively, so also the interventions and supports in the natural environment influence behavioral outcome after TBI. In their classic study of pediatric TBI, Rutter and colleagues found that the incidence of new (i.e., not preexisting) long-term behavior problems was more than 100% greater among children living in high psychosocial adversity settings than among comparably injured children in low psychosocial adversity settings (Brown, Chadwick, Shaffer, Rutter, & Traub, 1981). Similarly, Greenspan and MacKenzie (1994) found poverty to be a better predictor of long-term outcome than severity of injury in their cohort of children and adolescents with TBI. These results are supported by recent studies of the influence of family integrity and support on social and behavioral outcome after TBI (Klonoff, Costa, & Snow, 1986; Lucyshyn, Nixon, Glang, & Cooley, 1996; Taylor et al., 1995).

Taken together, these findings show convincingly that behavioral outcome after TBI involves a complex interaction of variables internal to the individual before the injury, those related to the injury itself, and those related to environmental supports available after the injury. Rehabilitation professionals must conclude from these findings that educating, training, and supporting everyday people in the injured person's environment is high on their list of professional responsibilities so that the long road after the injury is paved as effectively as it can be paved.

Delayed Behavioral Consequences

Investigators and clinicians have long observed that behavior problems tend to increase over the years after TBI in both children (Brown, Chadwick, Shaffer, Rutter, & Traub, 1981) and adults (Eames, 1990; Gaultieri & Cox, 1991; Jacobs, 1990). Although there are many exceptions, the phenomenon of escalating behavior problems merits its own discussion. In the immediately preceding sections, we described ways in which cognitive problems, communication problems, adjustment problems, poorly conceived treatments, and environmental stressors can contribute to gradually evolving long-term behavior problems in children and adults. In this section, our goal is to highlight themes in developmental neurology as a partial explanation for growing behavior problems in children and adolescents.

Delayed onset of symptoms, including behavioral symptoms, has become one of the major themes in the growing literature on TBI, and especially prefrontal injury, in children. Studies of outcome after prefrontal injury in experimental animals (Goldman, 1972; Kolb, 1995) and human children (Eslinger et al., 1997, 1992; Greenspan & MacKenzie, 1994; Marlowe, 1989, 1992; Thomsen, 1984, 1987, 1989) have seriously challenged the traditional assumption that young children enjoy a general advantage in outcome relative to adolescents and young adults with comparable injuries. Whereas the concept of neural plasticity of the immature brain, and associated superior outcome after injury, applies to some types of injury and some types of outcome, notably language outcome, there are major exceptions to this rule. Evidence to date suggests that early prefrontal injury can have not only serious and growing consequences on the development of self-regulatory functions, but that the effects on these executive functions may be more generalized than in comparably injured older people (Brown et al., 1981; Eslinger et al., 1997; Marlowe, 1992).

The neurological explanation for this troubling phenomenon is based on the slow and protracted anatomic and physiologic development of the frontal lobes and of their extensive connections to posterior regions of the brain (Thatcher, 1991; Yakovlev & Lecours, 1967), a process that continues at a decelerating rate through adolescence. Gradual physical development is mirrored by gradual development of executive control over cognitive, emotional, and social behavior. With this as background, it is easy to understand the common phenomenon of 2- or 3-year old children with focal prefrontal injury recovering well within the first few weeks or months after the injury, exhibiting a degree of impulsiveness, aggressiveness, egocentricity, lability, and unreflectiveness typical of their age. However, if the injury blocks ongoing development of the circuitry needed to support maturation in these areas, those children with early injuries are likely to appear seriously disabled when they begin grade school. Just this natural history was described in an interesting case study by Marlowe (1992). Similarly, a third grader with recently acquired prefrontal injury may evidence a degree of concreteness, egocentrism, inflexibility, impulsiveness, nonstrategic thinking, and need for externally imposed structure that is not unusual for third graders. However, without ongoing development of the frontal lobes and their connections, the same child may demonstrate those characteristics to a degree that creates substantial disability in middle school or high school.

Delayed consequences in adolescence have received less attention in the research literature than delayed consequences in early childhood. Our experience with large numbers of adolescents with frontal lobe injury associated with TBI suggests that clinicians must be alert to a parallel phenomenon with this age group. A template for guiding this cautious monitoring is provided in Table 6–1. If behavioral difficulties are allowed to spiral out of control, as was the case with Joe, described below, the effects on the individual and significant others can be immeasurable, and the difficulty of reversing the downward spiral grows with each passing year.

Having called attention to these neurobiological contributors to outcome, including delayed behavioral consequences, we wish to underscore an important reminder that we offered earlier. *Although certain types of brain injury play a major role in determining behavioral outcome and psychosocial adjustment, it is important not to overestimate that role.* A superficial reading of the neuropsychological literature on the topic of delayed consequences following frontal lobe injury in children (Eslinger et al., 1989; Grattan & Eslinger, 1990, 1992; Marlowe, 1989, 1992; Mateer & Williams, 1991) may lead one to anticipate these consequences as biologically inevitable. Far from being inevitable, delayed behavioral consequences are, in our experience, largely preventable and, if they are allowed to develop, this development can be reversed, but only with great effort (Feeney & Ylvisaker, 1995).

A FRAMEWORK FOR INTERVENTION

Traditional operant applications of applied behavior analysis have attempted to identify and manipulate functional relationships among antecedents of behavior, the behaviors themselves, and their consequences in an attempt to explain, predict, and control behavior (Skinnner, 1938, 1953, 1974). This analysis is typically coded as ABC analysis, depicted in Figure 6–1. In traditional applications, antecedents are often restricted to those that immediately precede the behavior (e.g., an instruction, presentation of a model for the individual to imitate, an immediate provocation). Consequences are

TABLE 6–1. Immediate and delayed consequences* of TBI in adolescence.

EARLY ADOLESCENCE

KEY DEVELOPMENTAL ISSUES

Social–emotional–behavioral issues

Emerging personality identity associated with short-term future goals, often involving physical accomplishments;

Emphasis on following a rigid code of behavior and on punishment in moral thinking;

Development of a cognitive map of social networks with primary emphasis on same-sex peers;

Emergence of fixed friendships, along with crowds and cliques;

External locus of control, with deference to the approval or disapproval of peers.

Cognitive–academic issues

Increase in abstract thinking and hypothetico-deductive reasoning;

Increase in ability to use organizing schemes deliberately to process large amounts of information (e.g., for reading texts and writing essays).

COMMON CONCERNS WITH TBI AT THIS STAGE

Social–emotional–behavioral issues

Social vulnerability, related to: separation from clique; socially awkward behavior (associated with frontal lobe injury);

Physical changes caused by the injury may precipitate role confusion and psychogenic problems ("I am not who I was");

Likelihood of behavior problems associated with vulnerability to environmental stressors (especially with frontal lobe injury).

Cognitive–academic issues

Increasing concerns with the academic curriculum associated with: cumulative effects of new learning problems; difficulty organizing large amounts of information; difficulty with increasingly abstract information.

COMMON DELAYED SYMPTOMS RELATED TO EARLIER INJURY

Social–emotional–behavioral issues

Behavior problems associated with decreasing external control and an inability to meet the expectation for increasing behavioral self-regulation;

Inability to meet increasing social demands associated with puberty.

Cognitive–academic issues

Increasing academic problems, associated with: cumulative effects of new learning problems; difficulty organizing large amounts of information; difficulty with increasingly abstract information.

MIDDLE ADOLESCENCE

KEY DEVELOPMENTAL ISSUES

Social–emotional–behavioral issues

Increasing awareness of changes associated with puberty; increasingly heterosexual social networks;

Increasing need to experiment and take risks;

Increasing ability to manage environmental stressors, profit from feedback, and make flexible and autonomous decisions;

Increasing ability to read social cues.

Cognitive academic–vocational issues

Decreasing egocentrism, resulting in increasing ability to communicate varied thoughts and feelings competently in varied social settings;

Emerging vocational goals and long-range goal planning.

COMMON CONCERNS WITH TBI AT THIS STAGE

Social–emotional–behavioral issues

Discontinuity of personal identification due to physical and cognitive changes; breakdown in social grouping associated with communication and other changes

Difficulty managing increasing environmental stressors; ongoing rigidity in responding; inability to profit from feedback;

Experimentation and risk-taking at dangerous levels;

Possible "hyper-egocentrism," with focus on the injury;

Difficulty reading social cues.

Cognitive–academic vocational issues:

Difficulty with increasingly demanding curriculum;

Possibly increasing incongruity between vocational goals and vocational potential after the injury.

COMMON DELAYED SYMPTOMS RELATED TO EARLIER INJURY

Social–emotional–behavioral issues

Continued rigidity and dependence on external control while peers become increasingly flexible and autonomous;

Hypersexuality;

Social withdrawal.

Cognitive–academic–vocational issues:

Increasing academic failure due to cumulative effect of new learning problems;

Difficulty achieving communicative effectiveness in varied social settings requiring varied social registers;

General difficulty with divergent thinking and flexible problem solving.

continued

168

TABLE 6–1. *continued*

LATE ADOLESCENCE

KEY DEVELOPMENTAL ISSUES	COMMON CONCERNS WITH TBI AT THIS STAGE	COMMON DELAYED SYMPTOMS RELATED TO EARLIER INJURY
Social–emotional–behavioral issues	***Social–emotional–behavioral issues***	***Social–emotional–behavioral issues***
Social networks loosen and shift, based on vocational and social needs;	Regression to rigid behavior, egocentric perspective, and dependence on external control; difficulty considering alternative perspectives;	Retention of concrete thinking and rigid responding;
Reduction in risk-taking;		Immature social skills; continued dependence on cliques while peers move on;
Increasing ability to identify source of stress and adjust behavior accordingly (self-management);	Inability to anticipate and recognize stressors and alter behavior accordingly;	Continued dependence on same sex peers for support; relations with opposite sex may be characterized by hypersexuality;
Continued reduction in egocentrism and growth in attention to the needs of others (a life-long process);	Loss of social networks; possible dependence on old social networks;	Possible perception of differences between self and others as representing a psychiatric problem.
Sexual relations move toward an increasing interest in companionship and love;	Sexual relations continue to focus on physical aspects.	
Solidification of communication styles.		
Cognitive academic–vocational issues	***Cognitive academic–vocational issues***	***Cognitive academic–vocational issues***
Solidification of vocational and academic goals; organization of behavior in pursuit of these goals;	Regression to rigid and concrete communication; loss of subtlety, abstractness, and flexibility in communication;	Possible failure in college or on the job due to the elimination of the supports provided in high school.
Increasingly mature understanding of academic and vocational potential.	Incongruity of previous academic/vocational goals and current abilities	

*"Delayed consequences" refer to symptoms associated with an earlier injury, usuallly incurred at a previous developemental stage, that are observed in individuals whose recovery had appeared to be generally good.

Source: Reprinted with permission from "Traumatic Brain Injury in Adolescence: Assessment and Reintegration," by M. Ylvisaker and T. Feeney, 1995, pp. 36–37. *Seminars in Speech and Language, 16.* Copyright 1995 Thieme Medical Publishers, Inc.

events that follow the behavior and either increase its likelihood of recurrence (i.e., reinforcers) or decrease that likelihood (i.e., punishers or no response). Although Skinner's early work justified an equal focus on antecedents and consequences in explaining and modifying behavior, elements of his later work (e.g., Skinner, 1969) and that of many practitioners, particularly those with a limited understanding of the theories guiding the field of applied behavior analysis, place disproportionate emphasis on consequences in the management of behavior (model 1 in Figure 6–1).

Practical interest in the antecedents of behavior increased with research on error-

less learning in animals (Terrace, 1963) and children with developmental disabilities (Bijou, Peterson, & Ault, 1968). Within this tradition, ample cues, along with stimulus fading and stimulus shaping procedures, are used to ensure that the individual successfully performs the target behavior with systematically decreasing antecedent support. The technologies of consequence and antecedent manipulation in behavior management and teaching have been successfully integrated into the armamentarium of intervention strategies in most teaching and helping professions. Although we recommend an approach to behavior management that extends far beyond manipulation

MODEL 1
A "Traditional" Approach

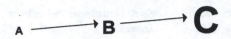

MODEL 2
A "Functional" Alternative

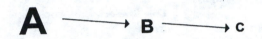

Figure 6–1. The ABCs of behavior: Antecedent-Behavior-Consequence.

of immediate antecedents and consequences, we do not intend to suggest abandonment of basic principles that have shown their usefulness over time and with varied disability groups, and must be considered a component of intervention for most people with behavior problems after TBI. The technologies of traditional applied behavior analysis are usefully summarized in Bijou and Baer (1978), Blackman and LeJeune (1990), and Martin and Pear (1996). These traditional technologies have been applied to TBI rehabilitation by a number of clinicians and investigators (Franzen, 1991; Parenté, 1994; Slifer et al., 1993, 1996; Silver, Boake, & Cavazos, 1994; Wood, 1987, 1988)

Until recently, there has been little systematic investigation of the manipulation of internal and external context variables (i.e., setting events) as a means to control behavior and ultimately help people control their own behavior (Michael, 1982, 1989). In our work with children and adults with TBI, attention to setting events and

other proactive procedures tends to bear more fruit than attention restricted to observable events that immediately surround the target behavior.

A Positive, Routine-Based, Antecedent-Focused Approach

In this discussion, we use the word *antecedent* in a broad sense that extends beyond the discrete events that precede and are temporally proximate to the responses that they influence. In this broad sense, antecedents include the events that immediately precede a target behavior and also all of the events and internal states that are described below under antecedent control procedures. With this as background, the approach to behavior management that we recommend for most individuals with TBI focuses predominately on antecedents (model 2 in Figure 6–1) and to a lesser extent on consequences.

The neuropsychological rationale for this approach was described in Chapter 2 and suggested earlier in this chapter. Available research and our daily work with individuals with TBI have led us to organize neuropsychological contributors to behavior problems into five broad categories. Together with common psychoreactive phenomena, they support a strongly antecedent-focused approach. Neuropsychological contributors, all of which fall on a continuum of severity, include:

1. Common orbito-frontal injury that results in some degree of disinhibition and impulsiveness (Damasio et al., 1991; Eslinger et al., 1997; Stuss & Benson, 1986). The greater the individual's disinhibition, the more important it is to support behavior through antecedent manipulation, as in the case of infants and toddlers.

2. Common dorsolateral frontal or mesial frontal injury that results in some degree of reduced initiation (Fuster, 1991; Stuss & Benson, 1986). The greater the individual's initiation impairment, the more important it is to support behavior through antecedent manipulation.

3. Common ventromedial prefrontal injury that results in inefficient learning from consequences (i.e., reduced attachment of somatic markers to stored memories) (Damasio, 1994; Eslinger & Damasio, 1985; Morgan & LeDoux, 1995). The greater the individual's impairment in this area, the more important it is to support behavior through antecedent manipulation.

4. Common dorsolateral and mesial prefrontal injury that results in impaired working memory (Baddeley, 1992; Brazzeli et al., 1994; Case, 1992). The greater the impairment in the individual's ability to manipulate multiple considerations prior to acting, the more important it is to support behavior through antecedent manipulation.

5. Common hippocampal damage that results in impaired declarative memory (Eichenbaum & Otto, 1992; Eichenbaum et al., 1994). Although it is possible for people with severely impaired declarative memory to learn from consequences, including people in post-traumatic amnesia, this deficit also lends itself to serious consideration of antecedent supports.

Many individuals with TBI are impaired in all of these areas of functioning, necessitating an approach that addresses problem behavior largely through antecedents (Feeney & Ylvisaker, 1997; Ylvisaker & Feeney, 1994, 1998; Ylvisaker, Feeney, & Szekeres, 1998; Zencius, Wesolowski, Burke, & McQuade, 1989). In addition, the emotional reaction to loss and repeated failure as the individual attempts to recreate a meaningful life after the injury argues for an approach to behavior that is as supportive as it can be, without creating learned helplessness (an important topic to which we return later).

In addition to this neuropsychological and psychoreactive rationale, a growing body of research literature in developmental disabilities supports a positive, proactive, antecedent-focused approach to problem behavior. Indeed, most of the proactive procedures described in the sections that follow have been validated in experimental work with children and adults with developmental disabilities and adolescents with behavior disorders (Carr, McConnachie, Levin, & Kemp, 1993; Carr et al., 1997; Conroy & Fox, 1994; Dunlap, Johnson, & Robbins, 1990; Halle & Spradlin, 1993; Horner et al., 1990; Horner, O'Neill, & Flannery, 1993; McIntosh, Vaughn, & Zaragoza, 1991).

The approach to behavior management of individuals with TBI that we describe in this chapter is based on all of the intervention premises presented in Chapter 1. We invite readers to review those premises as background for the current presentation.

Positive Setting Events

The concept of setting events has a long history in behavioral psychology (Kantor, 1959) and has recently enjoyed a lively revival in applications of applied behavioral analysis to management of children and adults with developmental disabilities and students with behavior disorders (Carr et al., 1994; Chandler, Fowler, & Lubek, 1992; Colvin & Sugai, 1989; Conroy & Fox, 1994; Fox & Conroy, 1995; Horner et al., 1997; Kennedy & Itkonen, 1993; Michael, 1982, 1989, 1993; Volmer & Iwata, 1991; Wahler & Fox, 1981). Setting events provide the external and internal context within which people act and which influences the behavior that follows a specific stimulus. Setting events include more than the immediate observable antecedents of a behavior (e.g., the teacher's instruction which preceded the student's outburst). They can include external events that are removed in time (e.g., a negative interaction with a parent at 8:00 AM might predispose a student to react negatively to a provocation in school at 2:00 PM) as well as internal events and states of the agent (e.g., pain, confusion, frustration). From the perspective of intervention, Baer and colleagues identified setting events as the conditions that determine whether a behavioral "intervention has maximal or minimal effectiveness" (Baer,

Wolf, & Risley, 1987, pp. 318–319) and called for clinicians to extend their intervention focus beyond the immediate antecedents and consequences of behavior. Table 6–2 presents a scheme for categorizing setting events (Feeney & Ylvisaker, 1997).

The influence of setting events on behavior is apparent in everyday life. The likelihood of negative behavior is increased by negative internal states, such as hunger, exhaustion, anger, sadness, anxiety, depression, confusion, or simply a "bad mood" and by negative external events, such as abrasive sensory stimulation, aggressive behavior of others, reception of bad news, failure at important tasks, and conflicts with others. Recent studies of aggressive behavior on busy highways support this thesis.

TABLE 6–2. Categories of setting events that potentially influence behavior.

INTERNAL STATES OF THE INDIVIDUAL

➤ **Neurologic states**
positive setting events: normal neurology
negative setting events: overactiveness of the limbic regions; seizures; neurotransmitter disruption, decreased cerebral blood flow

➤ **Other physiologic states**
positive setting events: rest, relaxation, satiation, appropriate levels of medication
negative setting events: pain, illness, exhaustion, hunger, over medication, under medication

➤ **Cognitive states**
positive setting events: orientation to task, familiarity with routine, adequate recall of relevant events, adequate recognition of things and people
negative setting events: confusion, disorientation, frustration, inadequate recall and recognition

➤ **Emotional states**
positive setting events: sense of accomplishment, success, achievement, acceptance by others, respect from others
negative setting events: anxiety, anger, depression, sense of loss and failure

➤ **Perception of task meaningfulness and difficulty**
positive setting events: belief that assigned tasks are meaningful and can be accomplished
negative setting events: belief that assigned tasks are meaningless, infantilizing, or impossible

EXTERNAL EVENTS AND CONDITIONS

➤ **Presence or absence of specific people**
positive setting events: presence of preferred people
negative setting events: absence of preferred people, presence of nonpreferred people

➤ **Recent history of interaction**
positive setting events: recent positive and pleasurable interactions
negative setting events: recent conflict or disrespectful interaction

➤ **Other environmental stressors**
positive setting events: appropriate and desirable environmental stimulation
negative setting events: irritating environmental stimulation; e.g., ambient noise, improper lighting, other distractors

➤ **Time of day**
positive setting events: alertness, best time of day relative to the individual's natural cycles
negative setting events: bad time of day relative to the individual's natural cycles

---

Setting events are of particular concern for people with brain injury because the setting events at any given moment are often predominantly negative and because the injury often reduces the threshold of tolerance for frustration and other negative stimulation. For example, the individual may routinely be confused, angry, depressed, in pain, hypersensitive to perceived threats because of an overactive or poorly regulated limbic system, and hypersensitive to annoying sounds or visual stimuli. TBI itself is a negative setting event. Furthermore, people with TBI face many tasks that are surprisingly difficult for them, they are often unsuccessful (relative to their preinjury standards), they may live in a restrictive setting that is not of their choosing, they often have unsatisfy-

ing social lives (relative to their preinjury standards), and, in general, they are expected to tackle the difficult task of creating a new life for themselves while actively mourning the loss of their old life. Taken together, these negative setting events understandably predispose individuals to negative behavior (e.g., refusal, withdrawal, aggression) when a difficult or unmotivating task is presented. This negative behavior may result in escape from the difficult task, which in turn increases the probability of the negative behavior over time. Negative setting events and the dynamic with which they are associated are depicted in Figure 6–2.

In contrast, positive setting events (e.g., rest, relaxation, good nutrition, recent exercise, clear orientation to task, understand-

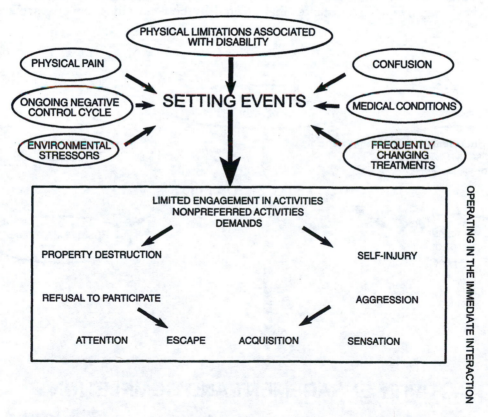

Figure 6–2. Illustration of the relationship between negative setting events and challenging behavior. (Reprinted with permission from "A Positive Communication-Based Approach to Challenging Behavior After TBI," by T. Feeney and M. Ylvisaker, 1997. In A. Glang, G. H. S. Singer, and B. Todis [Eds.], *Students with Acquired Brain Injury: The School's Response* [pp. 229–254]. Baltimore: Paul H. Brookes Publishing Company.)

ing of routines, feeling of competence, sense of control, a recent series of successes) increase the likelihood of engagement in and successful completion of difficult tasks. (See Figure 6–3.) That is, when people are feeling good physically, feeling good about themselves, and experiencing success with important tasks, they are in a better position to receive assignments that are difficult and to complete the task without reacting negatively. In all of the case illustrations that follow, one of our primary objectives was to help individuals with problem behavior after TBI and the significant people in their lives create daily routines in which considerable effort was devoted to inducing positive setting events before introducing difficult tasks.

Creativity and effort are often required to create positive setting events in the life of individuals with behavior problems after TBI. They often live in circumstances that

they object to, fail at most tasks they consider important, lack access to the activities that previously gave them satisfaction, and lapse into conflict with people around them at the slightest provocation. However, the more difficult it seems to induce positive setting events, the more important it is to try, because the behavior of people whose internal and external context of behavior is largely negative can be expected to worsen over time.

In our experience, many clinicians, using what they label an applied behavior analytic approach, neglect internal states or conditions, presumably because they are unobservable and beyond the reach of direct manipulation. The explosive developments in the neurosciences have rendered both of these theses untenable. First, internal states and processes are no longer the "black box" hypotheses they were once considered by behaviorally oriented psycholo-

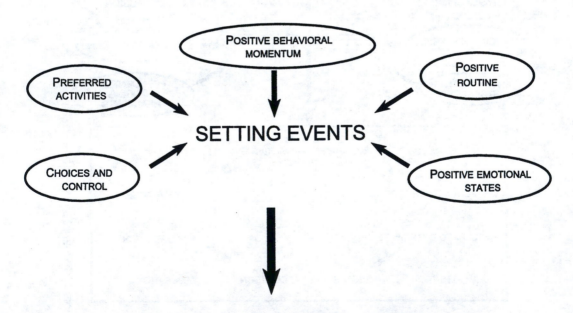

Figure 6–3. Illustration of the relationship between positive setting events and positive behavior. (Reprinted with permission from "A Positive Communication-Based Approach to Challenging Behavior After TBI," by T. Feeney and M. Ylvisaker, 1997, [pp. 229–254]. In A. Glang, G. H. S. Singer and B. Todis [Eds.], *Students with Acquired Brain Injury: The School's Response*. Baltimore: Paul H. Brookes Publishing Company.)

gists and philosophers. Much is known about the brain states and activities associated with mental phenomena. In addition, pharmacologic intervention is available for direct manipulation of at least some of the negative internal states that predispose a person to negative behavior. Indirect manipulation of these internal setting events includes developing positive behavioral momentum; ensuring that people have a satisfactory sense of control over their lives by giving them a reasonable domain of choices; engaging people in tasks that are respectful, interesting, and therefore motivating; helping people to develop a satisfactory sense of self and their role in life; desensitizing people to events that cause anxiety; helping people to manage their own setting events, including internal states; and ensuring that people have understandable daily routines that incorporate all of these principles of antecedent management. These approaches to managing setting events, including the indirect manipulation of internal setting events, are discussed in the sections that follow.

Positive Behavioral Momentum

The principle of behavioral momentum is one important component of the general principle of setting events and is equally plausible in everyday terms: Positive and successful behavior increases the likelihood of subsequent positive and successful behavior, whereas negative and unsuccessful behavior increases the likelihood of subsequent negative and unsuccessful behavior (Carr et al., 1995; Fowler, 1996; Mace et al., 1988; Mace et al., 1990; Mace, Mauro, Boyajian, & Eckert, 1997; Mace, Page, Ivanck, & O'Brien, 1986; Nevin, 1988, 1992). Closely related to pretask requesting (Kennedy, Itoken, & Lindquist, 1995), task variation, and embedding (Bambara, Koger, Katzer, & Davenport, 1995), the principle of behavioral momentum suggests that problematic tasks (i.e., those likely to induce negative behavior) be introduced in the context of successful and nonproblematic tasks. That

is, after enjoying success on a series of meaningful tasks, individuals are likely to accept new challenges, work hard, and succeed. We have depicted this principle in Figure 6–4 as a gas tank which, when full, enables a person to begin a long trip and, when empty, must be filled before beginning.

The principle of behavioral momentum is easily illustrated by common phenomena in everyday life. For example, every dieter knows that it is easier to continue a diet once the scale has begun to present good news than it is initially to reverse the course of overeating. Similarly, demanding exercise regimens become increasingly easy once one begins to get in shape and feel good about being in shape. Difficult academic tasks are easier to attack from a platform of uninterrupted academic success than from a platform of academic failure.

The principle of behavioral momentum has been validated in several studies of individuals with behavior problems associated with developmental disabilities (Davis, Brady, Hamilton, McEvoy, & Williams, 1994; Harchik & Putzier, 1990; Kennedy et al., 1995; Mace et al., 1988; Sanchez-Fort, Brady, & Davis, 1995; Zarcone, Iwata, Mazaleski, & Smith, 1994). However, in several studies highly artificial tasks were used to develop behavioral momentum (for example, momentum to deal with difficult math problems is generated by having the subjects successfully follow a series of simple gross motor commands, such as "Touch your nose, Touch your ear"). In our experience, most people with TBI need to experience success on tasks that are meaningful to them, not contrived tasks that bear no resemblance to the difficult tasks that tend to elicit negative behaviors (Feeney & Ylvisaker, 1995; Ylvisaker & Feeney, 1996, 1997).

Earlier we stated that it is often difficult to induce generally positive setting events in the life of a person with TBI. It is particularly difficult to generate a sense of positive momentum because people in both acute and chronic stages of their recovery fre-

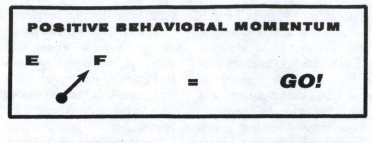

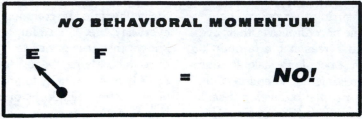

Figure 6–4. The principle of behavioral momentum, as illustrated metaphorically with a gas tank. (Reprinted with permission from "A Positive Communication- Based Approach to Challenging Behavior After TBI," by T. Feeney and M. Ylvisaker, 1997. In A. Glang, G. H. S. Singer and B. Todis, Eds. *Students with Acquired Brain Injury: The School's Response [pp, 229–254].* Baltimore: Paul H. Brookes Publishing Company.)

quently have great difficulty succeeding at meaningful tasks *in relation to their preinjury standards for success.* We emphasize the necessity of applying the individual's own standards of success. Engaging people in tasks at which they can succeed, but which they consider trivial or infantilizing, may generate increased frustration and sense of failure instead of the intended sense of success and momentum. Ideally, momentum needed to successfully attack a difficult academic task should be generated with academic tasks, momentum needed to approach social tasks confidently should be generated with success at social tasks, and momentum needed to approach physical tasks confidently should be generated with success at physical tasks. This principle of topographic similarity applies generally to all domains of behavior, remembering that the success needed to create momentum must be measured by the individual's own standards of success (Mace et al., 1997).

Vygotskyan scaffolding procedures are often helpful in generating positive behavioral momentum. That is, when a therapist, family member, teacher, or peer works col-

laboratively with the individual to enjoy success with meaningful tasks, momentum might be more easily achieved than when the individual is required to perform alone, thereby risking failure and frustration. The case illustrations presented below and in Chapters 4 and 5 include several descriptions of these scaffolding procedures in action. In each case, the scaffolding not only enabled the individual to succeed with the task at hand, it also helped undercut a potential downward spiral of failure breeding more failure, while generating a sense of positive momentum that served as a basis for ongoing effort and improvement.

Choice and Control

Like the principles of positive setting events and positive behavioral momentum, the principle of choice and control is familiar from everyday experience. Willingness to participate in activities, enjoyment of those activities, and positive behavior during the activities are more likely in self-chosen activities than in those imposed by others (Bannerman, Sheldon, Sherman, & Harchik,

1990; Brown, Belz, Corsi, & Wenig, 1993; Dunlap et al., 1994). This principle was strongly supported by a review of the developmental disabilities literature. Harchik and colleagues (1993) reviewed over 100 investigations of the effects of choice making on engagement in tasks, enjoyment of tasks, and reduction in challenging behavior in individuals with developmental disabilities. Despite some expected conflicts within this large body of research, the reviewers found that, in general, when people with developmental disabilities are allowed to choose activities and control aspects of those activities, they tend to participate more willingly, behave more appropriately, and rate the activity as positive.

In our experience, this principle is powerful when applied to people with acquired brain injury. In large numbers, people with TBI are adolescents or young adults who, prior to the injury, had begun to enjoy a great deal of freedom and control in their lives. In many cases they had a lively pretrauma history of taking risks and opposing others' attempts to control their behavior. In painful contrast, life after the injury is often dominated by externally imposed restrictions on choice and activities, including physical, social, academic, vocational, and recreational activities. These inevitable restrictions are often exaggerated by an overly protective posture on the part of parents and staff, and by an overriding concern that people with severe TBI are incapable of making sound choices for themselves.

Conviction on the part of staff or family members that the individual cannot make sound choices for himself or herself easily becomes a self-fulfilling prophecy as the two lock horns in pitched control battles. The classic downward cycle of control (depicted in Figure 6–5) can begin with a choice by the individual with TBI followed

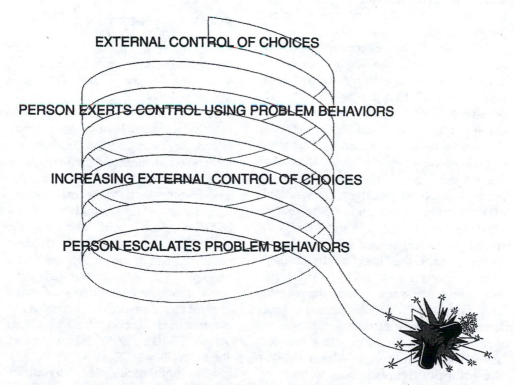

EXTERNAL CONTROL OF CHOICES

PERSON EXERTS CONTROL USING PROBLEM BEHAVIORS

INCREASING EXTERNAL CONTROL OF CHOICES

PERSON ESCALATES PROBLEM BEHAVIORS

Figure 6–5. Graphic representation of the negative cycle of control. (Reprinted with permission from "A Positive Communication-Based Approach to Challenging Behavior After TBI," by T. Feeney and M. Ylvisaker; 1997. In A. Glang, G. H. S. Singer, and B. Todis, (Eds.), *Students with Acquired Brain Injury: The School's Response* [pp. 229–254]). Baltimore: Paul H. Brookes Publishing Company.)

by a paternalistic refusal by the authority figure, or with a command from the authority figure followed by oppositional resistance from the person with TBI. In either case, what may begin as a relatively innocuous exchange (e.g., mother: "John, could you get your math done now, please?" John: "OK, I'll do it right after this TV show.") easily escalates into a full-fledged battle in which the original objective is quickly lost and replaced by a primitive need to exercise control over others and avoid being controlled oneself. Authority figures may leave this battlefield slightly bloodied and convinced that the individual is incapable of sound judgment and good choices—therefore requiring even more restrictions rather than fewer—when in fact responsibility for the battle may legitimately rest at the feet of the authority figure. Wisdom is typically on the side of giving as much opportunity for choice and control as possible and avoiding control battles, which typically worsen rather than improve a difficult behavioral situation.

To be sure, there are occasions for the exercise of authority and dogged persistence in that exercise. For example, it may be necessary to insist that the person with TBI take prescribed medications, refrain from driving, go to school, and the like, even in the face of resistance. Practice discriminating choice versus no choice situations may reduce conflict when external authority must be imposed, but there are inevitably occasions for battles. However, battles must be chosen wisely. When battles over trivial issues are waged and won by authority figures, the "loser" understandably regroups for the next battle, fueled in part by anger and resentment over the previous loss. People with serious behavior problems have a way of winning protracted wars, even though they may lose occasional battles within the war. Alternatively, if the authority figure chooses to do battle over a trivial issue and *loses*, then authority is quickly lost and problem behavior is likely to increase.

Interesting, Meaningful, Do-able Tasks

It is axiomatic that when people are allowed adequate amounts of choice and control in their lives, it is likely that they will choose a high proportion of activities that they identify as personally meaningful. It is also possible for staff and others to heighten motivation and thereby reduce the likelihood of refusal, conflict, and other behavior problems by ensuring that the individual is largely engaged in meaningful, respectful, and do-able tasks, including tasks that are chosen by staff. On the negative side, we have seen many adolescents and young adults with TBI become enraged when presented with assessment or treatment tasks that they considered disrespectful, infantilizing or overly difficult. In contrast, when activities are respectful of the person's interests, abilities, and sense of self, arrived at through a respectful process of negotiation, problem behavior is less frequent.

Positive Roles and Scripts

Connected to the theme of meaningful activities is the importance of positive roles and scripts for people with TBI. Before the injury, their positive behavior was maintained in part by scripts associated with positive roles, such as student, employee, friend, husband or wife, brother or sister, athlete/team member, musician/member of a music organization, and many more. These roles tend to be associated with scripts that dictate generally positive forms of behavior and social interaction. The development of social skills in children has recently been associated closely with the acquisition of internalized scripts tied to social roles, a theme that dominates the current literature on social-cognitive development in childhood (Hudson, 1993; Hudson & Fivush, 1993). We return to this theme in Chapter 7.

Meaningful social roles also contribute to a positive sense of self as a contributor and genuinely valuable person. Unfortunately, many of these roles are eliminated or rendered unsatisfying for people with chronic disability after brain injury. The new roles implicitly offered to a person with severe, chronic disability after brain injury are extremely limited. In the worst case scenario, staff or family members tacitly offer the individual a choice among two roles: compliant patient and defiant opposer. Given their pretrauma history and their legitimate need for a strong sense of self, many people with TBI choose the opposer role without hesitation—with serious consequences for their behavior.

The answer to this dilemma is not to coerce the individual into a compliant role, but rather to work with that person to establish as many positive roles as possible in life after the injury. We have frequently observed sudden transformations in behavior with changes in role and script. For example, we have worked with violently oppositional adolescents whose behavior changed from aggressive and defiant to positive and compliant when the staff person's communication changed from "I am determined to control your behavior" to "You have a contribution to make and I truly need your help."

We used a powerful but somewhat unusual application of this principle to manage a group of young adolescent males whose behavior had become nearly uncontrollable during dining times on an inpatient TBI rehabilitation unit. Meals were increasingly punctuated with teasing, disputes, food fights, food refusal, and similar oppositional behavior. A problem-solving discussion with these boys revealed that they had an adequate understanding of the dining time rules that staff wished them to follow. Therefore, traditional, role play based social skills training would have been a waste of time. The boys made it clear that their behavior was more a function of their desire to be "tough guys" than of a knowledge or skill deficiency. Therefore, we negotiated a dining "club" with them (the "Hans and Franz" club, named after the satirical Saturday Night Live skit that they enjoyed), worked with them to develop

their new roles and "code," and ate with them, playing one of the silly Hans and Franz roles. (We gradually introduced other staff into the Hans and Franz culture.) With this new script and these new roles in place, the boys began to support one another and eat in a way that was tolerable to others, while at the same time meeting their emotional need to be something more than compliant "good boys." For these young adolescent boys, the "manliness" theme of their new script helped them to feel better about themselves while also associating the "manly" themes of strength and control with their own self-control while eating. This script supported the development of a positive culture within which prosocial behaviors could be seen as attractive and, therefore, quickly established.

More generally, we attempt to help people establish *active contributor* roles for themselves to counteract the negative impact of the passive "patient" role implicit in most rehabilitation programs. Positive roles for children in a rehabilitation facility may include assisting with snacks, pushing others' wheelchairs, feeding pets, serving as a buddy, and introducing new patients to the program. In school, students with TBI may play contributor roles by assisting in teaching a brain injury curriculum in health class, serving as line leader, computer manager, sport manager, attendance monitor, snack manager, buddy for others, and other positive roles. Adults with significant disability may find meaning in volunteer roles through church, civic, or other organizations, serving as a mentor to others, and ideally having paid work, with or without support. Individuals with TBI and their significant others may also benefit from counseling designed to help them comfortably reestablish family and related relationships inevitably altered by the injury and subsequent disability (Singer, Glang, & Williams, 1996; Waaland, 1998; Williams & Kay, 1990).

In Chapter 8 we describe the important process of engaging individuals with TBI and possibly their family members in working with staff to produce a transitional/self-advocacy videotape. Among other benefits, this process often communicates a sense of empowerment to people whose dominant sense at the time may be powerlessness. We also try to engage people with whom we work in generating other training materials for the staff with whom they work. For example, an orientation group may devote 10 minutes each day to development of a manual on how to run an orientation group effectively and respectfully. A support group may devote some of their time to creating a manual or training videotapes on how to support people with TBI. There are many possibilities; the theme is that people with recent onset disability, as well as people with chronic disability who have not managed to create a satisfying life for themselves, generally need creative help in developing positive roles to replace the roles that were destroyed by the injury. Because these positive roles are associated with positive behavioral scripts, we include them in antecedent control behavior management.

Positive Communication
Alternatives to Problem Behavior

In Chapter 7, we discuss the important process of teaching positive communication alternatives to problem behavior. In an important sense, that entire chapter could be included in this section because teaching communication alternatives is one of the important proactive or antecedent-focused approaches to challenging behavior.

Self-Control of Antecedents

We sometimes hear professionals object to an antecedent-focused approach on the grounds that it artificially prevents problem behavior with extraordinary environmental manipulations, but does not truly address the training needs of the individual who, in all likelihood, will cease to behave in a tolerable way when those antecedent controls are removed in the real world. This objection raises important issues, but is misguided for three reasons.

1. Antecedent manipulations are often needed to prevent the evolution of problem behavior early after the injury and to give the individual ample time to learn satisfying, positive forms of behavior.
2. From the onset of intervention, our goal is to help individuals with behavior problems after TBI achieve the highest possible degree of *self*-control of behavior. In cases of organically based impairment of inhibition, initiation, or learning from feedback, self-control may take the form of self-management of antecedents (e.g., not entering interactions likely to result in loss of control; managing a system of support people and following rules for their use). In Chapter 4 we describe a young adult whom we helped to pull himself out of a tailspin after severe TBI by creating a daily routine that included an effective set of procedures designed to manage his own antecedents. Jason tells his own story in the epilogue to this book.
3. In cases of severe, chronic, injury-related behavioral impairment, antecedent-control procedures may be needed indefinitely. In this case, the work done by rehabilitation specialists to identify the most effective set of antecedent supports bears fruit throughout the person's life, in supported living and possibly supported work settings. In these extreme cases, it is support for the approach, not a criticism of it, that it "artificially" prevents problem behavior.

Daily Routines

A well understood and personally meaningful daily routine is by itself an antecedent-control behavior management procedure. That is, familiar and satisfying daily routines help to prevent confusion and disorientation, which contribute to behavioral disruption, and help to keep the individual focused and productive, which contributes to positive behavior. Well-organized routines are also the context within which all of the other procedures described in this section are applied. When we are asked to consult with staff who are having difficulty with a person with challenging behavior, our first task is to identify in detail the person's daily routine. Assuming there is a routine, our next task is to explore the degree to which the individual understands the routine and finds it meaningful. We then look for evidence of all of the antecedent-focused procedures described in this section. If they are not in place, we begin the process of helping staff to implement these procedures within the individual's everyday routines (while simultaneously working with staff to identify the specific variables that elicit and maintain the problem behaviors and the specific supports that may be needed to change the behavior). In an important sense, behavior modification is at its core modification of everyday routines in the individual's life, including the behavior of the people who interact with the individual in a daily basis.

The Role of Consequences

Value of Consequences

In our framework for behavioral intervention, we have emphasized the antecedents of behavior and a proactive versus reactive approach to behavior problems. There are several reasons for this relative emphasis, some based on the pathophysiology of TBI, discussed above. However, our comments are not intended to imply that consequences of behavior are unimportant or can be ignored. Some children and adults with TBI escape frontolimbic injury entirely and can therefore be expected to be as efficient at learning from consequences as their uninjured peers. Even those who are inefficient at learning from consequences benefit from a positive culture in which successful performance is greeted with encouragement and praise while failure and negative behavior are greeted with efforts to help the person succeed rather than with punishment that only tends to breed more failure.

Cautions About Consequences

The ability to learn from consequences and to guide future behavior on the basis of past consequences is a matter of degree, an observation clearly demonstrated by normal development. For example, an impulsive toddler has little self-control and therefore is in much greater need of antecedent control management procedures than a 5-year-old, who, in turn, is in much greater need of antecedent control than a 25-year-old. When people have limited neurologically based capacity for impulse inhibition, response initiation, learning from experience, and manipulation of multiple considerations at one time, they are candidates for behavior management systems that focus more on antecedents than on consequences. Many people with frontal lobe injury have exactly this set of deficits. In addition to these pathophysiological considerations, the following behavioral themes associated with consequence manipulation must be considered.

Natural and Logical Consequences

With the goal of helping people to succeed in the real world, rewards and punishments should be as natural and logically related to the individual's behavior as possible. For example, a good grade is a natural and logical consequence of effective preparation for a test; a raise or promotion is a natural and logical consequence of hard work on the job; an enjoyable social interaction is a natural and logical consequence of socially appropriate initiation. On the punishment side, cleaning one's room is a natural and logical consequence of "trashing" the room during a tantrum; receiving a poor grade is a natural and logical consequence of failing to prepare for an exam. In contrast, the following contingent responses are not related in a natural and logical way to the behavior and therefore not likely to help shape enduring positive behaviors: "Nice talking, Johnnie," "I liked the way you responded to Jeremy; I'll give you a point for that," and "That's not an appropriate way to request ice cream; you will not be able to go on the outing tonight."

The overall flavor of a behavior management system that employs natural and logical consequences is this: "Behavior B and consequence C are connected; I'll do my best to help you succeed and at the same time help you learn what goes with what in the real world." In contrast, the flavor of a system based on arbitrary consequences is this: "As an authority figure, I will dispense rewards of my choosing when you behave well and punishments of my choosing when you behave badly. These rewards and punishments may have nothing to do with the behaviors in question." The latter system fails to promote understanding of natural and logical relationships in the world and, at the same time, invites opposition to arbitrary authority, an invitation enthusiastically accepted by many naturally oppositional adolescents and young adults with TBI.

An additional problem associated with point systems and token economies frequently used in school and rehabilitation settings is that the provision of extrinsic rewards (e.g., points or tokens) for every positive behavior has the effect, in many people, of creating dependence on extrinsic rewards and thereby reducing intrinsic motivation. For example, we have worked with several children and adolescents whose special education programs before the injury used token economy systems to manage behavior and who, therefore, demanded points or tokens for every piece of work in rehabilitation after the injury, simply because they did not understand life under other circumstances. Questioning the value of traditional token economy systems is not to deny that some people, with a long history of challenging behavior, need frequent and powerful reinforcers to reestablish positive behavioral routines in their lives. It is rather to acknowledge the important long-term goal of establishing internal motivational systems within which some things are done simply because they are good things to do (e.g., helping friends, addressing others in a positive manner, completing

assignments in school and on the job), while others are done because of their natural long-term benefit (e.g., a good job later in life; a pay check).

"Time Out"

Used as they were originally intended to be used (Bijou & Baer, 1978), so-called "time out" procedures can be helpful for people with brain injury as well as others who have difficulty regulating their behavior. That is, many people need time away from a negative interaction to calm down and break a negative perseverative set. Unfortunately, the legitimate goal of time out can be easily subverted. When individuals are removed from an aversive situation after behaving in an unacceptable way (e.g., a painful physical therapy session is terminated), time out is transformed into reinforcement for challenging behavior—clearly an undesirable transformation. When time out is understood as a place and extended intimate interaction is required to get the individual to that place and keep him or her there, "time out from reinforcement" may be transformed into an extended period of reinforcing interaction with staff—again an undesirable transformation. Finally, when not carefully monitored, time-out procedures easily become punishment, particularly for individuals who are not well liked by staff. This dangerous transformation carries with it all of the cautions associated with frank punishment procedures, described below.

For a period of 3 years in a brain injury rehabilitation facility in which we worked, the time out rooms (one on each of the two TBI units) were never used. In contrast, "chill-out time" was a frequently used behavioral intervention, with the location being wherever was appropriate for the individual to be away from a negative interaction long enough to cool down and regain composure. Furthermore, for many of the children and adults with whom we have worked, learning to remove themselves from an out-of-control interaction (i.e., self-imposed chill-out time) was a high priority goal. For example, Ylvisaker and Feeney (1994) described an adolescent diagnosed with a severe behavior disorder prior to his traumatic brain injury that included severe, bilateral frontal lobe damage. After intensive training in self-removal from stressful situations, he returned to school in a less restrictive classroom setting than before the injury. His reentry plan included a right to remove himself from class at any time if he needed to reduce his anxiety or frustration. He implemented this plan with considerable success and, despite early predictions, based on the severity of his injury, that he would be unmanageable in community and school settings, his behavior proved to be less problematic than it was before the injury.

Crisis Management and Behavior Management

Unfortunately, many people understand behavior management to be restricted to a set of procedures that can be implemented after a person has acted. That is, when people behave in a positive manner, their behavior is followed by positive consequences; when they behave in a negative manner, their behavior is followed by negative consequences. In contrast, the approach offered in this chapter is one in which behavior management is largely understood to be a set of procedures designed to prevent people from acting in a negative way, to teach them to act in an effective way, and to enable them increasingly to control their own behavior. These positive, proactive procedures include all of the antecedent control procedures described above as well as the cognitive and executive system supports discussed in Chapters 4 and 5, and the communication teaching discussed in Chapter 7.

Despite well-conceived preventive efforts and positive teaching, behavioral crises do occur, necessitating intelligent responses from people in the environment. What follows is a list of Do's and Don'ts designed to

help staff and others regulate their own behavior during a behavioral crisis.

➤ **Remain Calm:** It is never helpful for people to respond to a behavioral crisis by going into crisis themselves. Anxiety tends to be infectious. An anxious person who engages in challenging behavior often transmits anxiety to other people in the environment, thereby reducing their effectiveness and reciprocally increasing the anxiety of the person originally in crisis. Conversely, a calm person tends to interrupt the spread of anxiety. It is often better to do nothing in a behavioral crisis than to act impulsively or react in anger. Therefore, critical competencies for people working with individuals with challenging behavior include maintaining a "stoneface" during a crisis and always *appearing* to know what they are doing, even when angry, frightened, or completely unclear about what to do. Repeating to oneself calming words like, "This too shall pass; this too shall pass" can help one through crises. The critical message to communicate to the person in crisis is, "I'm in control; I know what to do; I'm going to help you get through this and regain your control."

➤ **In the Early Stages of a Crisis, Use Redirection and Diffusion Procedures:** Individuals who are escalating but not yet out of control may respond positively to redirection procedures. This is particularly true of individuals who are still generally confused after TBI and who tend to perseverate. They may begin to yell or act aggressively for no apparent reason, and then perseverate or escalate because of confusion rather than genuine anger. Abrupt redirection to a completely unrelated focus of attention may break this confused and perseverative set. However, good judgment must be exercised when using redirection. If an individual who is acting out is redirected to a highly preferred activity (e.g., eating chocolate ice cream), the redirection may have the positive immediate effect of terminating the acting out behavior, but exacerbate the long-term problem by reinforcing that behavior (i.e., "I get it! When I threaten to hit people, I get ice cream"). Redirection should be to a neutral activity to avoid this unwanted consequence.

➤ **Keep Everybody Safe:** In most cases, attacks on property (e.g., overturning chairs and tables; throwing objects against the wall) should not be considered matters of extreme concern, mandating physical intervention. However, people must be protected. In most cases, safety is ensured by people in the immediate environment moving away from the person in crisis. In extreme cases, that person may need to be physically restrained to prevent harm to himself or others. Physical intervention must always be guided by the principle of least intrusive intervention and by agency protocols and state regulations regarding nonaggressive physical intervention.

➤ **Present Yourself as a Helper:** A few well chosen words like "What can I do to help?" or "Let's get through this" sometimes help the person in crisis regain control. At least this presentation is not likely to escalate the crisis, as do confrontations, threats, arguments, and physical intervention like physical restraint.

➤ **Help People in Crisis Identify Their Feelings:** People who are cognitively immature often have difficulty identifying their feelings. For example, a toddler may react the same way when excited and unhappy, requiring parents to comfort the child by saying something like, "Honey, it's OK. You're having fun! You got great presents. This is great—no need for tears!" People with cognitive impairment after brain injury sometimes have equal difficulty identifying their feelings and may react angrily when the emotion they are experiencing is really excitement or fear. In these cases, it is important to calmly attach words to the emotion that the person is feeling

at the time. For example, staff may say to a person who is beginning to threaten aggression, "This is scary. You're a little scared, but it's going to be OK."

➤ **Speak Clearly and Simply:** In an attempt to reduce the anxiety and agitation of the person in crisis, it is important to speak in a clear, simple, and confident manner. There should be no more than one spokesperson during a crisis. Repetition may be useful, but not if it appears to be nagging.

➤ **Choose Battles Wisely:** Before trying to win a control battle with a person in crisis, determine (1) that the issue is worth fighting over and (2) that you can win. If you choose to engage in a battle and then lose, you seriously increase the likelihood of future battles. If you choose to engage in battles over trivial issues, you lose authority when major issues arise and you create a generally negative social environment.

➤ **Reset to Zero:** In the event of ongoing behavioral crises with an individual, it is wise to "reset to zero," that is, to acknowledge that whatever behavior plan is in place is not working and to start again, but only after attempting to eliminate the crises with artificial means if necessary. This may entail reducing work expectations and providing unusually high levels of support. Staff who are frustrated with the individual may not be pleased with this proposal; however, it is generally wise to implement a new behavior plan and rebuild normal expectations for performance from a platform of no crises. Resetting to zero also entails trying to eliminate anger, resentments, and grudges so that everybody can start with a clean slate.

In addition to this list of positive rules of thumb for managing behavioral crises, there are problematic responses to crises that should be avoided, however natural they may seem at the time.

➤ **Avoid Attempting to "Teach Lessons":** After being threatened, hit, kicked, spat upon, or violated in some other way, it is tempting to say, "Look here, I'm about to teach you a lesson you'll never forget." Unfortunately, the history of punitive approaches to challenging behavior is not promising. Furthermore, a time of crisis is not a time for efficient teaching and learning. Typically, if learning does occur, it is pure "limbic system learning," that is, the memories that are retained tend to be "You are a threat to me and I need to avoid you" or "I hate this place and must escape." This is not the sort of lesson that people with brain injury need to be taught.

➤ **Avoid Planting the Suggestion of a Problem Behavior:** Instructions like "Do not hit me" or "Do not spit" easily have the effect of planting a suggestion in the mind of a person in crisis, or of laying down the gauntlet for an individual who is angry and looking for the most damaging behavior possible on that occasion. That is, the angry individual's response to "Don't you dare hit me!" is more likely to be "Oh, I hadn't thought of it, but thanks for reminding me" than "Sorry, how silly of me to consider hitting you." Suggestions can also be planted nonverbally, for example by attempting to protect things (e.g., one's earrings, glasses, papers on the desk) that had not yet been threatened.

➤ **Avoid Making Threats:** Threatening to impose consequences as a result of behavior during a crisis is problematic for three importantly different reasons. First, it is rarely effective. People in crisis are rarely in a position to control their behavior by reflecting on possible consequences of that behavior. Second, the threatened consequences frequently are not administered. This is particularly true if the threat is made by one person to be carried out by another (e.g., "If you do that, you will not get to go on the outing with John on Friday!" or "If you do that, your father will deal with you when he gets home!"). When threats are made, but not implemented, they quick-

ly become empty words and the authority of the person who issues the empty threats is diminished. Finally, many people with TBI cannot remember the original infraction at the time of punishment, resulting in a negative experience unrelated to the behavior that the punishment is supposed to eliminate.

➤ **Avoid Climbing Ladders:** Often staff members, particularly those who are insecure and easily threatened by loss of control, precipitate behavioral crises by engaging the individual in control battles that escalate out of control. Often the first rung of the ladder is a relatively innocent exchange, such as an instruction to finish the vegetables, followed by refusal. The staff person interprets the refusal as a challenge to his or her authority, and ups the ante by repeating the command firmly, possibly with a threatened consequence. The person with a history of behavior problems rises to the challenge and heightens his resistance, possibly with colorful language. The ladder continues to be climbed until the process reaches its inevitable conclusion, with both combatants falling off the ladder, locked in the grip of a behavioral crisis. "Avoid ladders" is closely connected to the positive rule, "choose battles wisely."

➤ **Avoid Pleading:** Pleading may take the form of explicit pleas (e.g., "John, *please* settle down") or more subtle pleas, often in the form of tag questions (e.g., "John, put that down right now, OK?"). In either case, pleading tacitly communicates to the person in crisis that he or she is in control of the situation.

➤ **Avoid Confusion:** Too much talk, more than one person talking, conflicting messages, and general commotion all conspire to escalate crises, rather than diffuse them. If people in the environment are not needed, they should be invited to leave the area. Teams of staff members should know in advance who will do the talking during a crisis. And the language that is used should be clear, to the point, positive, and not excessive, with adequate pause time for processing.

Physical Intervention

In our discussion of safety, we stated the principle, typically included in state regulations, that physical intervention during a behavioral crisis is justified only when the safety of the individual or others is at risk. There are rare exceptions to that important rule. For example, we have worked with individuals who, like infants, were calmed by a firm comforting embrace when they had lost control of their emotions and behavior. This procedure was most useful for children who were in the early-to-middle stages of cognitive recovery, were generally confused, and had a weak sense of their bodies in space. A firm, nonaggressive embrace appeared to help them regain a sense of position and of control. In every case, this behavioral intervention was prescribed in the child's rehabilitation plan and was associated with a program, coordinated by an occupational therapist with expertise in sensory integration and tactile defensiveness, to improve sensory integration generally, including responsiveness to touch. Furthermore, we made sure that physical contact (e.g., playful wrestling, hugging) was a frequent and positive event over the course of the day, and was not used only when the child's negative behavior began to escalate.

EVERYDAY POSITIVE BEHAVIORAL ROUTINES: CASE ILLUSTRATIONS

Case Illustration: Young Child Who Required Intensive Levels of Behavioral Supports

At the time of our behavioral intervention, Katie was a 5-year-old female who had been injured at age 4 when hit by a car.

Medical records indicated bilateral focal injury to the frontal lobes, the result of a depressed skull fracture and subdural hematoma. Acute care hospitalization lasted for approximately 5 weeks, followed by 3 months of inpatient rehabilitation.

Both prior to and after her injury, Katie lived at home with both parents and two older siblings. She was described by her mother as a bright, active, and "strong-willed" child who liked to dominate the play of other children, including her siblings. Despite her apparently domineering nature, Katie reportedly had numerous friends and was well liked by most of her peers in the daycare program that she had attended. There were no indications of motor, developmental, academic, behavioral, or emotional problems before the injury.

After her return from inpatient rehabilitation, Katie participated in a blended kindergarten-first grade classroom with the support of a paraprofessional aide. The professional staff from the rehabilitation center had attended numerous planning meetings and trained the school staff to provide an individualized and flexible educational program for Katie. When she returned to school, Katie did not have any of the common signs of a serious brain injury: Her gross motor functioning was within normal limits, she had no apparent fine-motor limitations, and her expressive and receptive language skills were similar to her same-age peers. Formal psychological and allied health testing indicated that her general information processing, memory, and general fund of knowledge were not impaired. Her WISC-III Full Scale IQ, derived in testing that occurred approximately 8 months after her injury, was reported as 102/100/102, Total, Performance, and Verbal, respectively

During the first few weeks back in school, there were no reports of serious behavioral challenges. However, over the course of the next 3 months, Katie became increasingly disinhibited and often challenged teachers, clinical staff, and her paraprofessional aide. In addition, staff noted slowly declining ac-

ademic performance and peer-related social skills. As a result, her teacher and paraprofessional aide provided an increased
amount of assistance to plan the steps of
each activity in advance and increased the
levels of ongoing monitoring and feedback
to ensure that she completed most of her
work and interacted with her peers in a
positive manner. As the prompting and cuing of staff increased, Katie's behavioral
challenges increased in frequency and intensity; she was extremely disruptive,
threatening and attempting to assault
teachers, clinicians, peers, and paraprofessionals who challenged her academically or
socially.

Katie's intervention included the following four critical components.

Photograph Routine

Because Katie was a concrete thinker whose
subtle difficulties with organization contributed to her apparently oppositional and
defiant behavior, we worked with her to
take photographs of her engaged in all of
the activities that she might choose or in
which she might be required to participate

during her day at school. She liked the photographs and the control she had in producing them. Furthermore, she quickly became comfortable with using a sequence of
photographs to guide herself through activities without reminders from her paraprofessional aide (which she perceived as
nagging). This supportive photograph routine was gradually faded over the course of
3 to 4 months to a spoken routine. (The
photos were successfully faded after the
data collection period depicted in Figures
6–6 and 6–7.)

Choice and Control

It was clear to staff and family alike that
Katie's challenging behavior was largely a
statement of her need to exercise control.
Prior to the intervention, staff—particularly
the paraprofessional aide who had the
largest amount of interaction with Katie—
understood that the issue was one of control, but chose to respond by routinely engaging Katie in control battles (or, more
accurately, allowed themselves to be drawn
into control battles by Katie). During the
period of active, planned intervention, staff

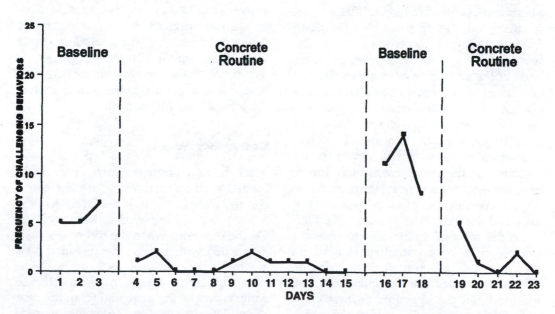

Figure 6–6. Frequency of challenging behavior: Katie.

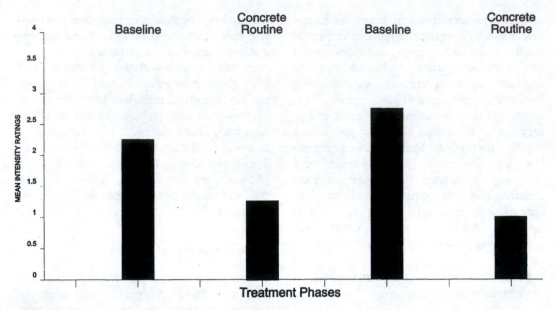

Figure 6–7. Intensity of challenging behavior: Katie. Key: 0 = not at all a problem; 1 = the behavior is a problem, but slight in degree; 2 = the problem is moderately serious; 3 = the problem is severe in degree (Aman & Singh, 1988).

began most activities by giving Katie a set of choices, often using photographs of Katie to present the choices. She was not allowed to dictate the activities of the class or group, but she routinely had choices about her participation within the activity.

Staff and family agreed that certain activities were nonnegotiable. These included attending school, riding the bus to and from school, dining times and the main foods eaten, and playground times. The words *choice* and *no choice* were routinely used at the beginning of activities. Once it was clear to Katie that she had a great deal of control over her school day, she accepted the no-choice components with few complaints.

Initially, the major obstacle to the implementation of the intervention was the reluctance of the paraprofessional aide to give the apearance of "caving in" to Katie. They were veterans of serious conflicts of will, and the aide simply could not understand the value of contributing to what she perceived to be a pathological need on Katie's part to be in control. Our work with the aide involved four components. First, we modeled the appropriate interaction with Katie so the aide could see a profes-

sional willingly relinquish some apparent control in the interest of gaining a more fundamental level of control. Second, we helped her to move beyond framing the interaction with Katie in terms of winning and losing. Third, we had many conversations about how this intervention would reduce Katie's long-term need to control adults and other children in an unacceptable manner. Finally, we coached the aide in some of the staff scripts (e.g., the flexibility script) that we describe in Chapter 8. The net effect of this change in staff interaction with Katie was a dramatic reduction in her "bossiness" (see Figure 6–6).

Contingency Plans

After the new photograph routines, richly loaded with opportunities for choice and control, were in place, Katie rarely refused to do what was expected of her in school. On the occasions when she did refuse, staff responded with a script that included (a) a reminder that she was refusing her own plan, (b) an invitation to her to change some aspect of the plan, and (c) in the case of continued refusal to participate, an invitation to Katie to let staff know when she was ready to resume her plan. This proved to be a successful script.

Goal-Plan-Do-Review

During the intervention period, all staff engaged Katie in a scripted executive system routine (see Chapter 4). Each activity began with staff asking Katie what she was trying to accomplish (Goal); they then engaged her in a discussion of how hard it would be or how much she could get done (Prediction); next they worked with her to make a plan (Plan); finally, after completing the activity, they helped her reflect on how well she had done, what worked, and what did not work (Review). Katie was a goal-oriented person who liked this format for structuring activities.

During the initial baseline period, Katie's frequency of aggressive behaviors ranged from 4 to 7 per day (Figure 6–6). During the period of active intervention, frequency declined rapidly. There were zero incidents of aggression or attempted aggression for the last 2 days. Frequency increased to over 11 incidents per school day during the return to baseline and then returned to zero incidents when the intervention was again implemented.

Intensity of her aggressive episodes is represented in Figure 6–7. For Katie, aggressive episodes were rated by educational staff as "moderately serious" during the initial baseline condition. Intensity decreased during both intervention conditions. Removal of the intervention for the second baseline phase resulted in an increase in the intensity ratings to a level slightly higher than the original baseline. In addition to these quantitative data, the reports of instructional staff indicated that Katie's social and academic behaviors improved as an apparent consequence of the intervention. After the period of intensive intervention, staff maintained the positive routines for Katie, gradually fading the use of photograph cues and gradually reducing the amount of overt control offered to Katie. At last report (2 years after initiation of the intervention),

Katie was succeeding in school, with no resumption of the seriously challenging behavior that motivated the intervention. She was fully participating in her third grade curriculum with resource room support for reading, but with no classroom paraprofessional support.

Case Illustration: Adolescent Who Required Moderate Levels of Behavioral Supports

Tom was 18 years old when he was injured in a motor vehicle accident after a party with some of his high school friends. He was a passenger in the open bed of a truck from which he was thrown. Before his injury, Tom lived with his mother, father, and younger brother and sister in a rural setting. He had been classified learning disabled prior to the injury and had been suspended from school for fighting on at least three occasions. He was a senior in high school, although he was several credits short of meeting the requirements for his diploma in order to graduate with his classmates. His relationships with his mother and siblings were always strong, although he openly fought with his father prior to the injury.

Tom was in coma for 2 weeks and remained hospitalized for another 4 weeks after regaining consciousness. He was then admitted to a rehabilitation hospital where he received acute rehabilitation services for approximately 3 months. Hospital records indicated a severe right frontal lobe injury with contrecoup damage to the left occipital regions.

Tom's physical recovery was slow; he used a wheelchair for mobility until several months after discharge from the rehabilitation hospital. Rehabilitation staff reported a significant impairment of organization and declarative/episodic memory. However, their primary concern was his reportedly severe behavior disorder. He routinely refused to participate in therapies and, when he agreed to attend physical and occupational therapies, he often became aggressive during therapy activities. On several occasions he attempted to leave the hospital. A consequence-focused behavior plan (i.e., a token-economy system) was implemented with no success during inpatient rehabilitation. Tom earned no tokens, which resulted in his being excluded from all outings. He expressed contempt for the behavior management system and no interest in the missed outings, in part because his parents consistently took him into the community on weekends.

Tom's repeated and insistent demands to leave the hospital contributed to his discharge to home earlier than staff had recommended. At that time (approximately 4 months postinjury), he received a Verbal IQ of 91, a Performance IQ of 87, and a Full Scale IQ of 89 on the WAIS, which was only marginally depressed relative to his preinjury FSIQ of 93 on the WISC III.

Tom returned to school in November with the expressed desire to graduate with his class that year. Hospital and school staff agreed that this was an unrealistic goal, in part because he was not a good student prior to his injury and now demonstrated significant cognitive and behavioral challenges beyond those evident prior to his injury. However, despite significant impairment of episodic memory and explicit memory, Tom was able to learn information and academic skills with repetition, thereby succeeding on examinations despite weak explicit memory for what he had studied. Supported by his mother, Tom persevered and confounded the experts by accumulating the needed credits and graduating with his class the following spring.

Tom's family was most concerned with his aggressive behaviors at home (e.g., hitting his sister, his girlfriend, and his father). When relaxed, he agreed with his family that nonaggressive methods of handling difficult or anger-provoking incidents were best, but he was unable to follow these procedures when provoked. Furthermore, he vehemently rejected any feedback about memory or organizational problems and often threatened to physically assault anyone who confronted him about these deficits. Therefore, efforts to help him compen-

sate for cognitive impairment (e.g., systems for remembering assignments) and succeed academically were indirect and discrete.

Functional analysis revealed that problem behaviors, including aggression, typically occurred when Tom failed socially or academically and was confronted about that failure. The following episode, involving Tom and his girlfriend, is illustrative of these negative communication routines, which occurred with school staff, family, and close friends.

Tom	"Pick me up after school." (forgetting that his girl friend worked until 3:30 and assuming that she would pick him up at school at 2:30)
Friend	"OK, I'll see you after school." (naturally assuming that he intended her to pick him up at home after she finished work)
Tom	(After waiting in vain at school for several minutes, Tom rode home with a friend, complaining violently about his girl friend.)
Tom	(confronting his girl friend when she finally arrived at his home) "You promised to pick me up! You're a damn liar! You were with somebody else, weren't you?"
Friend	"No, you told me to pick you up after work. You know I love you."
Tom	"You're lying!" (curses and attempts to hit her)
Friend	(runs off crying)

The intervention that we negotiated with Tom and his family and friends, included the following components, all of which involved modification of his daily routines and were formally accepted by Tom.

Daily Routine: Tom began his day with a planning routine. After dressing and eating breakfast, he invited his mother to review his plan for the day. The plan included transportation to school, after school activities, and evening activities. Tom then called his girlfriend to confirm his plans, after which he recorded them in a planning book, which he consulted periodically throughout the day. In most cases, plans were recorded as sequential (e.g., I will do X after completing Y) as opposed to chronological (e.g., I will do X at 3:30 PM) because violations of time expectations had become a source of agitation for Tom.

School Routine: Tom followed a similar procedure to develop his plan for the day at school. At the beginning of the school day, he and his resource room teacher negotiated his daily plan, which included identifying the mainstream classes he would attend that day, setting specific academic priorities, reviewing activities that would likely be difficult for him to complete without assistance, and creating a plan for obtaining assistance when needed (i.e., "When should I ask for help? Who will be the best help to me"). Tom then ended his school day by engaging in a "What worked?/What didn't work?" routine with his resource room teacher. Because of Tom's historical sensitivity to confrontation, this review session emphasized a growing list of his strengths (which he referred to as his "super list") and strategic procedures that he could use to succeed, in addition to the necessary identification of academic and social tasks with which he struggled that day.

School Accommodations: In a problem-solving meeting with the behavioral consultant, all teaching staff agreed to allow Tom to leave class whenever he indicated that he was upset or angry.

Communication Routines With His Girlfriend: Despite frequent confrontations with his girl friend, confrontations that occasionally included physically aggressive behavior, Tom wanted to maintain the relationship. To achieve this goal, he knew that there must be changes in their interaction. Although Tom insisted that he was not the cause of the problems, he agreed to negotiate a positive communication system with our help. The negotiated communication routine included the following proactive components:

➤ At the beginning of their interaction, Tom and his girlfriend reviewed his general mood and determined in advance the circumstances that would result in her need to leave.

➤ Initially, the girlfriend accepted responsibility for initiating escape communication (with the scripted words, "I need to stop this") when Tom's anger began to escalate. She would then leave.

➤ After a few weeks of successful use of these procedures (i.e., no physical confrontations), Tom began to initiate the escape communication (using the scripted words, "We need to stop this"). He reported that he used this escape communication strategy because he knew that she would come back sooner if he took responsibility for his behavior with her.

Because this communication strategy was successful, the behavioral consultant invited Tom's girlfriend to model the strategy for Tom's younger sister, who, in turn, used it with some success. Tom's sister continued indefinitely to take responsibility for initiating the escape communication.

Monthly Reviews: We met with Tom monthly to complete a "What's working?/What's not working?" review. These meetings were attended by family members or others, as relevant. In addition to helping Tom maintain his positive behavioral momentum, these meetings served a support function for family members who frequently felt attacked by Tom and therefore had difficulty maintaining their optimism and resilience.

After 2 weeks of baseline, this intervention plan was implemented. Figure 6–8 presents frequency counts of verbal and physical aggression at home and at school. Despite initially slow progress, ongoing fluctuation, and an inability to eliminate verbal and physical aggression entirely, Tom's behavior improved markedly. By the end of spring, after 6 months of intervention, Tom's family, his girlfriend, and staff at his school all reported that the intensity as well as the frequency of his aggression had improved to a level that they considered acceptable. Furthermore, they all reported that they now knew how to help Tom and were optimistic about their future with him.

Tom graduated with his class. Four years later, a follow-up visit with Tom and his

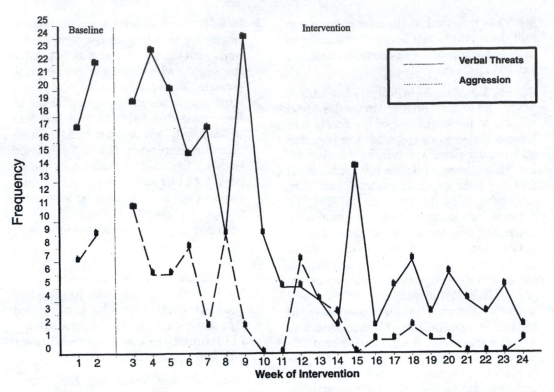

Figure 6–8. Frequency of aggression and verbal threats: Tom.

family revealed that he was living with a new girlfriend, had finished a job-training program, and was working as a landscaper. By report, he was getting along well with his family. Because of the nature of his injury, he remains vulnerable from a behavioral perspective and may be vulnerable for the rest of his life. However, Tom and the significant people in his life are competent in implementing antecedent-focused management strategies, which have enabled them to achieve a satisfying life together.

Case Illustration: Adult With Intensive Levels of Behavioral Supports

Al was walking on a dark stretch of road after an evening of drinking when he was hit by a car. Prior to the injury, he had lived alone and had prided himself on his independence his entire adult life. He had a history of service jobs, including gas station attendant, which he liked because he "loved to pump gas and help customers." However, he had lost several jobs in service stations because of unacceptable interaction with female customers. After losing a job, Al typically went on a drinking binge that lasted up to several weeks.

An MRI, completed 4 years after the injury, revealed right frontal lobe injury with specific dorsal focus and gross enlargement of the third and fourth ventricles. At that time, neuropsychological assessment resulted in a Full Scale IQ of 76 on the Wechsler Adult Intelligence Scale—Revised (Verbal IQ, 76; Performance IQ, 74). Following 20 months of acute inpatient rehabilitation, Al was discharged to a community reentry program that included support in one of their group residences. At that time, he spoke intelligibly, walked independently, but with an unusual gait (for which he was occasionally teased by peers in the program), and was independent in all physical aspects of daily living.

We were introduced to Al because of serious behavioral difficulties that had evolved in his community support program. He followed familiar routines without difficulty, but became disoriented and volatile when unexpected changes occurred in his routine. In addition, he frequently refused to participate in therapies and became belligerent when staff pushed him to do what was specified in his program. Specifically, he routinely refused to engage in prevocational programming. In addition, when residential staff engaged him in control battles about participation in the day program, he became verbally and physically aggressive. Al explained his resistance to the prevocational program by saying that he wanted to return to a service station job and that he was fully capable of doing this work.

With some encouragement, staff at the community support program finally chose to test Al's hypothesis, that is, to risk a trial placement for Al in a local service station. For the most part, his performance matched his predictions: He never missed work and demonstrated that he could manage the basic routine without help. Within 3 months of his employment, problems arose when Al started lingering after his work hours, frightening female employees. In addition, several female customers complained that he refused to terminate conversations with them, causing them to be concerned. When staff from the coordinating rehabilitation program counseled Al about these behaviors, he became upset, swore at the staff, and sometimes threatened physical aggression.

At that time, assessment of Al's relevant strengths revealed competence with specific vocational responsibilities, desire to succeed in the job, ability to follow routines, and willingness to work collaboratively with staff to solve problems and make plans for how to achieve his goals, but only when they raised the issues at the appropriate times and in a respectful and collegial manner. His weaknesses included serious episodic and declarative memory impairment (including difficulty remembering work assignments and day-to-day events), disorganized thinking and behavior outside the context of familiar routines, inflexibility and associated behavior problems with unexpected changes in his routine, difficulty interpreting the nonverbal communication of others, and generally weak social skills. Anecdotal reports of staff indicated approximately 15 episodes of negative interaction (including physically challenging behavior) with Al in his residence per week; Al's employer reported approximately 5 episodes per week of unacceptable interaction with coworkers or customers.

Assessment of staff communication competencies revealed frequent interaction with Al that was insensitive to his impairment. For example, disputes about past events were insensitive to Al's episodic memory impairment; office-bound counseling about behavior problems was insensitive to Al's need for change to occur in the concrete context of his daily routines; provocative accusations (which staff considered helpful verbal cues) were insensitive to Al's well understood disinhibition and dyscontrol. Al's interaction with staff in the community support program worsened as their need to address his socially unacceptable behavior on the job increased. The following pattern of negative interaction became increasingly routine:

Staff: (Informed that Al had intimidated a woman at work) "Al, what happened at work?"

Al: (curse) "You have no idea about my job."

Staff: "But Al, you know that you can't afford to get in trouble at work."

Al: (curse) "It's none of your business and my boss knows I'm a good worker."

Staff: "Al, your boss will not tolerate your behavior much longer."

Al: (curse) "You don't have any idea what it's like and how good a worker I am."

Staff: "It's inappropriate for you to stay around when they want you to leave."

Al: (more cursing) "Mind your own business!"

Staff: "You know if you keep this up, you're going to lose your job."

Al: (escalating) "Are you threatening me? My boss knows and if you say anything to him I'll beat you up." (curse)

Staff:	"That's unacceptable!"
Al:	(more cursing)
Staff:	(frustrated) "Al, you're not dealing with reality."

Intervention included the following components, each of which was negotiated with Al at a time when he was relaxed and able to focus on his goals and the means necessary to achieve those goals.

➤ **A daily planning regimen:** Each day began with Al dressing, eating breakfast, and then seeking out a staff person for review of the day's plan, made in writing and carried with Al in his daily planner.

➤ **A plan to deal with changes in the plan:** Al's plan to deal with unexpected changes in his plan or in his routines, which he referred to as his "shit hits the fan plan," included active solicitation of needed help. The cognitive script, which was written and which he followed explicitly, included the following sequence of self-prompts:

"What's the matter?"

"What should I do?"

"What are my choices?"

"Who can help me?"

"How will they help me?"

"OK, what's the new plan?"

It was critical that Al initiate seeking help when necessary, because his learned responses to unsolicited help from staff were negative.

➤ **Modification of Al's work contract:** We negotiated an arrangement with the work supervisor to modify Al's contract to include a social skills clause with two employee responsibilities:

1. After completing the work schedule, employees will leave the station.
2. After serving a customer, employees will thank the customer and then terminate the interaction.

The supervisor explained the modified contract to Al, reviewed the provisions once a week with Al for several weeks, and subsequently reduced the frequency of these reviews. The contractual obligation to refrain from unwanted social interaction with coworkers and customers was more meaningful to Al than the repeated "nagging" that had no effect in the preceding weeks.

➤ **Modification of staff interaction with Al:** Residential and professional staff were counseled to interact with Al in a manner that was consistent with his known deficits. This included sensitivity to positive and negative setting events, building positive behavioral momentum before confronting Al, and backing out of control battles before they escalate.

As of this writing, 12 months have passed with this plan in place. Al's employer remains generally pleased with his work. There have been few reports of challenging behavior at work (none over the past 3 months) and in the residence (one over the past 3 months). The residential staff report that the "shit hits the fan plan" has effectively reduced Al's level of disorganization and agitation during changes in routine. Although staff have ongoing difficulty allowing Al to make choices that they consider unwise, they are able to negotiate new plans with him. Al is currently seeking a job and living arrangements closer to home.

Behavior Change and Mutually Respectful, Collaborative Relationships

Having worked with several hundred children and adults with behavior problems associated with TBI, we believe that it would be disingenuous for us to assert or imply that successful intervention is exclusively the mechanical application of well-conceived management procedures. Many of the people with whom we have worked have reacted to professionals, initially including us, with an attitude ranging from skepticism to contempt. Many of the families and direct care staff with whom we have worked have been similarly suspicious of professionals, particularly those who propose modification of the familiar routines of their lives. In these cases, attempted intervention would likely have negligible results without the critical individuals coming to have respect for the professionals who are largely responsible for the proposals to modify routines.

It is no easy task to earn that respect or to describe the effort that goes into earning it. However, it is a step in the right direction to acknowledge that the first step in successful intervention is to earn the respect of the people whose behavior must change. In this section, we highlight what we consider important components of this effort, which are elaborated in Chapter 8.

Collaboration, Negotiation, and Experimentation

In interacting with individuals with challenging behavior, their families, and other important people in their lives, specialists in behavior and communication must present themselves as collaborators, intent on working with others to identify the most effective and, at the same time, the most comfortable intervention through a process of negotiation and experimentation. The interactive posture is not, "I will tell you what you must do to succeed," but rather, "How can I work with you to help you achieve your goals? What possibilities can we explore together in an attempt to change a negative situation into a more positive one?"

Respect

Implicit in an experimental and collaborative approach to intervention is respect for the individuals served. Respect is also tacitly communicated by engaging everyday people in the process of hypothesis-testing assessment described in Chapter 3. That respect can also be communicated more di-

rectly by frankly acknowledging that one is a "guest in their house," with no desire to impose mandates that are flatly unacceptable to the individuals served.

Effort

Implicit in respect is a willingness to work hard to help those who need help. For example, behavioral specialists who serve residential programs are invariably more successful if they willingly make themselves available at any time of night or day to help staff with behavioral crises. The point of this willingness is certainly not to engender helplessness in everyday people, but rather to create a solid working alliance with the people who make a difference. Similarly, individuals with behavior problems generally are able to distinguish between people who honestly try to help them and those who do their jobs in a less engaged manner.

Flexibility

Although the interventions described in this chapter share many common features, they also possess unique components created by applying principles flexibly to unique clinical situations. Flexibility is not only mandated by the uniqueness of each situation, it is also an attribute necessary to effective collaborative relationships.

Communication

The best plans in the world do not help if they are not communicated effectively to the people who need the plan. Many people with behavior problems after brain injury are adolescents and young adults from cultures and settings in which communication styles differ markedly from the style expected in rehabilitation hospitals, schools, and other professional settings. Therefore, specialists in behavior must possess the skill of communicating in a culturally sensitive manner, without appearing patronizing.

SUMMARY

In this chapter, we described the variety of possible contributors to behavioral outcome after TBI, factors that interact in complex ways, making prediction of outcome hazardous at best. We then presented an approach to behavioral intervention that emphasizes supports through manipulation of antecedents, with the goal of establishing positive everyday routines in which the individual with disability assumes as much control over his or her behavior as possible. A neuropsychological rationale for this approach is presented in Chapter 1. The chapter ends with case material representing varied ages and needs.

CHAPTER 7

Everyday Communication Routines

Our primary purpose in each of the intervention chapters of this book is to describe a functional and highly contextualized approach to helping people with types of disability commonly observed after TBI, in this case, communication disability. After a brief review of communication problems associated with TBI, we present the general themes that connect communication, behavior, and social skills, and review the rationale for intervention based on modification of everyday communication routines. Next we describe and illustrate with case material our approach to combined behavioral and communication disability and to social skills disability. Because the approach is equally applicable to children and young adults, we have selected cases representing a wide age range.

Earlier we cautioned the reader against separating executive function, cognitive, behavioral, and communication issues and interventions after TBI. For purposes of organizing a presentation of complex material, we have separated essentially inseparable themes into four distinct chapters. However, every individual used to illustrate intervention in each of these chapters had a disability that involved interaction among these four domains of human functioning. Therefore, individuals selected to illustrate themes in Chapters 4 through 6 could have been included in the present chapter, and those described here could have appeared elsewhere. We emphasize this integrative theme in part because it jus-

tifies a fiercely collaborative and integrative approach to intervention, in which varied professionals blend their assessments and interventions with one another and with the people who figure prominently in the routines of the person with a disability.

COMMUNICATION OUTCOME AFTER TBI

Virtually any combination of communication strengths and weaknesses is possible after TBI, depending on the individual's age and preinjury functioning, the nature and severity of the injury, and treatment and supports available after the injury. However, there are commonalities in the communication profiles of people with TBI, largely based on the frequency of prefrontal and frontolimbic injury. These commonalities are described in Chapter 2. In general, reviews of studies of communication outcome after TBI in children (Chapman, 1997; Chapman et al., 1995, 1997; Turkstra & Holland, 1998; Ylvisaker, 1993) and adults (Hartley, 1995; Sarno et al., 1986; Ylvisaker, 1992) have emphasized that communication profiles following severe TBI are typically quite distinct from those of adults with aphasia and children with congenital language disability. Specifically, linguistic knowledge may be retained, despite difficulties with the comprehension and appropriate use of language in the presence of cognitive stressors (e.g., demands for rapid processing or processing extended units of language) or social stressors on language processing (e.g., socially effective use of language in varied social contexts) (Chapman, 1997; Dennis, 1991, 1992; Dennis & Barnes, 1990; Dennis, Barnes, Donnelly, Wilkinson, & Humphreys, 1996; Dennis & Lovett, 1990; Groher, 1992; Hartley, 1995 ; Ylvisaker, 1992, 1993).

Organization and Language

During the past decade, several investigators have made effective use of discourse measures to identify subclinical language processing impairment in children and adults with TBI, particularly as that impairment is related to organizational difficulties (Biddle et al., 1996; Chapman, 1997; Chapman et al., 1995, 1997; Hartley, 1995; Hartley & Jenson, 1991; Liles et al., 1989; McDonald, 1992a, 1992b, 1993; Mentis & Prutting, 1991). Chapman (1997) reported that 75% of children with severe closed head injury demonstrated expressive discourse problems 3 years postinjury, which were frequently undiagnosed and untreated by the children's school staff. Impaired discourse may be evidenced in expressive language by disorganized and tangential conversations and monologues, imprecise language, or restricted output and lack of initiation. The same underlying organizational difficulty often results in word-retrieval problems. Receptively, organizational impairment may result in difficulty comprehending extended text or spoken language, detecting themes, and following rapidly spoken language. Some of these cognitive-language themes are addressed in Chapter 5. Ylvisaker, Szekeres, and Harbauer-Krupa (1998) presented a variety of intervention strategies for individuals with language-organizational impairment after TBI.

Language Processing and Flexible, Abstract Thinking

Linguistic and cognitive deficits also interact in producing commonly observed difficulties with abstract language, indirect language, and ambiguous language. Many children and adults with TBI interpret language concretely, fail to comprehend all but overlearned figures of speech and metaphors, and have difficulty shifting among alternate meanings of ambiguous words and sentences (Alexander et al., 1989; Dennis & Barnes, 1990). Concreteness in language processing can contribute to ineffective social interaction, particularly if the individual misinterprets as negative comments those that were intended to be sarcastic, ironic, or humorous, or in some other way had an intended meaning different from that received by the individual with brain injury.

Language and Memory

In Chapter 5 we explored the variety of memory and learning problems associated with medial temporal lobe damage (e.g., explicit and declarative memory) and prefrontal damage (e.g., strategic, deliberate learning). Children and adolescents with TBI return to school where they are expected to acquire new concepts and the language associated with those concepts. With significant new learning problems, children may increasingly fall behind their peers in knowledge, including language knowledge, over the years after the injury. Furthermore, if the control processes that facilitate strategic learning and strategic searches of memory are damaged, academic success is seriously jeopardized. The same observations apply to adults who return to college or vocational settings that require substantial new learining.

Communication and Behavior

Behavior problems after TBI, their etiology, and their long-term course were described in Chapter 6. Later in this chapter, we highlight the connection between communication and behavior.

Communication and Social Skills

As defined later in this chapter, social-interactive competence assumes adequate neurologically based capacities in many areas of functioning. Therefore, possible sources of disruption abound. From a neuropsychological perspective, orbitofrontal lesions are believed to be the primary contributor to the "pseudopsychopathic" characteristics (impulsiveness, aggressiveness, emotional lability, irritability, sexual excess, destructiveness) (Blumer & Benson, 1975) described in Chapter 2. In contrast, dorsolateral frontal or frontomedial lesions in adults, especially in the left hemisphere, have traditionally been associated with "pseudodepressive" characteristics, such as apathy, empty indifference, adynamia, loss of initiative, social withdrawal, slowness, and automatic responding in the absence of depression as a psychoreactive phenomenon (Blumer & Benson, 1975). Daigneault and colleagues (1997) recently presented the first known case of a young child with focal left hemisphere frontomedial damage and associated pseudodepressive symptoms. Both of these classical profiles are compatible with normal intelligence, language, and speech. Individuals with symptoms of the so-called pseudopsychopathic profile are typically diagnosed with a behavior problem, whereas those with symptoms of the so-called pseudodepressive profile are often said to have a social skills deficit or to be lazy or depressed. We highlight these two profiles because the frontal lobes are the most common site of focal lesion in closed head injury (Adams et al., 1980; Levin, Goldstein, Williams, & Eisenberg, 1991; Mendelsohn et al., 1992), the most common type of peacetime traumatic brain injury.

Social competence may also be weak for a variety of reasons not related to the injury. These reasons were described in some detail in Chapter 6. Many young people with TBI had checkered and sometimes unsuccessful social lives before their injury. Some experience severe psychological reactions to the injury and changes in life caused by the injury. Others grow progressively less socially competent because they have little opportunity to interact with others in varied social settings.

Taken together, these organic and reactive themes constitute what are often labeled personality changes after TBI: irritability, frequent loss of temper, impatience, emotional volatility, egocentrism, impulsiveness, anxiety, depression, loss of social contact, lack of interests, fatigue, and loss of initiation (Brooks & McKinlay, 1983; Brown et al., 1981; Jacobs, 1990, 1993; McKinlay, Brooks, Bond, Martinage, & Marshall, 1981; Petterson, 1991; Prigatano, 1986; Thomsen, 1984; Weddell et al., 1980). Most often, these personality changes present the greatest obstacles to satisfying family and community reintegration. Thomsen (1974) reported that 84% of family members surveyed complained of personality, behavioral, and emotional changes in their loved one with TBI. Furthermore, in adults with TBI, social-interaction challenges are associated with difficulty maintaining employment, living independently, and maintaining satisfying relationships with friends (Bond, 1990; Lezak, 1987b; Livingston & Brooks, 1988; Prigatano & Fordyce, 1986; Thomsen, 1984).

RATIONALE FOR ROUTINE-BASED COMMUNICATION INTERVENTION

Chapter 1 includes an extended explanation and justification of everyday routine-based intervention for cognitive, behavioral, and communication disability after TBI. In this section we highlight aspects of that discussion that are relevant to the current topic.

Transfer of Training

Historically, the nemesis of otherwise attractive communication, behavioral, and social skills interventions has been failure of transfer of training, that is, inadequate generalization and maintenance of newly learned responses or skills. In Chapter 1, we discuss transfer from both cognitive and behavioral perspectives. Reviews of the substantial efficacy literature in social skills intervention have highlighted the infrequency with which skills acquired in a training setting transfer to and have an impact on social interaction and social relations in natural environments (McIntosch, Vaughn, & Zaragoza, 1991; Vaughn, McIntosh, & Hogan, 1990; Wiener & Harris, 1998; Zaragoza, Vaughn, & McIntosh, 1991). Behavioral psychologists increasingly have addressed the problem of generalization by attending to features of the universe of instruction and implementing general-case instructional technologies in natural environments (DePaepe et al., 1994; Glang, Singer, Cooley, & Tish, 1992; Horner, McDonnell & Bellamy, 1986; O'Neill & Reichle, 1994; Pierce & Epling, 1995; Pierce & Schreibman, 1994). With the goal of effectively generalized and maintained positive communication behavior, the universe of instruction ideally includes a range of stimulus and response variation that adequately represents the individual's real world of interaction with others. That is, instruction occurs in the context of the people, places, activities, and stressors that are associated with challenging behavior or weak social skills. General-case instruction mandates the use of varied teaching opportunities and multiple critical examples from the initial stages of intervention. In these respects, current behavioral approaches to teaching have departed from the tradition within which instruction was initiated under training conditions that did not closely resemble the anticipated application environment, with generalization and maintenance targeted at a later stage, if at all. Cutting through a great deal of important detail, the more current approaches translate in our vocabulary into teaching communication and social skills as much as possible within the routines of everyday social life (Halle & Spradlin, 1994).

Time and Resources

In brain injury rehabilitation, a second and powerful rationale for everyday routine-based intervention is the dramatic reduction in funding for specialized rehabilitation. Managed care organizations place extraordinary pressure on rehabilitation specialists to effect positive functional outcomes with steadily decreasing reimbursed time to generate that effect. Under these economic conditions, wise management of resources dictates rapid identification of appropriate teaching routines and efficient training and orientation for everyday people so that they are in a position to effectively use these teaching opportunities as they arise over the course of the day.

Collaboration

When specialists in communication and behavior opt for everyday, routine-based intervention in dealing with challenging behavior, there is no escaping the need to collaborate with everyday communication partners from the beginning (Carnevale, 1996; Lucyshyn & Albin, 1993; Lucyshyn et al., 1996). This commitment to collaboration offers several important advantages. First, involving everyday communication partners as collaborators in assessment increases the number and variety of observations that can be made, while also orienting everyday people to an experimental approach to intervention (see Chapter 3). Second, when everyday people are actively engaged in assessment and decisions about intervention, the likelihood of their compliance with the intervention plan tends to increase. Third, involvement of everyday people in all stages of the process is an efficient training tool, increasing the likelihood that they will be able to creatively and effectively modify interventions and supports as new issues arise in the future. Fourth, with the involvement of everyday people from the early stages of intervention, potential obstacles can be identified and addressed, including rejection on the part of everyday people of the positive communication alternatives or social behaviors that have been established as treatment objectives, insufficient support for everyday people to implement the intervention in their natural environment, and others. Finally, involvement of everyday people from the beginning increases the number and variety of natural learning trials for the individual with disability, thereby facilitating more rapid acquisition of positive communication alternatives and more efficient generalization.

The Need for Practice

Implicit in the discussion of collaboration is the obvious point that abandoning a negative behavior or style of interaction that has been adequately successful and adopting a positive alternative typically requires considerable practice. Modifying communication routines of everyday life is one effective way to achieve adequate numbers of meaningful learning trials (Doss & Reichle, 1989; Halle, 1989). Whereas a person may have 5 or 10 or 20 learning trials in a specific interactive competency within an hour-long speech-language therapy session or social skills group session, that number can be multiplied by a substantial factor if everyday communication partners know how to create and appropriately use learning opportunities throughout the day.

Knowledge Versus Functional Use

Unlike many people with severe developmental disabilities, those with acquired brain injury typically retain knowledge of social rules, roles, and routines, and of the communication options considered positive alternatives to their challenging behavior (see later discussion of "can't do," "won't do," and "doesn't do"). That is, they may not need to be taught the repertoire of behaviors (e.g., words, gestures, social acts) considered positive communication in their social context. Rather, they require coaching and support in their everyday routines so that they routinely make functional use

of their knowledge of positive communication (Ylvisaker & Feeney, 1994). In these cases, it makes little sense to implement a lengthy and resource-intensive phase of intervention designed to practice behaviors out of communication context, behaviors that they do not need to learn (because they are already in the preinjury knowledge base), but do need to practice in social context. However, there is often value in exploring and negotiating communication alternatives to challenging behavior outside the context of everyday communication routines. Jack and Andy, whose cases are described later, are good illustrations of the value of this negotiation.

EVERYDAY COMMUNICATION ROUTINES: TEACHING POSITIVE ALTERNATIVES TO CHALLENGING BEHAVIOR

In the developmental disabilities literature, it has been well established that acquiring, generalizing, and maintaining a set of positive communication behaviors that are functionally equivalent to preexisting challenging behavior can have a profoundly positive effect on community integration for those with a history of negative behavior (Bellamy, Newton, LeBaron, & Horner, 1990). Not surprisingly, this awareness has spawned burgeoning clinical and research interest in the technology of teaching positive communication alternatives to challenging behavior (Burke, 1990; Carr & Durand, 1985a, 1985b; Carr et al., 1994; Durand, 1990; Durand & Carr, 1991; Reichle & Wacker, 1994). Although deceptively simple at its core ("If you don't like what he's doing, teach him a positive way to accomplish the same goal"), the process of teaching positive communication alternatives requires careful functional assessment of the problem behavior, thoughtful decisions about the communication alternative, and intervention that is well conceived and skillfully implemented. Furthermore, this approach to intervention invariably encounters serious obstacles along the way. Much of our work in brain injury rehabilitation has included flexible application of this technology to serving people with challenging behavior after their injury (Feeney & Ylvisaker, 1995, 1997; Ylvisaker & Feeney, 1994; Ylvisaker, Feeney, & Szekeres, 1998). Proactively teaching positive communication alternatives should be understood as a component of the antecedent-focused behavior management discussed and illustrated in Chapter 6.

Rationale for a Communication-Based Approach to Challenging Behavior

Functional communication training as an approach to behavior management is based on several straightforward premises. First, all behaviors, including the apparent absence of behavior, communicate (Burke, 1990; Carr et al., 1994; Durand, 1990). Whatever a person may be doing, it is possible to ask meaningfully, "I wonder what he is trying to tell us by doing that." Of course, this is not to say that all behavior is intentionally communicative. For example, mothers report that their newborns *tell them* that they are hungry, sick, tired, happy, and the like. However, newborns are not *trying* to communicate anything. Their reflexive behaviors combine with context cues to signal to familiar communication partners something about the infant's internal state. Furthermore, the behavior of people of any age and level of functioning can be and often is misinterpreted. Nevertheless, a starting point to positive behavior management is recognition that an individual's behavior is part of his or her communication system.

Specialists in functional communication training often group the socially motivated behaviors of people with challenging and unconventional behavior into two broad classes: *access-motivated behavior* (i.e., attempting to acquire the attention of others or a preferred activity, person, place, or thing) and *escape-motivated behavior* (i.e., attempting to escape nonpreferred demands, activities, people, places, or things) (Du-

rand, 1990; Durand & Crimmins, 1992). In many cases after TBI, challenging behavior functions as a declaration of *control*, possibly in the absence of specific access or escape intentions. Undesirable behaviors such as screaming, hitting, spitting, withdrawing, and others typically communicate one of these general messages. Some behavior is not socially motivated (e.g., laughing while watching TV alone, crying in pain, providing oneself with stimulation), although nonsocially motivated behavior can easily become socially motivated, depending on the response of communication partners (Carr et al., 1993, 1994; Taylor & Carr, 1992b).

Just as the communication behavior of an infant begins as unintended and gradually becomes increasingly deliberate as the child matures and learns to associate specific behaviors with specific effects, so also behavior that is purely reflexive in the early stages of recovery after brain injury (e.g., tugging at tubes, lashing out at others when confused and agitated) can become deliberately used communication behaviors if the individual learns over time that this is an efficient way to achieve important goals (e.g., gaining comforting attention from nursing staff, terminating a painful therapy session). Ylvisaker, Feeney, and Szekeres (1998) described a young man whose serious self-injurious behavior after TBI had just such a natural history.

Staff must be particularly alert to this possible evolution of challenging behavior in the case of individuals with TBI who are particularly impulsive. People with serious orbitofrontal injury may act in a reflexive, impulsive, and possibly perseverative manner, resulting in others interpreting their behavior as a call for help, or possibly as aggression, and responding in an overly positive way (e.g., by lavishing attention) or in an overly negative way (e.g., by punishing the individual or withdrawing). In these cases, which may be difficult to distinguish from cases of genuine learned aggression, the best intervention is redirection, as in the case of the reflexive and impulsive behavior of infants. The primary behavioral goal during the days, weeks, or months characterized by minimally regulated behavior of this sort is to ensure that staff and family responses to negative behavior do not have the effect of transforming it into learned behavior patterns that then become entrenched components of the individual's communication system. Unless this stage of recovery is prolonged, it may *not* be necessary to teach positive alternatives to negative behavior.

The second premise is more accurately a corollary of the first: There are few truly maladaptive behaviors (Carr & Carlson, 1993; Donnellan, Mirenda, Mesaros, & Fassbender, 1984; Taylor & Carr, 1992a). Although there are exceptions to this rule (e.g., extreme forms of self-injurious behavior associated with rare syndromes), it remains a healthy heuristic principle. Furthermore, it is dangerous to refer loosely to challenging behavior as maladaptive, because that label easily predisposes family and staff to attempt to extinguish the behavior without attempting to understand its communication function. If the behavior does serve an important communication function, it will prove difficult to extinguish, and if the extinction program is successful, an alternative behavior that may be more challenging than the original is likely to emerge. Therefore, identifying behaviors by their function serves an important practical purpose. On the other hand, if the behavior is purely reflexive or impulsive, it is best to label it as such, to help communication partners refrain from taking the behavior personally and responding punitively.

Our third premise follows logically from the second: If challenging behavior is used to communicate a message, then it is far preferable to offer a positive communication alternative than to attempt simply to extinguish the challenging behavior (Carr et al., 1994; Durand, 1990; Horner & Budd, 1985; Horner & Day, 1991). To be sure, it is a noble goal to help a person move beyond behavior that has a negative effect on social integration. However, teaching a positive alternative, if successful, guarantees improved social interaction, whereas successfully extinguishing the negative behavior without offering a substitute may or may not have a positive effect, depending on the new behavior the individual ultimately uses to communicate the intended message.

Our fourth and fifth premises were explained and defended in an earlier section of this chapter on routine-based intervention and in Chapter 1: The primary agents of change are everyday communication partners, and change in social behavior is most efficiently effected by modifying routines of everyday communication (Carr et al., 1994; Durand, 1990; Lucyshyn et al., 1996; Wacker et al., 1990; Ylvisaker & Feeney, 1994). These final premises imply that the primary responsibilities of specialists in communication and behavior are to coordinate, with everyday communication partners, a functional analysis of the individual's challenging behavior, collaboratively design an intervention plan with the components listed in the next section, educate, train and support everyday communication partners so that they are competent in providing contextualized teaching, monitor the effects of the intervention, and coordinate collaborative modifications of the intervention if it is not successful.

Procedures for Teaching Positive Communication Alternatives

The premises listed in the previous section as well as critical aspects of intervention are presented in Appendix B in a behavior plan jointly written by a speech-language pathologist and a behavioral specialist. We offer this plan as a model and as a way to underscore the importance of professional collaboration. If the communication (i.e., speech-language pathology) plans and reports are separate from the behavior plans and reports, it is likely that the intervention program will be fragmented and less effective than a fully integrated program. The model report (Appendix B) makes reference to most of the following six phases of teaching, which are often not as neatly distinguishable as they appear in our presentation of them. Furthermore, a given phase can require days or weeks of intensive collaborative effort or can be accomplished in a few minutes, depending on a variety of factors.

Collaboratively Interpret the Challenging Behavior

Chapter 3 presented an assessment framework in which relevant staff and everyday communication partners observe the individual in a variety of contexts, formulate hypotheses about the meaning or function of the challenging behavior, and test those hypotheses as deliberately and experimentally as possible. Applied to behavior, what we referred to as contextualized hypothesis testing is a form of functional assessment of behavior.

This functional assessment must be sensitive to the distinct possibility that a behavior may have multiple functions or meanings. For example, hitting may serve an escape function on some occasions and an attention-getting function on others. In behavioral terms, hitting would belong to at least two different response classes (Carr, 1988), requiring at least two different positive communication alternatives. Conversely, a variety of challenging behaviors may all serve the same function, that is, belong to the same response class. For example, a person may hit, scream, run, or withdraw to communicate a need to escape an activity or demand. In this case, it may be desirable to teach one positive alternative for the entire response class.

To help communication partners correctly interpret the individual's behavior, and therefore prompt the appropriate communication alternative, the recommendations for teaching in natural communication contexts may need to specify the behavior and surrounding context (Cooper, Walker, Sasso, Reimers, & Donn, 1990; Durand et al., 1993; Emery, Binkoff, Houts, & Carr, 1983; Kern et al., 1994; Sasso et al., 1992). For example, if a child appears ready to run or

scream after receiving a present (positive stimulus), the prompted communication alternative may be something like, "Great! This is great! Thank you." On the other hand, if the same behaviors seem likely midway through a difficult academic task (aversive stimulus), the prompted alternative may be, "Break? Can I take a break?"

The group of collaborators initially gathered together to interpret challenging behavior often includes the person with the disability. For example, Jack (described below) was invariably accurate in explaining why he acted in an aggressive way. In most cases, either he perceived an insult and intended to punish the perpetrator or he objected to a lack of control and chose to fight as a means of asserting his right to choose. In cases in which individuals lack insight into the purpose of their challenging behavior, therapeutic value may reside in engaging them in brainstorming about possible purposes, thereby perhaps bringing them incrementally closer to an accurate understanding of their behavior.

Collaboratively Decide When Escape and Access are Acceptable

People with a significant history of negative behavior require many learning opportunities if the teaching is to be successful (Berkman & Meyer, 1988; Horner & Budd, 1985; Horner et al., 1993). Therefore, if they are learning positive ways to communicate escape or access, they require many natural occasions for practicing this communication. Staff may need to terminate a therapy session in response to the individual's positive escape communication even though they know that the therapy is very important. At this point in the planning process, objections are invariably raised by staff or family members who resist allowing the individual the extent of escape or access that they believe is called for in the new plan. We offer solutions to this natural objection below. At this point, we wish to highlight two important points. If one or more members of the intervention team choose not to honor the individual's positive access or escape communication alternative, the likelihood that the individual will continue using the new behavior is thereby reduced. Worse yet, if a battle ensues and the individual ultimately wins by using the old challenging behavior (e.g., escapes an unwanted therapy by hitting the therapist), the probability of retaining the successful negative behavior is greatly enhanced. Therefore, basic agreement in goals of the program is necessary and it is critical to choose battles wisely.

Collaboratively Select a Positive Communication Alternative

The developmental disabilities literature contains important findings that pertain to the selection of a positive communication alternative (Carr et al., 1994; Durand et al., 1993; Horner & Budd, 1985; Horner & Day, 1991; Mace & Roberts, 1994). For the individual, the alternative must have the following characteristics:

➤ *Easy to Produce:* The positive communication alternative must be at least as easy to produce as the challenging behavior it is intended to replace. It is unreasonable to expect that people will abandon an effective and relatively easy mode of communication (e.g., screaming) if the alternative is difficult to produce.

➤ *Satisfying:* The positive alternative must be satisfying, meeting the individual's aesthetic and emotional standards. Jack (described below) illustrates this point. He needed an alternative to physical aggression to express his anger. However, he demanded that the alternative adequately express his feelings, which polite words failed to do. Similarly, we have worked with children and adults with TBI who rejected augmentative communication systems as their alternative communication (e.g., Ben, described below) on grounds that they did not like the voice, the device was too bulky and stigmatizing, or it was simply too difficult to use.

➤ *Effective:* The communication alternative must be at least as effective as the challenging behavior. It is unreasonable to expect that people will abandon an effective and relatively easy mode of communication (e.g., screaming) if the alternative is less effective in achieving their communication objective.

➤ *Promptable:* The alternative should be promptable. In the early stages of teaching, it is helpful to be able to prompt the alternative quickly and efficiently so that the teaching routine can proceed with normal pacing and without flirting with a return to the challenging behavior. This consideration supports the use of simple gestures or a communication display, both lending themselves to physical prompts. However, in many cases (e.g., Mark, described below), the positive communication alternative can be spoken words.

➤ *Interpretable:* If the alternative is not interpretable to most communication partners, it will not be routinely honored, will likely come to be associated with frustration and anxiety, and will therefore be rejected.

For communication partners, including strangers in the community, the communication alternative must be interpretable and must meet basic standards of acceptability. If the positive alternative is dysarthric speech that most people have difficulty understanding, success of the intervention is jeopardized. Similarly, if the alternative is objectionable to many people (e.g., touching or hugging as a way of requesting attention), the intervention is jeopardized (Durand et al., 1993).

An interesting variation on the theme of positive communication alternatives occurs when the alternative to challenging behavior is a self-directed communication. We have worked with many adolescents and young adults with TBI who react aggressively to even slight provocation from others. In this circumstance, it is common for hostile peers to deliberately provoke these reactions. Our job as communication and behavior coaches is to help the individual with TBI to recognize that hostile peers are successfully exercising control when he or she reacts strongly to their taunting. Therefore, the positive communication alternative to aggression, in an extended sense of the term, is a self-regulatory (subvocal) comment like, "I'm in control, not him; don't give him the satisfaction of a reaction."

Collaboratively Ensure a Large Number of Successful Positive Communication Routines Daily

Table 7–1 illustrates communication routines, some contrived and others naturally occurring, in which the student, Jon, either spontaneously or following a prompt, uses positive communication behaviors to communicate escape or access. The general form of the teaching routine, whether contrived or spontaneously occurring, is as follows

Person with TBI: The discriminitive stimuli for escape or access communication are present; the person gives the first signs of this intent.

Staff: Interprets the person's intent, based on context cues and the person's behavior. The person has not yet used challenging behavior.

Staff: Prompts the positive communication alternative (e.g., "Want to tell me you need a break?")

Person: Uses the communication alternative (e.g., "Break, OK?")

Staff: Rewards the positive communication (e.g., "Great, no problem. We can take a short break. Thanks for letting me know.")

Timing is critical in these teaching interactions. If the staff member waits too long and the person resorts to negative behavior, which may then be followed by a reward (i.e., escape or access), the teaching has an effect opposite of its intended ef-

fect—the negative behavior is strengthened. Second, these teaching interactions change over time as communication partners fade their prompts. Fading may be rapid or extremely gradual in the case of those who have longstanding patterns of negative communication and who rely on slow procedural learning because of significant memory impairment.

When we work as consultants with staff or family members, we typically draft sample scripts of the sort illustrated in Table 7–1 and urge the everyday communication partners to set as a goal 100 or more positive communication routines of this sort per day—or at least 10 successful communications with the positive alternative for each successful use of the challenging behavior. It is often helpful to videotape a familiar communication partner engaged with the individual in the positive communication routines. This video is then made available to others, with the request that they create as many of these positive routines as possible in their interaction with the person with challenging behavior. Furthermore, it is useful to ask everyday people to keep track—if only loosely—of the number of successful positive communication routines of the sort that have been scripted and videotaped. When staff and family members are asked to count *positive* routines (versus the more common request that they count episodes of challenging behavior), the likelihood increases that they will focus on their primary role, namely as facilitator of positive communication alternatives.

Gradually Reintroduce Normal Demands

During the early phases of teaching positive communication alternatives to individuals with longstanding use of challenging behavior, staff and family members must be prepared to honor many of the individual's requests to escape unwanted activities or demands and to access preferred activities and things (Carr et al., 1994; Durand, 1990). At some point—ideally sooner rather than later—normal daily routines and rea-

TABLE 7–1. Illustrations of positive communication routines for Jon.

Escape: Contrived communication situations

Context: Math instruction; assume that math is currently not a high priority and is not a desired activity.

Adult: "Here's your math book, Jon."
Jon: Looks unhappy, but hasn't yet acted.
Adult: "It looks like you don't want to do this now. Here, show me 'no' (or "break" or whatever)."
Jon: Is prompted to use positive communication alternative.
Adult: "OK! Thanks for telling me! Let's not do it now. We can come back to it later. It's great that you tell me that way that you don't want to do this. Let's do … OR Show me what you would like to do for a few minutes …"

This teaching sequence could be repeated several times during a 20–30 minute scheduled math period.

Escape: Natural communication situations

Context: Teacher wants Jon to carry his lunch box as he walks down the hall.

Adult: "Here Jon, carry your lunch box."
Jon: Reacts negatively, but does not yet fall to the floor or engage in any other negative communication.
Adult: "I bet you don't want to carry the box, do you? Why don't you tell me no?"
Jon: Is prompted to use positive communication alternative.
Adult: "Oh!!! Alright! I see you want me to carry it. Thanks for telling me so nicely. Of course I'll carry it when you ask like that."

Access: Contrived communication situation

Context: Jon is with other students and clearly wants to get a peer to interact with him. The peer has been alerted to respond when Jon uses the positive communication alternative.

Adult: "Jon, I bet you would like to talk with Tim. Why don't you tell him?"
Adult: Prompts the positive communication alternative.
Jon: Uses the positive communication alternative.
Peer: Responds to Jon's positive communication alternative: "Oh Hi Jon. I didn't see you. Thanks for letting me know you want to talk."

Access: Natural communication situations

Context: Jon is at home and it is time for him to do something he likes to do (e.g., watch TV).

Adult: "Jon, I wonder what you want to do. I bet you would like to watch TV. Can you let me know?"
Adult: Prompts the positive communication alternative.
Jon: Uses the positive communication alternative.
Adult: Responds to Jon's positive communication alternative: "OK, great, here's the remote. Thanks for telling me that you wanted to watch TV."

sonable demands must be phased back into the person's life. We have yet to be involved with intervention programs wherein this return to acceptable work expecta- tions was impossible. That is, individuals with whom we have worked never became persistent "escape monsters" or "access monsters" as a result of this approach to intervention. However, success in this early phase of teaching often mandates intensive use of the antecedent-focused procedures described in Chapter 6. Communication partners may need to be hyperalert to the presence of positive and negative setting events, may need to create considerable positive behavioral momentum before demanding performance of difficult or non-preferred tasks, may need to provide ample opportunity for choice and control in the individual's daily routine, and may need to be hypervigilant about the difficulty level of the individual's tasks.

With these cautions and procedures in place, we are invariably confident that normal routines and expectations for work can be reintroduced. Most often, successful implementation of this intervention results in the individual accomplishing more rather than less productive work. In contrast, if the individual's setting events are generally negative, if he or she perceives life as unacceptably restrictive, or if tasks are routinely perceived as too difficult to accomplish, then the intervention is unlikely to be successful.

Monitor and Modify

Finally, success of all behavioral interventions requires careful monitoring, with possible recycling of the entire process in the event of failure. This monitoring should use real-world indicators of success. In their review of the efficacy literature in the field of positive approaches to challenging behavior, Meyer and Evans (1994) lament the infrequency with which investigators select adequate dependent variables in investigating the effectiveness of their interventions. Meaningful monitoring includes documentation of increases in positive interaction and decreases in negative interaction in varied real-world communication contexts, a measure of the effort and supports needed to achieve and maintain the positive outcome, and a measure of satisfaction—on the part of the individual with disability and communication partners—with the new communication routines. Psy-

chometrically validated data collection forms are available to meet some of these objectives (e.g., Durand's Motivation Assessment Scale [MAS]; Durand & Crimmins, 1992). However, others may require ad hoc program monitoring systems, possibly including thoughtful (subjective) judgments from relevant individuals.

Obstacles to Success and Strategies for Overcoming the Obstacles

In attempting to implement functional communication training as an approach to behavior management for individuals with challenging behavior, we routinely encounter combinations of the following obstacles. We are convinced that each obstacle can be successfully removed; however, skilled salesmanship and a collaborative spirit are often required to do so.

Staff Commitment to the Overriding Importance of Their Discipline-Specific Goals

Often therapists, teachers, vocational specialists, and others object that their specific goals and objectives are too important to be jeopardized by a communication and behavior program that may require them to honor the individual's request to terminate work or to engage in less productive activities. This commitment to discipline-specific goals and objectives is admirable and should not be slighted in the negotiation process. However, the following observations are often sufficient to convince staff to work with the communication and behavior program.

➤ Often the individual's participation in therapies, instruction, or vocational activities is limited by the challenging behavior prior to the implementation of the behavioral intervention. Success in the functional communication training program typically results in a net increase in productive time in these settings.

➤ Positive escape or access communication in a therapy or work setting can often be honored with a short break or brief engagement in a preferred activity (e.g., 3 to 5 minutes), without seriously jeopardizing therapeutic efforts in those settings.

➤ If the behavior problem is significant, staff and family may need to be reminded of its devastating long-term effects on the individual and communication partners.

➤ If discipline-specific objectives have overriding importance, then those sessions can be identified as *no choice* times (see below).

Staff and Family Concern That the Individual Will Exercise Unacceptable Levels of Control

In our work, we anticipate the objection that this intervention will turn the individual into an "escape monster" (e.g., "He'll never do another minute's work the rest of his life!!") or an "access monster" (e.g., "He'll be bossing me around all day!"). This reaction is natural and must be respectfully addressed. When a long history of conflict between staff or family and the individual exists, the objection may be an expression of frustration or of a more problematic sentiment, namely, a refusal to give the individual the satisfaction of any victories in any power struggles. In this case, the response to the objection may need to have more of a counseling component than that described in the next paragraph. In addition, it may be helpful to model interaction with the individual, showing reluctant staff members how they can *win* even though (or, better, *because*) they are enabling the individual to make choices and thereby feel competent and in control.

In other cases, staff and family members are less concerned with control and more concerned with the individual's long-term well being. For these people, the short and somewhat cavalier sounding reply to their objection is that it simply does not happen; people do not turn into escape or access monsters. This reply must be expanded to include all of the cautions described earlier in the section "Gradually Reintroduce Normal Demands." That is, normal demands must be reintroduced in an environment in which staff and family members attend to all of the proactive procedures explained in Chapter 6. In addition, an experimental spirit is helpful for skeptical staff. The intervention can be introduced as a test of a hypothesis, empowering staff to modify or terminate the approach if their fears materialize.

Staff and Family Concern That Some Activities Are Mandatory, Others Forbidden

Related to the last objection is the natural concern that there can be no choice about some components of the individual's routine. For example, medication may be critical; going to school or work may be necessary, despite the individual's objections; the person must eat and bathe. The appropriate response to this concern is that it is absolutely correct. About some demands, there will be no negotiation. In these cases, it is useful to teach communication partners and the individual with challenging behavior a *no choice* script (e.g., "No choice, John. You will get on the bus and go to school. But you can choose which seat you want to sit on.") to contrast with the *choice* script that he knows is more frequent (e.g., "Choice time, John; do you want to do A, B, or C?"). In addition, the antecedent-focused procedures described in Chapter 6 can be used to increase the likelihood of compliance with *no choice* activities. Staff and family members should make every effort to ensure that *choice* times heavily outweigh *no choice* times.

Staff and Family Conviction That Behavior Management Is Somebody Else's Job

In our experience, most professionals recognize that specialists in behavior management play a critical leadership role in developing, implementing, and monitoring behavioral programs, but that everybody who interacts with people with challenging behavior on a routine basis is essential to the effectiveness of the intervention. In those rare cases in which team members refuse to embrace their role in behavior management and functional communication training, the approach may be through the supervisory system or may directly target the reluctant staff person. Supervisors are well advised to ensure in staff job descriptions that cross-disciplinary areas of functioning, like communication and behavior, are approached in an appropriately collaborative manner. Ylvisaker and Feeney (1998) listed communication and behavior competencies that could be added to the job description of any staff person who comes in regular contact with people with communication and behavior impairment after TBI.

Persuasive conversations with reluctant staff and family members emphasize the importance of positive communication and behavior patterns that enable the person to achieve a satisfying community life, along with the brutal reality that generalization and maintenance of positive communication behaviors are unlikely in a setting in which expectations for and interaction with the individual substantially differ from partner to partner. Therefore, the responsibility for implementing the intervention is necessarily distributed among everyday people in the person's life.

Staff and Family Difficulty With Timing

In our earlier brief description of teaching routines, we highlighted the importance of timing. If communication partners wait too long for positive communication behaviors, the individual with disability is likely to resort to challenging behavior, which in all likelihood will be reinforced in some way. Written scripts (e.g., those presented in Table 7–1) are useful training tools. However, more useful is a videotape of a competent communication partner modeling these incidental teaching routines. We like to use family members or direct care staff as the models for several reasons: They are often among the most competent facilitators of positive communication; if they are not, then making the video holds the potential to improve their competence; using these people as models is a statement of respect; and the implicit message in using a family member or aide as the model is that this teaching is everybody's business!

Case Illustrations: Communication Alternatives to Challenging Behavior

Case Illustration: Child With Aggressive Behavior Requiring Moderate Supports

Background. At the time of our intervention, Mark was a 7-year-old boy who was injured at age 5 in an automobile-bicycle accident. Medical records indicated that Mark suffered multiple-site skull fractures with an associated closed head injury resulting in focal right frontal injury, presumably combined with widespread diffuse injury less easily detected by CT scan. He received treatment in an acute care hospital for 2 weeks before transfer to an inpatient rehabilitation facility, where he remained for an additional 2 months. School and medical records indicated no preinjury history of neurologic, developmental, learning, or behavior problems.

At the time of his injury, Mark was in a half-day kindergarten program and was described by his teacher as a bright child who "easily mastered every part" of the curriculum. Despite the fact that he was the youngest child in his class, Mark was said to be socially mature and had many friends before his injury. His family, which was and continued to be supportive, included two parents and three siblings in the home.

At age 7 (2 years postinjury), Mark evidenced significant residual physical disability. He was able to use a rolling walker to navigate smooth surfaces for short distances but typically required a wheelchair for mobility throughout the school. He also had a severe communication disability, including speech which was halting, dysarthric, and unintelligible to unfamiliar persons. He demonstrated impaired memory, including difficulty remembering daily events and academic instruction, and reduced information processing capacity, being able to follow only simple familiar one-step commands. However, once information was well understood and encoded, he retained it well and could effectively retrieve the information when cued recall or recognition memory tasks were used. Planning and organizational difficulties were evidenced by extremely disorganized personal effects (e.g., cubby area, tote bag) and frequent forgetting of things and classroom routines. His WISC-III full scale IQ was reported to be 79, which was significantly depressed relative to preinjury estimates.

After returning home from the inpatient rehabilitation center, Mark completed his kindergarten school year with home instruction and home therapies. His parents reported no noteworthy behavioral difficulties during this period at home. Mark returned to the school and participated in a first grade class the following academic year. Despite the help of a one-to-one paraprofessional aide, he had difficulty meeting the academic and interpersonal demands of the class, largely because of his severely slowed processing and memory problems. With significant academic accommodations and schedule changes, he managed most of the demands of the classroom. However, challenging behaviors emerged during this first year back in school, almost 2 years postinjury. When confronted with tasks that were cognitively demanding (e.g., a weekly spelling quiz) or physically demanding (e.g., walking with minimal support of others), Mark responded with physical aggression, including hitting and throwing objects at people (but not in a way that was dangerous). Initially he only hit his aide, but he subsequently also hit peers who came close to him when he was

acting out. The assumed purpose of the negative behavior was to escape from tasks that were threatening or unpleasant. Unfortunately, the unintended result was increasing social isolation, emerging attitudes of helplessness and self-pity, and many removals from the classroom. Mark generally accepted help when he recognized the need for it; however, when help was offered in the absence of this recognition, he responded with intense and sustained aggressive behavior.

Intervention

Intervention occurred in a first grade classroom of a small rural elementary school. Mark's class included 10 female students, 14 male students, 1 teacher, and 1 paraprofessional aide assigned to Mark, who was the only student identified as needing special education services. Prior to initiating the intervention, Mark's daily routine began with a teacher or paraprofessional aide reminding him of his schedule and assignments. Reminders were then intermittently given throughout the day, often when provoked by Mark's off-task, inappropriate, or oppositional behavior. For this reason, they probably were perceived by Mark as nagging, thereby increasing the likelihood of a negative response.

Closely monitored and integrated behavioral, cognitive, and communication intervention, which lasted for slightly over 3 weeks, was offered in the context of tasks at the same level of difficulty and delivered by the same educational staff as during the baseline period (with some support from us). The intervention was designed to improve Mark's behavior and communication by modifying the routines that had become contributors to his negative behavior, thereby increasing the likelihood of a positive functional outcome which would be maintained in Mark's school life.

Four substantive changes were made in Mark's classroom routines: His daily routine was negotiated, made more explicit, and designed to be sensitive to the need for positive setting events; staff helped Mark learn a positive communication alternative to his negative behavior; staff gave Mark cognitive support with photograph cues; and staff initiated an executive system routine that gave Mark a greater sense of control and served as additional cognitive support.

Daily Routine. Mark's daily routine was collaboratively task analyzed by instructional staff, consultant, and Mark. This group then made decisions about the minimum amount of work that needed to be completed (for Mark to accomplish his goals). The sequence of tasks to be accomplished was negotiated between Mark and the instructional staff. In some cases, the sequence of activities was nonnegotiable (e.g., lunch, certain group activities). However, the goal of negotiation was to ensure that Mark was engaged in planning and decision making, and also to ensure successful performance. Furthermore, an attempt was made to place an activity Mark preferred (i.e., a positive setting event) before every mandated or nonpreferred activity to increase the likelihood of compliance.

Escape Communication. A critical component of the intervention was a concerted effort on the part of staff to teach Mark a positive communication alternative to aggression as a means of communicating the need to escape. Because the functional analysis of Mark's aggressive behavior indicated that he was trying to escape or avoid some aspect of the classroom activity, it was important to teach an alternative that communicated the concept "stop" or "I don't want to." The positive communicative alternative (saying "I'm done" or "I'm finished") was easy for Mark to use and was easy for the staff to prompt.

Despite reservations, classroom staff agreed to implement this plan because they were keenly aware that their current plan was ineffective. Furthermore, the new plan resulted from guided negotiation and was understood to be the first in a set of options that they would try in sequence (another was removal to a self-contained special education class). That is, staff did not believe that they were acting under duress or that they lacked the authority to change the plan if it proved to be ineffective. Importantly, we spent several days in the classroom modeling the intervention for the teacher and paraprofessional staff, showing them that their primary fear—that Mark would do no work at all if he had the right to escape by saying "I'm done"—was groundless. That is, Mark frequently said "I'm done," but invariably, after no more than 5 minutes, returned to the activity. Some staff remained unhappy about Mark routinely "being let off the hook," but were persuaded to implement the program because of its resounding success in eliminating aggression.

Classroom staff used the following procedures to teach Mark to use his positive communication alternative when he wanted an activity to end or felt a need to reject an activity. At the end of each fully completed activity, the staff prompted Mark to verbalize "I'm done" or "I'm finished" before terminating the activity. That is, staff helped Mark create a routine in which saying "I'm done" or "I'm finished" preceded termination. In addition, when Mark began to appear upset, angry, or frustrated within an activity, staff quickly created a natural point of transition (e.g., finishing a math problem, finishing reading a sentence, finishing painting with one color), then modeled the key phrase ("I'm done" or "I'm finished") and prompted Mark to imitate the model. This was done in a nonthreatening, conversational manner so as not to create yet one more demand that might elicit an oppositional response from Mark. When he said "I'm done" or "I'm finished," Mark was allowed to leave the activity area. If he did not say the words, staff presented one more model; if Mark still did not respond, staff then said, "Great, thanks for telling me you're done" (pretending that Mark had spoken the last modeled utterance) and moved on, thereby avoiding a confrontation and still procedurally connecting "I'm done" with termination of activities.

With staff and parents, we also negotiated *choice* and *no choice* times. The nonnegotiable (i.e., no choice) activities were riding the bus in the morning and afternoon (which Mark hated), lunch, and PT (which the team considered extremely important for Mark). With ample opportunities for choice (for example, initially he was free to say "I'm done" in the middle of academic activities), Mark had few sustained difficulties with the *no choice* activities. However, within PT sessions, Mark had ample opportunity for choice. During the active intervention period, Mark refused a *no choice* activity (PT) only once. On that occasion, he later negotiated a make-up time with his aide and completed the requisite PT exercises.

Prior to the intervention, typical interactions between Mark and classroom staff had the following structure:

Staff:	(approaching Mark to tell him that it's time to begin an academic activity) "Mark, come over hear and begin your reading."
Mark:	"No way, I'm not gonna do that, I don't want to, I can't read anyhow."
Staff:	"Now you know that we've got to learn to read, and it's *our* reading time now."
Mark:	"No, no, no! I'm not! I won't! I hate you! (lots of cursing)."
Staff:	"Now Mark, that's inappropriate language for school, and you know that *we* don't talk like that in school."
Mark:	(more cursing and attempts to hit the staff person, resulting in removal from the classroom)

A component of Mark's intervention was planning time at the beginning of the day. He used photographs to keep himself organized. During planning time he also practiced his escape communication. The following exchange is typical of the early morning interaction during planning time.

Staff:	(looking at pictures of Mark engaged in specific classroom activities) "OK, Mark, let's look at the day, first there's

Show and Tell Circle—what's your job?"

Mark:	"I need to sit and wait for my turn, and then talk when it's my turn."
Staff:	"Right, now what happens if you're having a hard time in the Circle?"
Mark:	"I tell you that I'm done."
Staff:	"Yep, then what happens?"
Mark:	"I go to my chair until I'm ready."
Staff:	"You got it!" (Flipping to the next picture) "Then it's Computers—what's your job here?"
Mark:	"I get to turn on all the computers and pick the program."
Staff:	"Yes sir, and remember what happens if you're having a hard time?"
Mark:	"I know, I know."
Staff:	"OK, great."

This continued until the plan for the day was made.

The following teaching interaction is typical of the help he received when frustrated or angry during the intensive intervention period and continuing as part of Mark's ongoing classroom routine:

Staff:	(approaches Mark, showing him his reading photograph) "Mark, I see that it's time for reading."
Mark:	"I see. I know."
Staff:	"O.K. pal, what are you reading?"
Mark:	"Five Dancing Ducks."
Staff:	"Great book, I laughed, I cried, I loved it."
Mark:	(begins to flip through the book) "I hate this! I don't want to do this. I'm done."
Staff:	"O.K. buddy, you know what to do."
Mark:	(goes to his seat)
Staff:	"Let me know when you're ready."
Mark:	(after a few minutes passes, he approaches the teacher) "How much do I have to read?"
Staff:	"Let's look at the book and you tell me. Is this a hard book or an easy book for you?"
Mark:	"Easy."
Staff:	"Oh yeah, you've read it before then, right?"
Mark:	"No!"
Staff:	"Oh really, then how'd you know it's easy?"
Mark:	"I don't know, I just know!"

Staff: "Gee, let's go through it together and then we can figure out how hard it is to read."

Mark: (sits next to staff and attempts to read a page with great difficulty) "I hate this book!!"

Staff: "It looks like a pretty hard one to read."

Mark: "Yeah, it's hard."

Staff: "So how much do you want to try before you're finished?"

Mark: "Five."

Staff: "OK, you'll read five pages and I'll help if it gets tough. Then you're done with this activity; sounds like a plan."

Mark: (reads the book)

Mark's parents eagerly implemented the escape communication program at home. They were concerned about the attention that Mark was receiving for negative behavior and were understandably upset about the disruption of family life caused by Mark's aggressive behaviors and tantrums. We also spent time with Mark's older brothers who expressed some resentment about Mark's special treatment. With this assistance, the brothers came to appreciate that the communication training would ultimately result in Mark contributing more rather than less to family life.

Cognitive Support: Photograph Cues. Because Mark's difficulty with complex tasks was related in part to his organizational impairment, classroom staff and the consultant recognized the need to provide him with organizational support that would not appear to Mark to be unwanted nagging. Therefore, they experimented with photograph cues as advance organizers for complex tasks. Fortunately, Mark liked this procedure and it helped him to stay on task. He invited peers and his aide to take photographs of him engaged in a variety of tasks. In some cases, the activity materials were sufficient cues and Mark took a picture of those cues (e.g., he took a picture of his cubby to represent the concept "hang up your coat and put your backpack away"). The pictures served as both advance organizers and ongoing references. All photos were held in a small binder. Mark selected the photographs that he particularly liked and used them proudly

This cognitive support was a critical component of the plan to teach positive communication alternatives to challenging behavior. As long as Mark's work was perceived by him as overwhelming, he would be likely to continue the aggressive behavior that had successfully enabled him to escape hard work in the past, or he would use his new escape ticket "I'm done" in response to the presentation of most tasks, and staff would consider the experiment a failure. Therefore, his work had to be doable and the photograph cues contributed to making the work do-able without the "helpful verbal cues" of his aide, which were often perceived by Mark as nagging.

Executive System Routine. Additional cognitive support took the form of a planning or executive system routine. Using a Planning Form similar to the Executive Function Routine Form described in Chapter 4, the instructional staff helped Mark to create a concrete plan at the beginning of his activities and to review his performance after completing the activity. Both planning and reviewing were as simple and conversational as possible. This planing routine included the following elements:

1. an initial decision about or choice of a goal ("What are you trying to accomplish?");

2. a decision about how easy or difficult it will be to accomplish the goal ("Is this going to be hard or easy?");

3. development of a plan to achieve the expressed goal ("What materials do we need? Who will do what? In what order do we need to do these things? How long will it take? What kind of help might you need?");

4. a quick review of the goal, plan, and accomplishments at the end ("What were you trying to accomplish? How'd you do? How'd you do it?"); and

5. a summary of what worked and what didn't work, a summary of what was easy and what was difficult, and why.

Outcome

During the week of observation before the intervention began, Mark's frequency of aggressive behavior ranged from 8 to 11 episodes per school day. Four of the 5 days, the frequency was 10 or 11 episodes. The frequency and intensity of these behaviors were considerably higher than that of the other students in the classroom. However, the staff and peers in the classroom were committed to Mark's success, so their level of tolerance was high. During the 2 weeks of intensive intervention with a routine that included photograph cues and staff facilitation of positive communication alternatives to aggression as a means to communicate escape, Mark's frequency of aggression decreased to zero in 4 of the last 6 days. Frequency increased to six or more episodes per day when staff reinstituted the nonsupportive classroom routines that were in place for Mark before the intervention. This

return to baseline convinced staff that the intervention was instrumental in improving Mark's behavior. Therefore, they resumed the intervention and Mark's frequency of aggression rapidly returned to low levels. These data are presented in Figure 7–1. Staff subsequently continued the supportive routines for the remainder of the year, with steadily decreasing need for them to prompt positive communication alternatives and a correspondingly decreasing frequency of Mark's escaping academic or other tasks.

In addition to frequency counts, the intensity of Mark's negative behavior was measured using the disruption elements of the Aberrant Behavior Checklist (Aman & Singh, 1994). Before intervention, Mark's frequent episodes of aggression were rated on average as moderately severe. During the intervention period, the infrequent episodes of aggression were rated as mild. During the subsequent brief withholding of the intervention, severity ratings increased to their preintervention level. This was followed by reinstatement of the intervention and a return to acceptable levels of intensity of behavior.

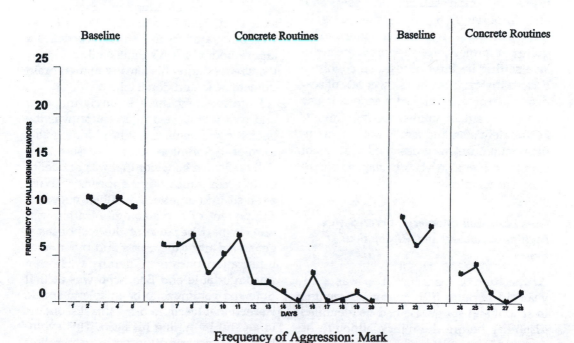

Frequency of Aggression: Mark

Figure 7–1. Mark's frequency of aggression during baseline and intervention periods.

Interviews with staff following the short-term intervention indicated strong positive impressions of its effects. There was consensus that the intervention was educationally relevant, that the procedures were helpful in the reduction of challenging behaviors, and that the procedures contributed to an increase in work-related behaviors. At the end of the school year, the school team and Mark's family reported that problem behaviors were not a concern for them any longer, and, because of his increased levels of positive behaviors, he was much better accepted by his peers. The classroom teacher specifically commented on Mark's increased levels of work following the initiation of the photograph routines. To their credit, the first grade teacher and Mark's paraprofessional aide initiated interaction with the second grade teaching staff to ensure that Mark's cognitive, communication, and behavioral supports would be in place for him the next year. The first grade staff offered three training sessions to the second grade staff. A follow-up interview found that Mark had adjusted well to his second grade class and new peers and, most importantly, that there were no significant behavioral issues. He continued to require paraprofessional support in the inclusive setting because of residual cognitive deficits that resulted in a slower rate of academic learning. Mark had a serious injury and may remain vulnerable indefinitely. Fortunately, staff and family know that implementation of well-designed systems of support can enable Mark to succeed socially and academically.

Case Illustration: Adolescent With Severe Multiple Disability and Self-Injurious Behavior

At the time of his injury, Ben was a 10-year-old popular fifth grader, succeeding in school and sports. He had no identified disability before the injury, although he was said to be rather stubborn. He had two siblings and divided his time between his divorced parents, one of whom, his mother, was remarried. In the spring of fifth grade, Ben was delivering newspapers when he was hit by a car. His multiple injuries included severe bilateral frontal lobe injury as well as diffuse damage throughout the brain. His right frontal and parietal regions were almost totally obliterated by the impact and subsequent surgery. Ben was in an acute care hospital for 6 months, 6 weeks in intensive care and a total of 4 months in coma.

Ben's inpatient rehabilitation, which began 6 months after the injury, was marked by frustratingly slow progress. As he emerged from coma, he began to touch the right side of his skull with his right hand, presumably because of the itching or discomfort associated with the healing process. Videotapes made at the rehabilitation hospital indicate that staff focused on this behavior, trying to extinguish it with verbal prompts (e.g., "No, Ben, your hand must stay here on the tray") or by physically holding Ben's hand away from his head. When Ben persisted and the interaction escalated into a conflict, staff occasionally responded by terminating their therapy session with Ben. To be sure, the staff was well-motivated in this strategy because a large amount of Ben's right skull was gone, thereby rendering his already injured brain vulnerable to additional injury.

Unfortunately, this seemingly innocent and well-intentioned intervention was the beginning of Ben's use of head hitting as a form of communication. In his case, an initially reflexive behavior that was not deliberately communicative appears to have evolved into an effective, albeit negative, component of Ben's communication system, in part because of the responses it generated from therapists and other communication partners. Therapy was often uncomfortable and Ben, who was at that time and continues to be unable to speak, learned that he could bring this discomfort to an end by hitting his head. This evolution of communication gestures parallels the gradual emergence of illocutionary communication acts in early child development, similarly associated with the pattern of responses of everyday communication partners.

After 3½ months of inpatient rehabilitation, Ben's parents removed him from the program, against professional advice, because they were impatient with his slow progress. At that time, he was quadriplegic, unable to walk, and unable to talk or use his arms and hands effectively as a result of severe oral and limb apraxia. He was fed through a gastrostomy tube because of a pharyngeal swallowing disorder that was gradually resolving. He was alert and comprehended simple language directed at him, but had no expressive communication modality other than gross, undifferentiated vocalization and gestures.

Over the next year and a half, Ben's rehabilitation and special education program evolved from home therapy and tutoring (3 months) to a developmental disabilities classroom, then to a classroom for children with severe behavior problems, then to a classroom for students with autism, and finally to a private school for students with behavior problems. In each setting, staff attempted to manage Ben's escalating self-injurious and aggressive behavior with consequence-oriented procedures that they were accustomed to using with their other students. For example, in the first classroom placement, the behavior management system focused exclusively on consequences (token economy, including response cost [i.e., Ben lost points for bad behavior]). When Ben refused to participate in assigned activities, staff attempted to force compliance physically. His challenging behavior escalated. At the same time, school staff attempted to have Ben resume oral eating, using contingency procedures (e.g., loss of privileges for refusing food). This program was unsuccessful and contributed to Ben's increasing use of challenging behavior to communicate his desire to escape from demands and undesirable activities.

Subsequent classrooms similarly relied on contingency management, including punishment, with steadily increasing use of physical intervention. Many staff asserted that Ben's behavior was unrelated to his injury. They perceived his negative behavior to be willful, necessitating forceful measures to teach him that he must comply with the instructions and rules of authority figures. In each setting, his behavior worsened. This worsening was exacerbated by Ben's clearly indicated distaste for the social and developmental mix of students in these classrooms, for the infantilizing tasks he was required to perform in the developmental disabilities classrooms, and for the system of rewards (e.g., stickers, points) and punishments (e.g,. denial of privileges) that he considered insulting.

By 2½ years after the injury, Ben was 13-years-old and his self-injurious and aggressive behavior had reached such a level of frequency and intensity that his parents sought a second inpatient rehabilitation program, despite their deep suspicions of rehabilitation professionals. It was in this program that we came to know Ben and his family. On admission, his behavior was characterized by frequent and severe self-injury (hitting himself in the head), aggression toward objects (e.g., overturning chairs and tables), and infrequent aggression toward people. The positive, antecedent-focused, communication-based interventions described in Chapter 6 and earlier in this chapter were initiated during this admission, with the effect of increasing positive, socially acceptable communication and, as a consequence, completely extinguishing self-injurious and aggressive behavior. With periodic consulting support, this approach to intervention was reinitiated at important points over the subsequent 8 years after Ben's discharge.

A simple experiment confirmed that Ben's head hitting served an important communication purpose, namely escape from undesirable tasks or situations. In half of Ben's therapies and instructional sessions, the staff was instructed to look for the first sign of escape-motivated behavior. They then took his hand (before he had a chance to hit himself on the head) and quickly shaped it into a gross gesture for "stop." Staff then thanked Ben for telling them that he wanted a break and respected his wishes (i.e., discontinued the activity). In those therapies, the frequency of head hitting was quickly reduced to zero. In the therapies and instructional sessions in which staff did not prompt and respect the "stop" communication, Ben's frequency of head hitting remained high. Two weeks after his admission, a facility-wide program was implemented to teach Ben to use his hand gesture for stop as an alternative to head hitting as an effective way to communicate his desire to escape a demand or activity. Subsequently, the teaching program was expanded to include other communication situations and other communication acts. The general assumption was that Ben's negative behaviors were communication acts and that, with few exceptions, they communicated either *escape* (i.e., a desire to escape an activity, demand, person, or place) or *access* (i.e., a desire to gain access to an activity, someone's attention, a place, or simply increased stimulation).

Some staff members voiced the concern, invariably expressed at this stage of teaching positive communication alternatives, that this teaching would turn Ben into "an escape monster." That is, if staff and family members could escape any task he wished to escape? The concern is a natural and legitimate one. Fortunately, it has—and had in Ben's case—a relatively simple answer. Teaching communication alternatives to challenging behavior does not produce "escape monsters" or "access monsters" (i.e., people who get whatever they want when they use positive request communication), *if the teaching is accompanied by other positive intervention procedures and by a clear distinction between choice and no choice situations*. In Ben's case, it was critical to add intensive use of other antecedent control procedures (including positive setting events, positive behavioral momentum, and choice).

With all of these management procedures in place, the staff was able to reintroduce less desirable and more difficult tasks. For example, Ben did not like potentially painful physical therapy procedures. During the period of intensive teaching of his gesture for "stop," staff invariably respected this gesture and Ben escaped the difficult PT tasks. Once the positive escape communication had been learned, staff reintroduced PT exercises by preceding them with high success tasks (behavioral momentum), by ensuring that Ben was in a generally good state (setting events), and by giving him a choice of PT exercises (choice). Ben still had a sense of control and knew that if he persisted in gesturing "stop," his wishes would be respected. Within a relatively short period of time, all of Ben's therapies and instructional sessions had been resumed, with a higher level of productivity than before the intervention, when he routinely protested with self-injurious and aggressive behavior. The staff was understandably pleased with Ben's heightened engagement and the associated increases in effectiveness of their interventions.

This teaching process was repeated when Ben's behavior deteriorated after several months back in school. Later, staff and family members added a variety of other communication gestures for escape (no, quit, leave me alone) as well as communication acts for requesting access to things, activities, and people (e.g., raise hand for access to people's attention). Subsequently, additional communication gestures and more complex messages were added to Ben's repertoire.

In addition, staff and family devoted considerable effort to helping Ben understand and discriminate between *choice* and *no choice* situations. For example, going to school or—in Ben's current situation—going to work may be a *no choice* situation, whereas within the school or work day, there may be many opportunities for choice and many occasions when staff know that they should honor positive escape or access communication. During his inpatient rehabilitation, with a primary focus on teaching communication alternatives to challenging behavior, Ben was always given choices regarding activities and places in which to engage in those activities. When he returned to school, staff routines included presenting embedded choices along with no choice demands. For example, Ben had no choice about getting on the school bus, but he was routinely reminded of the choices he had once on the bus (e.g., where to sit, what music to listen to, and the like).

Figure 7–2 presents an instructive 10-year history of Ben's alternation between periods of generally positive and generally negative behavior. We have carefully analyzed the circumstances of Ben's life and have discussed this history with Ben's mother, who has a deep understanding of her son and the influences on his behavior. In our judgment, two critical factors explain the profound pendulum swings in his life: (1) the degree to which he is actively and respectfully engaged in personally meaningful activities and (2) the use of proactive as opposed to reactive behavior management procedures.

Engagement in Meaningful Activities. Ben's early behavioral deterioration after returning home following his first rehabilitation admission appeared to be related in large part to his perception that the activities assigned to him in school were infantilizing and meaningless (e.g., highly repetitious drills with preschool-level tasks). Furthermore, none of his new peers fit his preinjury understanding of an appropriate social group. In retrospect, his classroom placements and curriculum were probably chosen with insufficient attention to Ben's strong sense of self, which was shaped by his successful preinjury life. In fairness to the educational decision-makers at the time, Ben's profile of abilities seemed to be consistent with their decisions. However, a critical lesson to be derived from Ben's story—and those of many children and adults like him—is that decisions about intervention and support must account for the individual's sense of self.

Ben's vocational experiences illustrate the positive impact of personally meaningful activities. He began vocational training in a supported work environment 7 years after his injury. Over the following 3 years, his behavior at school fluctuated. There were periods of admirable compliance followed by periods of noncompliance and aggressive behavior, depending on the way in which staff related to him and tried to manage his behavior. However, through all of these fluctuations at school, Ben had no episodes of negative behavior at work. He liked his job (which included manual tasks, such as cleaning and stocking shelves in the back room of a bagel shop) and indicated that it gave him a sense of competence. Furthermore, his paycheck provided strong validation of his sense of personal worth, despite severe ongoing disability.

Proactive Behavior Management. Retrospective analysis of Ben's 10-year history clearly reveals that traditional, consequence-oriented behavior management systems were associated with steadily deteriorating behavior. In contrast, implementation of positive, antecedent-focused, communication-based management procedures, described in Chapter 6 and the current chapter, invariably succeeded in turning the negative behavioral tide and creating positive communication and behavioral routines. As of this writing, Ben is 10-years postinjury, maintains a part-time job with minimal support, continues to receive some functional academic instruction through his school district, and is beginning to prepare for a move to supported living.

The series of arrows in Figure 7–2 is both ominous and encouraging. The arrows are ominous in that they reveal how vulnerable Ben remains in relation to environmental stressors and traditional management procedures. His life could easily take a turn for the worse and, without an alert person to put intervention and supports back on a positive track, spiral out of control. Furthermore, the series of alternating arrows

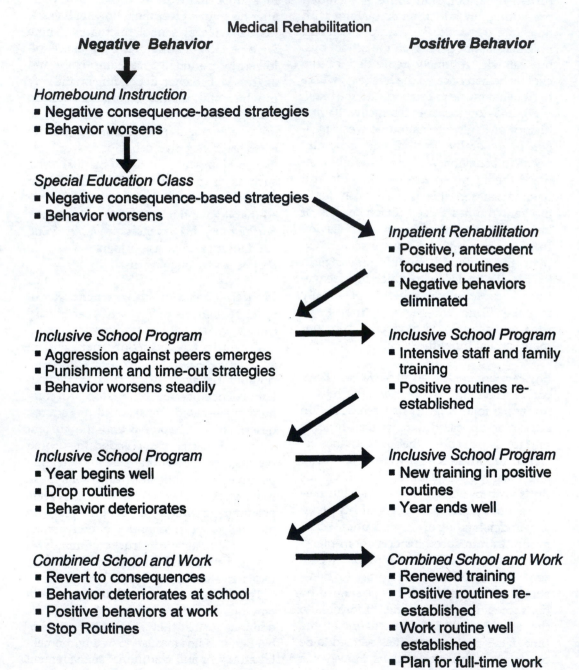

Ben

Severe TBI

Medical Rehabilitation

Negative Behavior

↓

Homebound Instruction
- Negative consequence-based strategies
- Behavior worsens

↓

Special Education Class
- Negative consequence-based strategies
- Behavior worsens

Inclusive School Program
- Aggression against peers emerges
- Punishment and time-out strategies
- Behavior worsens steadily

Inclusive School Program
- Year begins well
- Drop routines
- Behavior deteriorates

Combined School and Work
- Revert to consequences
- Behavior deteriorates at school
- Positive behaviors at work
- Stop Routines

Positive Behavior

Inpatient Rehabilitation
- Positive, antecedent focused routines
- Negative behaviors eliminated

Inclusive School Program
- Intensive staff and family training
- Positive routines re-established

Inclusive School Program
- New training in positive routines
- Year ends well

Combined School and Work
- Renewed training
- Positive routines re-established
- Work routine well established
- Plan for full-time work program

Figure 7–2. A 10-year history of dramatically alternating behavioral conditions in an adolescent with TBI.

bespeaks a system of intervention in which insufficient attention is given to "passing the torch" to the next level of care or the next stage of education. At several points in his educational career, Ben's staff had developed solid competence in interacting with him and managing his behavior. However, in some cases they neglected to provide sufficient orientation and training to the next team, with the sad—but avoidable—consequences depicted in Figure 7–2.

On the other hand, there is great encouragement implicit in the ongoing possibility of halting such a downward behavioral spiral. In Ben's case and in others (e.g., Feeney & Ylvisaker, 1995), we have found it possible to effect positive communication and behavioral outcomes in the face of great pessimism based on gloomy neurological predictors and on a lengthy history of negative behavior and undesirable communication routines.

Case Illustration: Young Adult With Aggressive Behavior Requiring Intensive Supports

We include the following brief case illustration to underscore the cultural conflicts that frequently arise when teaching positive communication alternatives to challenging behavior. Jack was 19 years old when he received a severe closed head injury in a motor vehicle accident. Early neurodiagnostic reports indicated multiple right frontal subdural hematomas with descending glial lesions, diffuse bilateral temporoparietal hematomas, and contrecoup injury to the left cerebellum. Jack was reported to be a bright, but somewhat unmotivated student before his injury, receiving Bs with little effort. There was a history of substance abuse, including alcohol and marijuana. His mother reported that he had a fierce temper, willingly accepted invitations to fight, and received multiple suspensions from high school for fighting. He was taking classes at a community college at the time of the injury.

Jack's 8 weeks of acute-care hospitalization were followed by 4½ months of acute inpatient rehabilitation. As he became increasingly alert during his rehabilitation admission, he also became increasingly aggressive. His preinjury tendency to resolve conflicts physically was seriously exacerbated by the volatility and lack of inhibition associated with his frontal lobe injury. He frequently challenged staff verbally and physically and, on more than one occasion, was accused of assaulting another patient on his unit.

Staff and family agreed that Jack needed a way to express his anger that stopped short of physical aggression. Jack agreed, but insisted that polite options (e.g., saying something like, "I'm sorry, but I find that very upsetting") were out of the question. This was simply not the way he communicated with anybody; it was not natural or satisfying and he would not do it. Furthermore, he claimed, and his family confirmed that, if he left the hospital communicating in this way, he would be an outcast in his social world. After some negotiation, Jack agreed that he would try to express anger with a readily interpretable middle finger gesture rather than physical aggression. Some staff vehemently objected to this proposal on grounds that the proposed "positive communication alternative" was itself unacceptable behavior. However, they reluctantly agreed with the plan after a long conversation about cultural relativity at this level of values and about the goal of rehabilitation, which is to reenable a person with disability to succeed in his or her chosen setting and culture.

The speech-language pathologist accepted primary responsibility for helping Jack to habituate the finger gesture as a substitute for aggression. Sensitive to problems surrounding transfer of training, she accompanied Jack to the nursing unit, dining area, and other common areas in and out of the facility. When she sensed that Jack was becoming angry at somebody (based on previous interaction with Jack in similar circumstances), she modeled the finger gesture and encouraged him to imitate the model. Furthermore, she accompanied the model with words like "I'm not going to let that jerk get to me" or "I'm a winner; he's a loser; blow him off." The goal of the intervention was to practice behaviors, including self-instruction procedures, in real communication contexts so that they would become automatic, knowing that procedural memory was a considerably stronger memory system for Jack than declarative memory. Furthermore, when Jack directed the gesture at his therapists, their scripted response was to say something like "OK, you need a break; cool." They would then return to the task when Jack no longer appeared agitated.

After 2 weeks of this intervention, reported incidents of physical aggression were reduced to zero, although Jack continued to have serious difficulty with anger control, including frequent verbal challenges. As a result of ongoing functional communication intervention, verbal aggression was eventually reduced to acceptable levels. At that point Jack was transferred to a postacute rehabilitation facility for additional rehabilitation in a less restrictive setting. Although staff at the new facility were fully oriented to his short temper, his need for control, and the importance of his self-selected communication options, they chose to set different goals for him—goals that they considered more appropriate. Furthermore, they employed traditional, consequence-oriented behavior management systems (e.g., token economy, level system) that Jack considered infantile and to which he responded in a predictably explosive manner. The frequency of Jack's physical aggression, by their report, increased rapidly under these conditions and remained high throughout his admission to that facility. After 8 months of participation in this program with minimal progress, his family removed him from the program.

Jack's story illustrates many important themes in communication and behavior. First, Jack's cognitive profile, like that of many people with TBI, mandated teaching

of the communication alternative in real communication contexts and within the framework of procedural versus declarative memory. Second, rehabilitation professionals must recognize that they are helping people to succeed in their own cultural milieu, which might value very different communication patterns from those considered acceptable in a rehabilitation hospital. Furthermore, positive communication alternatives to challenging behavior are unlikely to succeed if the alternative is unappealing, emotionally unsatisfying, or difficult to produce. Negotiation is often the key to selection of the alternative. Finally, the high risk group for TBI—risk-taking adolescents and young adults—is filled with people like Jack who respond violently to attempts at overt external control. Jack was completely clear about his need to feel in control. This need was respected in the negotiated, antecedent-focused program in his acute rehabilitation facility. Unfortunately, the need for control was not respected in the postacute facility, with negative consequences for Jack and staff alike.

EVERYDAY SOCIAL ROUTINES: TEACHING SOCIAL SKILLS

Social skills include the general competencies and situationally relative behaviors that enable a person to be accepted and possibly liked in chosen social settings. Socially skilled people are able to affect others positively and with the effect that they intend to have and are capable of being affected positively by others the way others would like to affect them. These broad definitions imply that the domain of social skills intervention is extensive and that the characteristics and behaviors that constitute social competence must be identified in relation to specific contexts, cultural values, and communication partners. Taken together, these two axioms of social skills intervention convincingly legislate against the logistically simple but overly simplistic approach within which a limited set of skills is selected as a curriculum and taught exclusively by means of role playing in a training context.

As depicted in Figure 7–3, socially skilled people have adequate awareness of their own interactive strengths and weaknesses, are reasonably comfortable with themselves as social agents, posses adequate knowledge of relevant social rules, roles, and routines, are able to correctly perceive and interpret the social behavior of others, communicate their intentions effectively and in ways that are considered situationally appropriate by others and flexibly shift communication styles to meet changing social demands. They also know how to enter into interaction with others, comfortably maintain that interaction, and negotiate conflicts. They dress and groom themselves in ways that are considered appropriate in their social milieu, and are understood and accepted by members of the social groups with which they choose to affiliate.

Reflection on the domains of functioning listed in the last paragraph and illustrated in Figure 7–3 leads inescapably to the conclusion that many helping professions have a legitimate stake in the delivery of social skills intervention, including psychology and social work, education and special education, speech-language pathology, occupational therapy, vocational rehabilitation, nursing, and family counseling. By itself, this multiplicity of helping professionals mandates vigilant attention to integration of services and supports. Acknowledgment of the internal fragmentation characteristic of many people with severe TBI intensifies this need for vigilance.

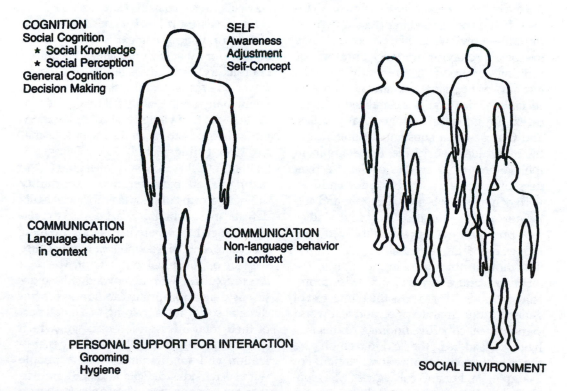

SOCIAL SKILLS

COGNITION
Social Cognition
★ Social Knowledge
★ Social Perception
General Cognition
Decision Making

SELF
Awareness
Adjustment
Self-Concept

COMMUNICATION
Language behavior
in context

COMMUNICATION
Non-language behavior
in context

PERSONAL SUPPORT FOR INTERACTION
Grooming
Hygiene

SOCIAL ENVIRONMENT

Figure 7–3. Components of social interactive competence. (Reprinted with permission from "Social Skills Following Traumatic Brain Injury," by M. Ylvisaker, T. Feeney, and B. Urbanczyk, 1992. *Seminars in Speech and Language,* *13*[4], 308-321.)

Shortcomings of Traditional Social Skills Intervention

For over 25 years, social skills intervention has been a staple in the delivery of services to individuals with developmental and educational disabilities, motivated in large part by deinstitutionalization in developmental disabilities and mainstreaming in special education. Individuals with weak social skills are at risk for a variety of failures, including underachievement, dropping out of school, juvenile delinquency, and vocational and relationship problems (Strain, Guralnick, & Walker, 1986). With the popularizing of pragmatics as a domain of speech-language pathology in the 1970s, social skills intervention came to be understood as a central component of language therapy. In the 1990s, several reviews of the efficacy literature in this field have appeared, focused on a variety of disability groups (McIntosh, Vaughn, & Zaragoza, 1991; Wiener & Harris, 1998; Zaragoza, Vaughn, & McIntosh, 1991). The general impression derived from these reviews is that, whereas change in social behavior under laboratory or training conditions is eminently possible, few studies objectively document change in social behavior that is generalized to natural communication settings, that persists, and that makes a substantial difference in the individual's social life. For example, in their review of 27 studies of the effectiveness of social skills training for children with behavior problems, Zaragoza and colleagues (1991) identified only four studies that provided evidence of improved peer ratings following the training.

Although not surprising in light of the historical failure of many otherwise promising interventions to pass the litmus test of generalization, maintenance, and real-world significance, sobering findings of this sort have led leaders in the field to reemphasize the need to contextualize intervention. For example, Walker and colleagues (1994) concluded their review of social skills intervention for school age children by proposing 11 cardinal rules for conducting social skills training. Only 2 of these 11 cardinal rules related to traditional social skills intervention, namely identifying skills that the person should master and teaching those skills in a training context using scripted role-play activities. In contrast, at least six of the cardinal rules related to contextual issues in assessment and intervention (skills to be taught must be selected based on needs dictated by demands in the individual's specific social context; context factors affect learning; generalization from acquisition context to application context is questionable, threatened by well known obstacles; effective learning must include response opportunities and feedback in natural contexts; effectiveness of intervention must be measured by documentation of functional use of social skills in natural settings). This relative emphasis on real-world context is especially noteworthy because Walker and his colleagues are responsible for developing two popular direct-instruction-based curricula for social skills training.

Emphasis on role-play training outside of a natural social context is doubly questionable for most individuals with acquired brain injury. Not only is failure of generalization an ever-present threat, but more to the point, many people with TBI retain the requisite social knowledge that role-play training is designed to teach (Eslinger & Damasio, 1985; Eslinger et al., 1997; Eslinger & Grattan, 1993)! Walker and colleagues (1994) distinguished between two importantly different groups of people with social skills deficits: those who *can't do*, because the relevant social competence is not in their repertoire, and those who *won't do*, because they are oppositional and defiant. The *can't do* group, those with a knowledge base deficiency, are appropriate candidates for traditional social skills training as a small part of their total intervention package (which also includes substantial efforts at generalization and maintenance). Many people with social skills deficits after TBI are neither *can't do* nor *won't do* people. Rather, at the core of their social-interactive weakness is the set of frontal lobe themes, including disinhibition, lack of initiation, and impaired social perception, that we have emphasized throughout this book. They have adequate knowledge of social rules, roles, and routines, and they would like to interact in positive ways, but often do not. As Hans Teuber (1964) wisely observed, the "riddle of the frontal lobes" is just this curious disassociation between knowing and doing.

As consultants in TBI rehabilitation facilities, we have frequently endured the painful experience of observing social skills training sessions punctuated by shrill objections from group members that they already know how they are supposed to act, that what they are practicing is silly, that the group leader knows nothing about their social group, or that they are simply bored. To be sure, there is a place for out-of-social-context role playing in TBI rehabilitation. For example, we frequently use brief exploratory role-play sessions as part of negotiating with individuals about what they should do to succeed in difficult social situations (as in the cases of Mark and Jack, just described). In Andy's case (described in the next section) group interaction was used as a source of peer support and problem solving. We have profitably used social skills groups to videotape staged social interaction for purposes of careful video analysis of the interaction, with the goal of helping the members identify what is and what is not working for them. In the case of adults who truly need controlled practice in using specific social skills, but who react negatively to typical social skills group activities, we have engaged them in developing a social skills manual or demonstration videotapes, thereby according them respect as adults and defining them as contributors, but at the same time ensuring intensive practice and discussion of skilled social interaction. However, when all is said and done, the lion's share of the intervention is delivered in real social contexts and involves modification of social routines.

The increasingly rich research base in the field of social skills intervention combined with our experience with a large number of children and adolescents with TBI and with the philosophical premises articulated in Chapter 1 has led us to embrace an approach that is guided by familiar premises: (a) Intervention begins with careful differential diagnosis of the problem (noting possible environmental contributors and the contribution of executive system, cognitive, perceptual, and linguistic deficits) and functional analysis of troubling behaviors; (b) intervention focuses more on antecedents than on consequences (see Chapter 6); (c) social skills intervention may require provision of cognitive supports; (d) effective intervention occurs largely in social-communicative contexts and is designed to influence routines in those contexts; and (e) everyday communication partners are often the most effective providers of the intervention.

Case Illustration: Socially Withdrawn Child With Initiation Impairment Requiring Moderate Supports

Background. Deb was injured at age 9 in a motor vehicle accident. Early neurodiagnostic reports indicated a complex depressed skull fracture with left dorsofrontal and left parietal bruising. A left parietal craniotomy was performed to elevate the skull fracture. Reportedly, Deb lost consciousness for no more than a few minutes at the scene of the accident and was alert and oriented on her arrival at the emergency room, where she had three tonic-clonic seizures, but regained consciousness after each seizure. She was admitted to the pediatric unit where she remained for 3 days before discharge to home. Her mother was told by the attending physician that Deb would be fine and that the parents should not worry.

Deb was the youngest of five siblings in a very active family. All the children participated in sports and other community activities. The family was well-liked in the school and community, in part because both parents were leaders in school and community organizations. According to her mother, Deb was the shy child in her family, but once she was convinced to participate in sports and social activities, she was an active participant. She was in third grade at the time of her injury and academic records indicted she was an excellent student, placed in the top group for all academic content areas.

Almost immediately upon her return home, Deb demonstrated severe lability. Her mother reported that she spent hours crying in her room. When she returned to school, Deb indicated that she could not remember what to do and hated being in the classroom. She spent most of her time huddled in the corner crying and refusing to interact. Her mother was frequently asked to leave work to take Deb home. Following a referral to the special education committee at approximately 2 months postinjury, the school psychologist evaluated her using the WISC-III. The results of IQ testing (Verbal, 107; Performance, 110; Full Scale, 108) led the school psychologist to the erroneous conclusion that Deb's problems were not the result of her brain injury. Therefore, counseling was recommended, which was increased in frequency to twice daily, but with no demonstrable effect as Deb became progressively more socially withdrawn. By the end of that academic year, Deb engaged in minimal social interaction and maintained adequate grades only with intensive tutoring from her parents at home.

At a scheduled follow-up visit the following summer, the neurosurgeon agreed with the diagnosis of posttraumatic stress disorder and recommended a quiet summer at home, a plan that probably exacerbated Deb's withdrawal. When she began fourth grade in the fall, she was withdrawn and uncomfortable initiating any social interactions with peers, preferring to walk in the halls alone, to sit alone at the lunch table, and to play alone on the playground. She reported that she was afraid of the other kids. In addition, she demonstrated difficulty remembering academic content and was falling behind academically. Deb told her teacher that she felt "all mixed-up" all the time.

Intervention. When we were invited to consult with the school staff, we were impressed that the neurodiagnostic information, combined with the chronic symptoms of withdrawal, suggested an initiation impairment (the classical "pseudodepressive" personality, historically associated with left hemisphere dorsolateral frontal or dorsomesial frontal lesions; see Chapter 2) along with additional cognitive difficulties. Therefore, our initial negotiation with staff and family emphasized Deb's probable need for social supports to interact socially and for cognitive supports to succeed academically. Because Deb's social and academic condition was worsening, staff were willing to explore an alternative approach.

Deb's social supports included the following:

1. A Circle of Friends was identified, along with a rotating set of peer buddies. Buddies were selected on the basis of their willingness to participate and general social competence. The friends and buddies were oriented to Deb's difficulties initiating and maintaining social interaction after her accident. The peers were taught how to initiate and maintain interaction with Deb in a natural manner. Initially, the peers' special efforts served to compensate for Deb's impaired initiation. Later, their contribution evolved more toward being models and facilitators of competent social interaction for Deb.

2. The teacher was encouraged to use group work as much as possible to accomplish academic tasks. This gave Deb several natural occasions daily to interact with peers, who were trained to include her in the interaction. Furthermore, daily interaction around academic topics gave Deb and her peers sufficient conversational material to continue their interaction during social times at school, provided that peers initiated the interaction. Peers were trained to use play-

ground and lunchtime interaction to chat with Deb about what they were working on in class.

3. The classroom paraprofessional aide was trained to facilitate Deb's reacquisition of specific social skills (e.g., initiating interaction, maintaining interaction, taking turns, responding contingently to others) using specific strategies in social context. During group activities, the aide (a) modeled the target behaviors for Deb; (b) indirectly prompted Deb (commenting on the interaction), and (c) directly prompted Deb (e.g., "Deb, why don't you ask Robert if he knows how to do this problem?"). In addition, after a group activity, the aide reviewed with Deb what she had done that worked and what seemed difficult. In the case of persistently problematic social skills, they made a plan for how to accomplish the task the next time.

4. Recognizing the potential for Deb to grow dependent on her support, the aide worked with peers to turn over her role as facilitator of Deb's social interaction to them. The peers quickly learned how to play this role.

5. During planning times with the teacher or aide, Deb rehearsed scripts that she could use to initiate interaction with peers during social times (e.g., "Have you finished the science assignment?" "Do you like the story we are reading in class?"). In this respect, direct instruction was used as a component of the intervention. However, these role-play sessions were brief and explicitly directed at implementation in natural communication. Deb enjoyed practicing these scripts with her teaching staff; more important, they noted that she used the scripts to help her interact with peers.

6. Deb was allowed to select the times and places for implementing her scripts.

Outcome. This intervention began around Thanksgiving. For the first 2 months, the classroom aide served as an active coach of Deb, initially during structured, academic groups, and later during unstructured social times. She also helped to orient and train peer buddies. Deb became increasingly interactive, more so when her task was to respond to others than when she was expected to initiate. The aide gradually faded her involvement.

By the end of fourth grade, the paraprofessional aide had been entirely removed from the classroom. Deb remained shy, but within tolerable limits. She followed interaction initiated by others and occasionally initiated interaction herself. No overt withdrawal or crying was observed. However, fifth grade began much as had the previous year, with crying and withdrawing. Unfortunately, the school had done nothing to train the fifth grade staff in strategies for meeting Deb's needs. Using a consultant teacher familiar with the previous year's intervention, the plan was again implemented and, within a few weeks, Deb had returned to the level of competence achieved the previous spring. Since then, no special supports or consultants have been used. At 3 years postinjury, Deb continues to be perceived as shy, presumably related in part to her preinjury personality and in part to the injury. She continues to have difficulty initiating, particularly in the context of fluid, unpredictable activities such as conversations. However, her mother reports that she remains good at following scripts: When she knows a script, she uses it. Most importantly, she gets along well with peers in school and has two good friends who spend a great deal of time with her, in school and at their homes.

The keys to success for Deb's social skills intervention included social supports initially designed to compensate for her most significant disability (e.g., peers trained to initiate and maintain interaction with her), procedures designed to ensure that Deb and her peers shared interesting information about which to communicate (e.g., group academic work), frequent opportunities to practice her skills in real social contexts, brief direct instruction, situational coaching, and natural reinforcement.

Case Illustration: Adult With Social Skills Impairment Before and After TBI Requiring Intensive Levels of Support

Background. Andy was 36-years-old when he rode his motorcycle into a bridge abutment at high speed. He was intoxicated at the time. Prior to the injury, he lived in a mobile home in a rural area. His formal education ended at age 16 when he dropped out of high school. At age 18 he took Graduate Equivalency Courses, with the goal of earning a diploma and enlisting in the Navy, but ultimately failed the examinations. His vocational life was characterized by a series of unskilled jobs that he typically lost due to drunkenness or arguments with his boss or others. He had a history of serious alcohol and drug abuse and had spent a total of 8 years in jail and prison for offenses that included bar fights, domestic violence, and felonious assault with intent to kill.

Records indicate that Andy was unresponsive for approximately 3 weeks and acutely hospitalized for a total of 5 weeks, which was followed by 4 months of inpatient rehabilitation. An MRI scan completed during acute hospitalization indicated bilateral frontal subdural hematomas associated with a depressed skull fracture. Secondary to the severe left frontal injury was ischemic damage to left parietal and temporal regions.

Reports from the rehabilitation hospital indicate that Andy willingly participated in all therapies and in counseling sessions, in which he committed himself to giving up drugs and alcohol, saying that the accident had been a wake-up call for him. It is noteworthy that Andy's site of focal injury is consistent with a diagnosis of adynamia (the "pseudodepressive personality"), which may have contributed to his compliance and apparently improved behavioral adjustment, relative to preinjury patterns, during the early months after the injury. However, this diagnosis was not made at the time. When he was discharged from the rehabilitation hospital to a local nursing home

at 5 months postinjury, Andy had significant right hemiparesis (which has persisted) and right visual neglect. Neuropsychological evaluation at that time documented significant long- and short-term memory impairments, an inability to maintain attention for periods of time greater than 2 to 3 minutes, and difficulty following basic verbal requests. Aphasic symptoms gradually resolved into significant word-retrieval problems, difficulty with language organization (discourse), and difficulty following complex or abstract spoken language. His WAIS scores at that time were VIQ: 79, PIQ: 76, and FSIQ: 76.

After discharge from acute rehabilitation, Andy was admitted to a traditional nursing home where he remained for 2 years. During those 2 years, he experienced gradual physical recovery, although he remained significantly disorganized, with serious associated problems with memory and verbal expression. After discharge from the nursing facility, he married a practical nurse who had worked with him there. She and her two young children moved into Andy's mobile home. Within 2 months, Andy resumed heavy drinking and use of drugs, which was followed by a series of altercations with his wife and another man with whom his wife had become involved. Andy was subsequently arrested for assault, found guilty, and sentenced to treatment in a residential substance abuse program for individuals with a history of TBI, which is where we met him and began to work with him.

Current Intervention Program. When treatment in the dual diagnosis TBI-Substance Abuse program began, Andy could follow familiar routines, was motivated to do meaningful work, enjoyed helping others, and often interacted with others in an engaging and playful manner. However, he continued to evidence serious cognitive and behavioral disorganization, memory impairment (including both declarative and procedural memory deficits), difficulty applying the knowledge that he had retained, word-retrieval problems, and weak comprehension of extended or complex language. In addition he had a very negative self-perception, often perseverating on how he had damaged many lives. He wanted to please others and be liked, but had a short temper and was often manipulated by peers who enjoyed seeing him lose control and engage in destructive behavior.

Early in the intervention process, the following interaction occurred in a group therapy session that included seven peers and a group leader with little experience in TBI rehabilitation. We present this interaction as an illustration of Andy's preintervention social interaction and social problem solving when provoked. In this case, the provocation was a peer who had scribbled an accusatory obscenity on the wall of Andy's room. Andy entered the group session late and was visibly angry.

Andy: (cursing) "That guy, I've had it, I'm not taking his crap anymore; this is it! He's going down tonight."

Staff: "Andy, what's the matter?"

Andy: (cursing) "I told you he's going down: I'm not taking it; he can't do this to me no more!" (begins to pace, clench his fists, and hit the walls)

Staff: "Calm down, Andy! We're in group."

Andy: (cursing) "No way I've had it; you have no idea; I try and try!"

Staff: "I said calm down. Now stop it; the yelling and swearing are inappropriate and you sure aren't going to be aggressive. It's not acceptable, not in this group, not in this program. Ever!"

Andy: (walked out of the room and started a verbal fight with the peer who had angered him)

After we engaged staff and Andy in several brainstorming sessions, they all agreed to an intervention program that included a number of components described below. A critical feature of this intervention was the use of peers to help Andy compensate for his cognitive and social-interactive weaknesses. Problem-solving interaction with peers served two purposes: It often result-

ed in social decisions that were acceptable to Andy and were preferable to decisions he would make impulsively. In addition, the problem-solving interaction was itself an occasion for Andy to practice skilled, satisfying, and socially reinforced social interaction. The following illustrative episode occurred 1 month after the interaction quoted earlier. The group sessions had come to be called Community Meetings to emphasize the value of peer support and the active role of all community members in solving problems. In this case, the staff person was a consultant with extensive experience working with individuals with challenging behavior after TBI. Two other staff members were present as part of their apprenticeship program. Andy entered the group late and was visibly agitated.

Andy: (cursing) "I'm so mad, I'm going to kill him. He did it again!"

Staff: "Andy you *are* mad! Who did what?"

Andy: "You know, Jack. He always does this kind of stuff!" (cursing)

Staff: "I hear you. He can be a real jerk."

Andy: "You know it (cursing). You know, I've had it! I'm going to wait till tonight and when I see him—POW!"

Staff: "What happened this time?"

Andy: (cursing) "He wrote my name all over the wall and said (sexually explicit graffiti). I've had it. I'm a good guy; I don't need his (cursing). I'm killing him. I can, I've really hurt people in the past."

Staff: "I suppose that's an option. Hey guys, Andy's ticked off; he wants to kill Jack. That's understandable, I'd be ticked too. Anybody got any ideas about what he can do?"

Peer 1: "Cut him open with a sharp knife!"

Staff: "OK, he can do that; then what'll happen to Andy?"

Peer 2: "Jail; somebody's wife in jail."

Staff: "Yep, you want that, Andy?"

Andy: "Hell no, I've been in jail; I ain't going back. But I'm getting Jack, I don't care."

Staff: "OK guys, any other ideas?"

Peer 3: "Blanket party—you know, we all go after him in the dark and beat him. I hate him too, Andy!"

Staff:	"Then what happens?"
All:	"Jail!"
Staff:	"Any other ideas?"
Peer 4:	"Andy, you know, you can just ignore him."
Andy:	(cursing) "No way!" (more cursing)
Peer 4:	"Well, we can help you. We can let him know that we're all tired of his (curse) and if you hurt Andy, you hurt us. Ain't no way any of us deals with you, Jack, until you do right by Andy. That's what we'll tell him."
Peer 3:	"Yeah, he hates to be left out. He's gotta have his attention." (curse)
Staff:	"So, what's the plan then?"
Group:	[Together they formulated the following plan: Andy and Peer 4 would go to Jack at dinner, let him know that what he did was unacceptable, and that he was not welcome to participate in card games and other activities that the guys did on their own until he apologized to Andy and washed off the graffiti.]
Andy:	"Yeah, that's good. That's it; I don't have to be an (curse) like him; this will drive him crazy not to see me go off. Yeah, let's do it!"

After the meeting, the staff member and Andy sat down and wrote out the plan, clearly delineating in sequence what Andy was going to do, with some contingency plans depending on Jack's reaction to Andy's confrontation. The plan included simple scripts for Andy. He and Peer 4 then followed the plan in confronting Jack, who became upset and stormed off. Later that night when the guys were playing cards and Jack tried to enter the game, they said no. Jack cursed at them and sat down, expecting to play. The guys then got up to leave (following the script), causing Jack to storm out of the room. Ten minutes later, Jack returned, apologized to Andy in front of all the peers, got some cleaner, and cleaned up the graffitti.

We do not wish to suggest that one or a small number of experiences of this sort hold the potential to change the social life of a person with significant impairment after TBI in substantial ways. However, we do wish to suggest that these experiences, *if they can be made routine in the person's life*, have the power to substantially and positively influence social life. This is precisely what happened in Andy's case. He was pleased with the outcome of his conflict with Jack and with the support that he received from peers and staff. With some initial encouragement from staff, Andy developed a habit of bringing troubling social issues to the Community Meeting. On each occasion, peers and staff worked with Andy to produce effective solutions to social problems or plans for difficult interaction. Over the course of the next year, Andy made use of this social forum and support about once a week, with an associated dramatic decrease in negative social interaction with peers and staff and a corresponding increase in positive interaction.

From the perspective of social skills intervention, the features of what came to be Andy's routine are the following:

➤ **Meaningful Social Issues:** In each case, problem solving and scripting were focused on issues that were *important to Andy at that time*. They were not hypothetical problems, the use of which always risks failure of transfer, and discussion of the problems was not deferred, risking later irrelevance because of Andy's memory problems.

➤ **Contextualized Intervention:** In each case, the planning occurred in a social context and the execution of the plan, with staff or peer coaching, occurred in real social context.

➤ **Peer Involvement and Support:** With some guidance from staff, peers in the program learned how to support Andy and became a reliable source of good advice for him. Knowing that they could play this role well reciprocally yielded a significant benefit to Andy's peers.

➤ **Respect for Individual Values:** In each case, the positive communication scripts offered to Andy as an alternative to his violent inclinations were negotiated with him and acceptable to him within the framework of his values. At no point was the message to him, "You must behave like us; you must be a good boy." Andy was a veteran of thousands of these messages in his life, and they served only to alienate him from the person who delivered the message.

➤ **Natural and Logical Consequences:** Andy had experienced many natural negative consequences of his behavior, but rarely positive natural consequences, at least on a sustained basis. A feature of his social skills program was that success was rewarded by socially satisfying experiences. On the negative side, when he failed to complete assigned work, the natural consequence was that he had more work to do. During much of Andy's life, his fortunes were dictated by people who he believed exercised arbitrary authority over him. He had learned to react with habitual opposition to those who wielded arbitrary authority. In contrast, his fortunes in the program were directly related to his choices, with satisfying social rewards directly flowing from his positive social behavior.

➤ **Cognitive Support: Scripts:** Andy had difficulty making good decisions about how to act and what to say when under stress. Therefore, he had a history of turning minor disagreements into major altercations as a result of poorly conceived responses. His scripts, created and rehearsed at a time when he was calm, enabled him to successfully negotiate potentially treacherous interactions.

➤ **Emotional Support: Scripts:** The scripts were also emotionally supportive because they gave him a voice that he valued and because they often generated an outcome that he found satisfying.

➤ **Integration of Cognitive, Behavioral, Social Skills, and Counseling Intervention:** We have included Andy in the section on social skills intervention because of the social nature of the issues. However, the approach also has elements of cognitive rehabilitation, behavior management, and counseling. For example, many aspects of this intervention could legitimately be called cognitive rehabilitation. Group exploration of alternative possible solutions to problems and identification of their consequences is a contextualized exercise in divergent and convergent reasoning. Writing scripts, including anticipation of responses, is an exercise in social cognition and divergent thinking. Making a plan and implementing it at a later time is an exercise in planning and prospective memory, possibly including practice using needed prosthetics. However, unlike exercises in cognitive rehabilitation workbooks, Andy's exercises were not just exercises; he was processing information to meet an important and personally meaningful goal, thereby enhancing his learning efficiency and eliminating the threat of no transfer of training.

From the perspective of behavior management, Andy's intervention could be understood as antecedent control, with extensive use of positive communication alternatives to negative behavior. Most of the components of antecedent-focused behavior management described in Chapter 6 were present in Andy's social skills intervention.

Finally, Andy has received counseling in various forms in several professional settings, all of which have resulted in his verbally committing himself to changing his behavior, but with no actual changes in the way he conducted his life. In contrast, Andy's routine of seeking support from peers and successfully implementing negotiated social-interaction plans has clearly been effective in meeting the traditional objectives of counseling. He has come to trust others and has a dramatically higher opinion of his own competence and worth than he had when the majority of his interactions with others were negative or unsuccessful. Like many people who experience an unrelenting series of failures in life, Andy was unable to think in a positive way about himself without experiencing genuine success, which this social intervention enabled him to experience.

In all of these respects, social skills intervention for Andy resembled the behavioral intervention described in Chapter 6 as the Hans and Franz Dining Club. In that case, the young adolescents initially used an artificial script, complete with roles and assigned names, to break out of established negative patterns of interaction and practice positive alternatives. However, in both cases, the intervention addressed personally meaningful social issues, was delivered in real social contexts, made essential use of peer support, communicated respect for individual values in negotiating acceptable communication scripts and strategies, used only natural and logical consequences for reinforcement and feedback, combined the cognitive support of scripts with the emotional support of satisfying roles, and integrated a variety of rehabilitation perspectives in one natural intervention.

General Intervention Strategies. Andy's social skills intervention was a component of a larger rehabilitation plan that included a daily routine much like Bill's, described in Chapter 5. (Andy and Bill were peers in the dual-diagnosis program.)

➤ After dressing and eating breakfast, Andy would find a staff person to review his goals for the day and his plan for achieving the goals.
➤ Unlike Bill's plan, which was based on specific time frames, Andy's was based on a sequence of activities without specification of times for completion. In Andy's case, it was more important to complete what he began and to reduce anxiety associated with time pressure than to accustom him to a rigid, real-world time schedule, which was Bill's goal.
➤ As was the case with Bill's routine, the morning planning session included identification of activities that would be difficult for him to complete independently. He then negotiated a plan for asking for help (e.g., "When should I ask for help? Who will be the best help to me?").
➤ Like Bill, Andy's goals included using others efficiently in making good decisions and formulating effective plans. Unlike Bill, Andy chose to use the daily Community Meeting as his primary source of support and feedback. However, his routine also included a script, "Upset? Get help!!!" Andy used staff help more frequently than Bill because of the concreteness of his thinking and associated need for staff help in interpreting social events.
➤ At the end of each day, Andy met with a staff person to review his day and identify positive and negative events. Staff encouraged him to focus on his successes and jointly make a plan to deal with problematic events and interactions.

Outcome. As we write this chapter, it is about 2 years since we began to help Andy learn how to control his social interaction so that he could lead a more satisfying life in a setting of his choosing. He remains in the residential treatment program as mandated by his sentence. However, he now tolerates others saying negative things about him and he typically manages his anger in an adequate way. For example, over the course of 2 years, the frequency of episodes of uncontrolled anger decreased from a range of two to three episodes per day to less that one per month. For several months, he worked with support as a janitor in a hotel. Supervisors reported that he was a reliable and conscientious worker. However, he was removed from the job at the request of the probation department due to the nature of his criminal past. Andy reports that he is happier than he has been for many years and sees his life moving in a positive direction. Of great significance in relation to the ultimate goal of social skills training, he has two good friends in the program.

Andy continues to have difficulty interpreting the social behavior of others within the context of social roles. For example, he is inclined to interpret friendly behavior of female coworkers as a social invitation. Fortunately, he now seeks out and welcomes help from staff and peers to correctly interpret social behavior of this sort. This change has dramatically reduced awkward social situations based on misinterpretations and conflicts with those who would seek to correct those misinterpretations.

SUMMARY

In this chapter, we have described two closely associated types of intervention for individuals with communication and psychosocial problems after TBI, namely, teaching communication alternatives to challenging behavior and facilitating improved social skills. We presented an intervention framework and illustrated its application to individuals ranging in age from young children to adults, in severity of disability from severe multiple disability to apparently full recovery, in preinjury problems from significant social and behavioral concerns to none, and in types of social-communication problems from aggression to withdrawal. The themes of this chapter apply to a wide variety of individuals with disability after brain injury, and to other disabilities as well. These themes include providing intervention in the context of people's everyday routines; delivering services as much as possible through everyday communication partners, including peers; planning intervention through careful functional analysis of the communicative value of behavior and analysis of the behavior of communication partners; respectfully collaborating with everyday communication partners and the individual with disability in planning intervention; integrating cognitive, behavioral, social, and communication supports in the intervention plan; and influencing the individual's social success through modification of everyday routines.

CHAPTER 8

Collaboration and Apprenticeship: Creating a Network of Competence, Confidence, and Support

At age 16, a sophomore in high school wrote the following observations in an English paper on the assigned topic of personal values and their origin:

"What did you learn in school today, Ben?" I can still hear my father's voice coming out of my grade school years, every day, wanting to know what I had learned. One of the most important things that my parents taught me was to take a critical look at myself. This questioning set up an important pattern of self-examination. I naturally wanted to please my father, so I would start thinking about what I *had* learned that day, even before he asked the question when I got home. As I matured, I started to think about more things than what I had learned that day: What did I do? How did I do it? How did I feel? To this day it is virtually impossible for me to do anything and simply forget about it; I have to mull it over for days afterwards. And it's all because I was taught early in life that examining one's thoughts is a good thing to do—and I learned this from example and conversation, not from explicit teaching.

Over the course of several hundred simple, everyday, dinnertime conversations on the topic of the day's learning, Ben had gradu-

ally internalized the question and a sense for its importance so that it became a part of his own thinking, of his automatic self-governance system. He subsequently generalized this form of reflectiveness to domains of activity other than learning. Repeated conversations in early childhood had become higher levels of cognitive and executive functioning. What began as an interpsychic process—dinnertime parent-child conversations—had become an intrapsychic process. So we have come full circle in this book, returning to the theoretical framework of Vygotsky with which we introduced many of our themes in Chapter 1.

Having presented a theoretical framework in the introductory chapter, a discussion of the themes in TBI outcome to which this framework applies in Chapter 2, and illustrations of assessment and intervention procedures within this framework in Chapters 3 through 7, we now turn to the practical issue of procedures for creating alliances with individuals with disability and with those people who are the critical contributors to the positive, everyday routines we have illustrated so that the routines of everyday life can be made to be as positive and therapeutic as possible.

In this chapter and in the entire book, we use the term *everyday person* both descriptively (i.e., these are the people who interact regularly with the person with disability) and honorifically (i.e., these are the people who hold the potential to contribute most significantly to the rehabilitation and quality of life of the person with chronic disability after TBI). In our vocabulary, this is a term of high praise. For many people, the everyday people who make the greatest difference in their lives are family members. Others who may deserve this important title include friends, work supervisors, coworkers, teachers, assistant teachers, personal care attendants, direct care staff, and other support personnel. After offering a rationale for creating working alliances with everyday people and with individuals with TBI, we describe obstacles to this everyday approach to rehabilitation and suggest procedures for overcoming the obstacles. This chapter should be read as continuous with the book's epilogue, which presents a vivid illustration of many of the intervention themes contained in the chapter and in the book as a whole.

CREATING COLLABORATIVE ALLIANCES WITH PEOPLE IN THE EVERYDAY WORLD: RATIONALE

In an important sense, this entire book is a rationale for specialists in rehabilitation to devote a great deal of their time and effort to creating mutually respectful working alliances with people who figure prominently in the everyday routines of individuals with disability. In most of our case illustrations, the positive outcome was a product of implementing changes in everyday routines, changes that necessitated some modification of the behavior of the people involved in those routines. Collaborative alliances with the everyday people were the key to these successful outcomes. The central theme of this book is that people with chronic disability in the areas of executive functions, cognition, behavior, and communication are most effectively served by ensuring that

the routines of their everyday lives are designed to facilitate success and improvement in functioning in their area of need.

To be as supportive as they can be, people who figure prominently in everyday routines should be knowledgeable about the issues facing the person with disability, competent in everyday interaction and in facilitation procedures, optimistic, flexible, creative, mature, and nondefensive. Ideally they are also enthusiastic and effective problem solvers. Many of those who play important roles in the everyday life of people with disability after TBI possess large quantities of all of these characteristics. They need no help from professionals; indeed, specialists in rehabilitation are well advised to take lessons from these people. Other everyday people may be in a position to benefit in one or more of these areas from the support of specialists or others who are in a position to provide that support. This chapter presents procedures for providing such support.

More specifically, creating a collaborative alliance with everyday people is justified because it is an expression of respect; it yields benefits in assessment; it increases the intensity, consistency, and duration of services; it facilitates generalization and maintenance of treatment gains; and it helps to ensure that rehabilitation is functional, that supports will be in place over the long run, and that community inclusion is a focus of intervention throughout the process.

Respect

Respect is at the same time a reason for creating a collaborative relationship and a product of that relationship. A natural posture of defensiveness often exists in people with little or no formal education in rehabilitation when they interact with specialists who may be perceived as unapproachable or even condescending and disrespectful. One of the most effective means of breaking through such an obstacle is for specialists to communicate clearly to family members, direct care staff and others that, in the long run, they—the everyday people—are the most critical contributors to the individual's rehabilitation. Engaging these people as collaborators in assessment and intervention, and ensuring that they have the support they need to effectively play their collaborative role, is an effective way to communicate this message (Gans, 1987; Giangreco, Cloninger, & Iverson, 1993; Hilton & Henderson, 1993).

Use of Observations and Insights of Everyday People

In Chapter 3, we presented an approach to functional assessment that includes a variety of assessment activities, including collaborative hypothesis testing in a variety of contexts. To be successful, this process must engage the observational powers of as many people in as many settings as possible. In addition, the hypothesis-generation phase of this process benefits from the insights of people who interact regularly with the individual. Experienced clinicians recognize that it is often these people who have the clearest understanding of the behavior of complex children and adults with TBI, and certainly the most thorough understanding of the individual's interests, motivators, goals, and personal history, all critical to a thorough assessment and an effective rehabilitation plan.

Intensity, Consistency, and Duration of Services

In a rehabilitation hospital, specialists in the cognitive or communication domains of behavior may each spend 5 or so hours per week with a patient. Those 5 hours probably account for less than 5% of the individual's waking hours. In most cases, it is possible to multiply that 5% severalfold, but only if everyday people in that setting are clearly oriented to what they can do with the individual at other times to facilitate progress in the clinician's domain of specialization. We do not recommend turn-

ing all of life into serious work. The point is rather that virtually any activity, however recreational or relaxing it is (e.g., evening conversations or games) and however mundane it appears (e.g., self-care activities), can be used to achieve some therapeutic goals (Mount & Zwernik, 1986; Timm, 1993). Furthermore, collaboration with everyday people helps to ensure that everybody is "on the same page" in areas of intervention (e.g., behavior management) in which reasonable levels of consistency are important (Kaiser & McWhorter, 1990; Landis & Peeler, 1990; Self, Benning, Marston, & Magnusson, 1991). In the absence of such collaboration, a confusing and fragmenting cacophony of interventions is the likely result (Dunst, Trivette, & Deal, 1988; Dunst, Trivette, Gordon, & Fletcher, 1989; Dunst, Johanson, Trivette, & Hamby, 1991). Finally, well-oriented and supported everyday people hold the potential to prolong brain injury rehabilitation services from the few weeks that is the norm in today's funding environment to many years.

Generalization and Maintenance of Treatment Gains

In Chapter 1 we highlighted the centrality of generalization and maintenance as factors in outcome from the perspective of executive functions, cognition, behavior, and communication. Professionals at both ends of the theoretical dimension we plotted out in that chapter (i.e., the Wimbledon Approach and the Mom and Pop Approach) recognize the extraordinary importance of planning for generalization and maintenance of treatment gains. In many areas of rehabilitation, the Achilles heel of otherwise well-conceived intervention plans is the classic failure of generalization and maintenance (Kaiser & McWhorter, 1990; Powers, Singer, Stevens, & Sowers, 1992; Self et al., 1991; Singley & Anderson, 1989; Stokes & Baer, 1977; Timm, 1993). We have argued that an intelligent response to the crisis of generalization is to provide rehabilitation services (in our areas of focus) as much as possible within the context of everyday routines so that generalization to functional contexts is reduced as an issue (i.e., the improvements in functioning are facilitated in those contexts) and so that the likelihood of maintenance is increased because everyday people are well oriented to their ongoing role in facilitating maintenance.

Infusion of Reality, Common Sense, and Functional Goals into Professional Practice

In our professional practice, many of the most powerful lessons we have learned have come from the people we have served. For example, Linda's Law ("Nobody's gotta do nothin!") was taught by a woman with diagnoses of mental illness and severe psychopathic behavior. Her point—that it is impossible to coerce anybody into doing anything that he or she is willing to resist doing—has had a fundamental impact on our clinical practice since the fateful day many years ago that she articulated her law during a life-and-death behavioral crisis. Linda's Law has been a primary consideration for us in shaping the everyday routines of people with serious behavior problems.

More generally, ongoing collaboration with family members and nursing assistants in a rehabilitation hospital, or other everyday people in other settings, forces specialists to relate their work to the real-world needs of the people they serve. This point was well made, unfortunately with a negative model, by the mother of an adolescent who had pulled him out of a cognitive rehabilitation outpatient program in which he spent large amounts of time playing chess with a clinician. The mother said, "If Jim needs to play chess to get better, we can play chess with him 10 hours a day. But all this chess playing is not making him any better or more strategic in his school work or social activities. It's absurd!" Early collaboration between the clinician and the mother may have helped the clinician focus her efforts in a more positive and functional manner.

Community Inclusion: Creating Networks of Community Support for the Long Term

The time that people with TBI spend in rehabilitation hospitals as inpatients or in outpatient or day programs can be intense and powerfully effective. However, when placed in context with the remainder of the person's life, the active rehabilitation phase recedes into minor significance. In the long run, the lives of people with chronic disability are primarily influenced by community supports. Children may spend weeks or months in a rehabilitation setting, but years in schools. Adults may spend weeks or months in a rehabilitation setting, but years in work or volunteer settings. Both children and adults spend decades with family and friends after the injury, ideally supported within networks of community supports that are readily available and sufficiently flexible to meet changing needs over time. From this perspective, it is easy to understand what individuals with disability and their families repeatedly point out, namely that their primary need is for ongoing community supports, including meaningful activities for the person with disability and ongoing emotional support and guidance for everyday people who may have a difficult role to play in supporting the person with disability.

From this real-world, long-term perspective, rehabilitation professionals serving children are well advised to devote energy and resources to creating collaborative relationships with the school staff who are the long-term providers of rehabilitation for school-age children and adolescents. The analogous commitment for rehabilitation professionals serving adults is to orienting and supporting employers or coworkers in the case of adults with TBI returning to work, or to facilitating alternative meaningful activities, such as those provided within the Club House movement (Jacobs, 1997) for those unable to return to work. Often the rehabilitation hospital is the first in a series of many transitions from one setting or service provider to another. Each transition carries with it the potential for breakdowns in continuity and associated regression in the individual's function. Professionals in the early stages of rehabilitation cannot be expected to anticipate later settings. However, they can set in motion a training chain in which each setting—each link in the chain over time—acknowledges its responsibility for providing adequate orientation and training to the next setting. Furthermore, intensive early collaboration with family members and other natural support people puts them in a position to play an effective role in ensuring positive transitions as *de facto* case managers for their loved one (Elkinson & Elkinson, 1989; Landis & Peeler, 1990; Smull & Harrison, 1992; Stainback & Stainback, 1990; Timm, 1993; Wetzel & Hoschouer, 1984).

Managed Care: Limitations on Professional Resources

All of the considerations in this section are magnified by the crisis in brain injury rehabilitation created by dramatic reductions in resources associated with managed care. Many rehabilitation hospitals report that their average length of inpatient stay decreased by more than 50% from the mid-1980s to the mid-1990s. Under these circumstances, the collaborative activities undertaken with a vision of the long run (promoted in the preceding paragraphs) move from their status as good ideas to necessary ideas. If costly labor- and time-intensive direct professional services are curtailed by draconian cuts in funding, then rehabilitation specialists are constrained to identify alternative ways in which they can positively affect functional outcomes over the long run. A necessary component of the alternative service delivery system is intensified collaboration with everyday people so that the ongoing routines of life supported by those everyday people are well designed and well implemented in relation to positive rehabilitation outcomes.

CREATING COLLABORATIVE ALLIANCES WITH INDIVIDUALS WITH TBI: RATIONALE

In the preceding sections, we advocated collaborative alliances with the people who play a role in the everyday routines of individuals with chronic disability after TBI. In this section, we argue for an analogous collaborative alliance with the individuals themselves. The importance of such a collaboration with people with disability was underscored by Wehmeyer and Schwartz (1997), who presented results of a major follow-up study of young people with learning disabilities or mental retardation. Their interest was in identifying a possible contribution of self-determination to positive adult outcomes. They defined *self-determination* as including four critical components:

➤ *Self-realization:* possession of a reasonably accurate awareness of one's strengths and limitations, and use of that awareness in capitalizing on strengths to compensate for weaknesses.
➤ *Psychological empowerment:* a settled disposition to believe in one's capacity to act in a way that positively influences important outcomes in one's life.
➤ *Self-regulation:* a pattern of behavior characterized by thoughtful planning, careful monitoring and evaluation of the effectiveness of the plan, and strategic revisions in the plan in the event of difficulty.
➤ *Autonomy:* action based on personal preferences and choices, free from undue external interference.

Eighty students from four states participated in the study, half with identified learning disabilities (mean IQ: 93.1) and half with mild mental retardation (mean IQ: 61.43). They divided the 80 students into a high self-determination group and a low self-determination group, based on performance on *The Arc's Self-Determination Scale* (Wehmeyer & Kelcher, 1995), administered during the student's last year in school. Interestingly, the high self-determination group (mean IQ: 75) did not differ significantly in intelligence from the low self-determination group (mean IQ: 72). However, the two groups differed in important practical ways when followed 1 year after leaving school. In the areas of working for pay, having a checking account, and having a savings account, members of the high self-determination group were superior to the low self-determination group by a factor of approximately 2:1.

Based on these striking findings, Wehmeyer and Schwartz (1997) called for educators to focus greater attention on the following skills and attitudes: choice making, decision making, problem solving, goal setting, self-observation, self-awareness and knowledge, self-evaluation, internal locus of control, and positive attributions of efficacy. The authors concluded their discussion with a recommendation that educators teach students with disabilities to advocate for themselves, including learning how to be assertive (without being aggressive), how to negotiate, compromise, and persuade, and how to be an effective team member.

In light of the frequency of frontal lobe injury and associated executive system impairment after TBI, these themes take on special urgency. Unfortunately, rehabilitation specialists all-too-often assume responsibility for all of the executive dimensions of tasks (i.e., the components of self-determination). In Chapter 4, we operationally defined executive functions as follows:

➤ **Self-Awareness of Strengths and Limitations:** Clinicians characteristically take responsibility for all aspects of the individual's assessment and interpretation of that assessment.

➤ **Goal Setting:** Clinicians characteristically take responsibility for setting goals for their patients, students, or clients.

➤ **Planning:** Clinicians characteristically take responsibility for planning how to achieve the goals.

➤ **Initiating:** Clinicians characteristically take responsibility for motivating their clients and ensuring that they initiate activity toward achieving their goals.

➤ **Inhibiting:** Clinicians characteristically take responsibility for ensuring that their clients retain their focus and do not lose control.

➤ **Self-Monitoring and Self-Evaluating:** Clinicians characteristically take responsibility for monitoring and evaluating their clients' performance and documenting that performance in necessary reports.

➤ **Problem Solving and Strategic Thinking:** Clinicians characteristically take responsibility for solving problems that arise over the course of their intervention and developing alternative strategies if they are needed.

In highlighting this sobering clinical reality, we are clearly not recommending that rehabilitation specialists suddenly and completely abdicate all responsibility for these critical functions. Indeed, many people with disability require a great deal of support for an extended period of time before they are in a position to assume major responsibility for the components of executive functioning. Our point is rather that self-determination, as defined earlier, or improved executive functioning, must always be embraced as a goal, with procedures in place, from an early age in the case of children and from early in recovery in the case of adults, to facilitate development in these critical areas. When clinicians fail to collaborate with the individuals with whom they work and do not systematically turn over responsibility for the executive dimensions of tasks, the likely consequence is learned helplessness in the individuals thus improperly served or a growing adversarial relationship or both.

The everyday, contextualized executive system routines described in Chapter 4 are a useful context within which to facilitate development of the components of self-determination. Ylvisaker, Szekeres, and Feeney (1998) provided elaboration of these intervention themes for work with children and adolescents. From the perspective of self-awareness and self-knowledge, the self-assessment and negotiated assessment procedures described in Chapter 3 are useful. We also routinely engage people with whom we work in planning and producing a self-advocacy or transitional videotape (described later). One of the many goals of this procedure is to help individuals with disability identify their strengths and needs, their goals, the intervention procedures and supports most useful in helping them to achieve their goals, and the type of interaction with others, including specialists, that are positive and effective for the individual. The process is from beginning to end a collaborative process, with some combination of rehabilitation specialists, the individual, family members, and possibly others working together to create a product that holds the potential to play a self-advocacy role, as well as serve as a training tool for staff who work with the person with TBI.

CHARACTERISTICS OF EFFECTIVE EVERYDAY COACH-PARTNERS

In Chapter 2, we cited studies that have shown that the long-term functional outcome of both children and adults with TBI, particularly behavioral, psychosocial, and vocational outcome, is strongly influenced by the people who play a prominent role in their lives, including family members, work supervisors, and school staff in the case of children. This should be no sur-

prise. With this finding as background, the critical questions are: What are the characteristics of everyday people that enable them to have a positive impact on outcome? and What are the most effective procedures for improving those characteristics if they need improvement? The following list of characteristics represents our best attempt to answer the first question: knowledge, interactive competence, competence in facilitation procedures, optimism, flexibility, creativity, problem-solving enthusiasm and skill, and maturity.

Knowledge

Understanding the consequences of brain injury and the principles and procedures associated with relevant intervention approaches is in general helpful for everyday people in the world of an individual with TBI. However, in placing knowledge first in our list of critical characteristics of everyday coach-partners, we do not wish to miscommunicate that it is most important. People who are knowledgable, but pessimistic, inflexible, uncreative, immature, and incompetent problem solvers are far less useful in rehabilitation than those with the opposite profile. Training vehicles designed to impart information often include informational inservice sessions, reading materials, and videotapes. In our experience, although these options are useful, they should be complemented by elbow-to-elbow collaborative work with specialists in an apprenticeship relationship (see below) to ensure practical integration of the information.

Interactive Competence

Communicating effectively with people with disability is critical for several reasons. First, it is through positive communication that a relationship of trust is created, enabling the everyday communication partner to identify problems, give honest feedback, and set high expectations. When people with disability lack a relationship of mutual respect with the people charged with serving them, they are unlikely to benefit from that person's feedback or to be motivated to meet that person's standards.

Second, many important cognitive objectives can be achieved through practice that takes the form of positive interactive routines. For example, socially co-constructed narratives can be the context within which cognitive organization and strategic memory can be practiced (see Chapter 5). Similarly, the social interaction that precedes and ends any activity can be the context for rehearsing executive functions (see Chapter 4). Finally, because challenging behaviors are often acts of communication that are used because they have been successful in communicating intentions to communication partners in the environment, those interactions are the appropriate context within which to teach positive communication alternatives (see Chapter 6).

Because communication competencies are critical for staff and for other everyday communication partners, we have historically placed considerable emphasis on training and support in this area. Ylvisaker, Feeney, and Urbanczyk (1993b) presented a comprehensive staff and family education program designed to facilitate communication competencies within the broader context of a positive communication culture in rehabilitation, a program that we have implemented in flexible ways in many settings.

Appendix C lists the communication and behavioral competencies that we believe should be possessed by people who work with individuals with cognitive, communication, and behavioral disability. The communication competencies are grouped under five headings: *content* of communication, *form* of communication, *environment* for communication, procedures for *encouraging the communication partner*, and procedures for *communicating respect*. We have included staff competencies for communicating with *individuals with disability*, for communicating with *family members*, and for communicating with *other staff*. Each of

these three domains is critical in creating a positive communication culture for rehabilitation. In one of the rehabilitation hospitals in which we worked, these competencies were included as a component of the job description for all rehabilitation staff.

Ylvisaker, Feeney, and Urbanczyk (1993b) also presented a detailed outline for a 2- to 4-hour competency-based training session focused on these competencies and several sample vignettes that could be used in the training session. Having conducted many of these training sessions, we are enthusiastic about their possibilities, but also realistic about their limitations. Staff or other everyday communication partners who are particularly weak in any of the areas of communication or behavior management are unlikely to become competent as a result of a 2- to 4-hour group training session. They need follow-up, ideally using situational coaching within an apprenticeship relationship. Furthermore, if they are employees, the competencies listed in Appendix C should be part of the job description on the basis of which their job performance is evaluated.

Optimism

Individuals with chronic disability are best served by staff and family members who have a positive vision of the individual's progress and life in the near and distant future and who rejoice in response to the small indications of progress toward that vision. Some people are naturally optimistic and routinely put a positive spin on events that could be interpreted negatively, even when progress is frustratingly slow and it becomes hard to remain optimistic.

Other people are easily discouraged and require support to retain the resilience necessary to play their role in rehabilitation effectively. Such support and encouragement are best provided by people who are respected and who can speak about life after TBI with personal authority (Condeluci, 1991). Family members might receive the encouragement they need from a support group sponsored by the local chapter of the Brain Injury Association. Others say that people with whom they have a personal relationship, such as a relative or religious leader, are more effective. In either case, rehabilitation specialists have a responsibility to ensure that family members have some source of support and encouragement for those dark moments when the future seems gloomiest.

Staff members also deal with troubling emotions when working with individuals whose progress is slow or who engage in challenging behavior. In most workplaces, the natural stress associated with clients with challenging behavior is exaggerated by other workplace stressors, such as long hours and insufficient staff. Under these circumstances, it is common for staff to lapse unconsciously into a *negative scanning* mode, actively seeking out conflicts and problems as the focus of their attention and overlooking potential sources of optimism. At such times, the people who figure prominently in the everyday lives of individuals with disability should be brought together to practice *positive scanning*, that is, surveying realities in the world of the individual and identifying everything in that world that is positive. Although such scanning may seem artificial at times, it can be a useful antidote to the potentially dangerous negative scanning mode that grows in momentum as people become increasingly tired, discouraged, and depressed. If negative scanning is allowed to spin out of control, it becomes increasingly difficult to reverse.

Flexibility, Creativity, and Problem-Solving Ability

Throughout this book, we have described the powerful role that can be played by the people who are active in the everyday routines of individuals with chronic cognitive and behavioral disability after TBI. However, a certain amount of flexibility, creativity, and problem-solving skill is required to shape the routines of everyday life in a positive way. Many everyday people and reha-

bilitation specialists have these attributes in abundance and therefore require little assistance in this domain. In our experience, these characteristics are not associated with formal education.

Other people are relatively rigid, not particularly creative, and far more enthusiastic about fixed solutions to problems than about open-ended problem solving. Ylvisaker and Feeney (1998) offered routines or scripts that can be practiced by people who fall into this category, but who nevertheless need to contribute to a world that is flexible, creative, and capable of generating fresh solutions to unpredictable problems. It might seem oxymoronic on the surface to present flexibility routines and creativity routines. After all, flexibility and creativity seem to be the opposite of routine.

Our point is that people who are not by nature flexible, creative, or enthusiastic about solving problems are unlikely to acquire these attributes with training. Routines of the sort we present here can at least give these people the comfort and security they need in a context that calls for flexibility, creativity, and open-ended problem solving. Although they are following a script, they still manage to avoid the confrontation that often attaches to rigidity and present the individual with TBI with opportunities for practicing flexible, creative, and strategic thinking. We have worked with many staff and family members who have practiced and internalized these scripts, thereby reducing the frequency of conflict with the person with TBI and at the same time increasing the frequency of satisfying, generative interactions. Respectful adult illustrations of these scripted routines can be easily created.

Flexibility Routine With a Child with TBI

Adult:	(present activity or plan)
Child:	resist (e.g., "No, I don't want to do that!")
Adult:	routine response: "OK, maybe you're right; maybe it's not a

good idea. Let's think of some other way to get this job done. Any ideas? ... How about ...? How about ...?"

Creativity Routine With a Child With TBI

An issue arises; the child becomes upset.

Adult: "We need to think about this." (i.e., create thinking time)

Child: "OK." (or perhaps no response)

Adult: "What are you trying to accomplish here?" (i.e., focus on the goal)

Child: "I want to finish this and I can't; I'm angry."

Adult: "You've done some good work here; that's great; and I know we can figure out some way to get this done." (i.e., focus on the big picture and the availability of support)

Child: (grumbles)

Adult: "How can I help you? Let's think about it together." (i.e., communicate helpfulness and openness to alternatives).

Child: (grumbles)

Adult: "Are you ready to try? I'm not sure I will come up with anything good, but let's brainstorm. I know we can get this done."

(If in group) "Let's all think about this."

(If no good ideas emerge) "Is there somebody we can talk to who might have a good idea?"

Problem-Solving Routine With a Child With TBI

Child: (is having a hard time doing something)

Adult: "Boy, Fred, that looks like a hard thing to do."

Child: (continues unsuccessfully to do what he wants to do)

Adult: "I wonder what would make that go easier"

Child: "I don't know."

Adult: "Let's see, maybe you could do (A) or (B) or maybe (C)."

Child: "I'll try (A)."

Adult: "OK, you could do that. But hold on; let's think about this for a minute. If you do (A), will it solve the problem? Take a lot of time? If you do (B) will it solve the problem? Take a lot of time? (etc.)?"

Child: "Don't know."

Adult: "Let's think. (A) would take all day. (B) might not get the job done. (C) is easy and quick and would probably be successful. What do you think?"

Child: "I'll do (C)."

Adult: "Good choice. This was hard to figure out, but we thought of several possibilities and I think you chose the smartest one. Good thinking!"

Maturity, Nondefensiveness

People who work with children and adults with chronic disability after TBI must be sufficiently mature that they do not react defensively to mood swings, angry outbursts, and possible aggression from the person or to anger and frustration expressed by family members, both of which are naturally associated with this disability. In addition, supporting the individual's growth in independence necessitates withholding positive solutions to problems while the individual works on his or her own solution. Finally, people who provide support must seek to reduce dependence on that support even if the individual's dependence on them may be personally gratifying. Performing these functions well is a mark of maturity.

Some staff need their own support system to maintain a mature and nondefensive posture in relation to these sources of stress. In particularly stressful work environments, managers are well advised to create time for staff to vent their frustrations, to remind one another that they are doing good work, and to reflect as a group on the reasons for the stressors, reasons that typically have nothing to do with the effort or quality of work of the staff. To help staff disengage and avoid creating overdependence on them or unhealthy enmeshment with clients, managers should see to it that signs of independence and emotional distance are celebrated rather than mourned, as they often are when staff develop an unhealthy need to be involved in the lives of the individuals with whom they work.

COLLABORATING WITH EVERYDAY PEOPLE: OBSTACLES

There is no shortage of potential obstacles to collaborative relationships between rehabilitation specialists and the people who are contributors to everyday routines. In this section, we highlight some of these obstacles and suggest means to overcome them.

Distrust

In unhealthy work environments, distrust often exists in relations among staff. The classic example of this is the frequently observed adversarial relationship between therapists and nursing staff in a rehabilitation hospital. Therapists often complain that nursing staff fail to follow through on orders and recommendations, while nursing staff complains in turn that therapists are wholly unrealistic about work responsibilities on the nursing unit and about the extent to which nurses are available to serve the therapists. It is difficult to reduce these tensions without creating opportunities for elbow-to-elbow collaborative work. Flexible scheduling of therapists, including

occasional early hours to interact with night staff, late hours to interact with evening staff, and weekend hours to interact with weekend staff, may be necessary. In our work in inpatient rehabilitation, we found that collaborative efforts of this sort were necessary to create an environment in which nursing staff respected and were respected by therapists, in which therapists had a realistic understanding of the role that nursing staff could play in relation to specific therapy goals for their patients, and, as a consequence, in which everyday routine activities on the nursing unit were effectively used to facilitate functional gains in the individuals served.

Distrust is unfortunately common also in relationships between family members and staff. Rehabilitation specialists may complain that family members lack a realistic perception of their loved one's disability and prognosis, while family members may complain that specialists are overly negative; insufficiently committed to the recovery of their loved one; and unappreciative of the knowledge, competence, and insight that family members bring to the rehabilitation process. As in the case of therapy staff-nursing relationships, distrust is most effectively overcome when therapists create opportunities to work collaboratively with family members, clearly communicating that both parties can benefit from the collaboration.

Professional Self-Perception

Ylvisaker and Feeney (1998) presented a lengthy discussion of professional self-perception as an obstacle to collaborative intervention. In summary, their contention was that many rehabilitation professionals have one or more internalized metaphors that drive their thinking and values in relation to their work. These professional metaphors, or models of clinical activity, may have been acquired early in the professional's education program, but are often held without conscious awareness of their presence or power. Ylvisaker and Feeney explored the meaning of the following clinical metaphors for the work of rehabilitation professionals:

Surgeon-Patient Metaphor (Medical Model): The clinician diagnoses impairments in the person with disability and sets about to cure the impairment (i.e., a deficit model). It is an expert model in that the clinician sets the goals and makes all of the decisions. The relationship is paternalistic and the setting for delivering services is typically a clinical setting.

Animal Trainer Metaphor (Behavioral Model): The clinician identifies the trainee's weaknesses and implements a hierarchy of training exercises designed to extinguish undesirable behaviors and build desirable behaviors (i.e., another deficit model). This is also an expert model, with the clinician setting the goals and making the decisions. The relationship is paternalistic; the setting is typically a specialized training setting.

Teacher-Student Metaphor (Educational Model): The clinician identifies knowledge and skill deficiencies and attempts to remediate the deficiencies. This is also an expert model, with the clinician setting the goals and making the decisions. The relationship is paternalistic; the setting is typically a specialized educational setting.

Master Craftsperson-Apprentice Metaphor: The clinician identifies the skills that the apprentices wish to acquire and works collaboratively with them on practical projects, showing them how to be successful and systematically turning over more and more responsibility to the apprentices as their competence increases (see discussion of Vygotsky in Chapter 1). This begins as an expert, paternalistic model, but quickly changes as the apprentice gains sufficient competence to function with growing independence. The context is typically one in which the to-be-acquired competence is naturally used.

Coach-Athlete Metaphor: The client lets the clinician know what skill he or she wishes to improve and the coach teaches skills and guides performance under systematically increasingly gamelike conditions. The relationship is largely paternalistic; the setting is as much like ultimate application settings as possible.

Consultant-Client Metaphor: The client selects a consultant to assist him or her in overcoming obstacles to self-determined goals. The relationship is not paternalistic: power and decision making are retained by the client. The setting is any setting in which the client wishes to overcome obstacles.

Counselor-Client Metaphor: The client selects a counselor and an issue to work through. The counselor accepts the client's goals, and attempts to help the client in actively overcoming personal obstacles that block progress. The relationship is not paternalistic in that the counselor attempts to empower the client to take responsibility for his or her growth. Setting is not a critical component of the metaphor.

Parent-Child Metaphor: The clinician identifies threats to the client's successful performance or sense of well being and acts to protect the client from failure and frustration. The relationship is paternalistic or maternalistic; the setting is not a critical feature of the metaphor.

These do not exhaust the set of possible metaphors that are capable of enfleshing a skeletal concept of the work of rehabilitation professionals. We have heard professionals say that they frequently think of themselves as cheerleaders, drill sergeants, or guardian angels. In our education programs, we were largely taught (implicitly of course) to act like animal trainers in our work with people with developmental disabilities and to act like surgeons in our work in medical settings with people with acquired brain injury. Evidence of the former was the comfort with which professionals in developmental disabilities settings said things like, "I have decided that the trainee must master such-and-such skill; I will start training on level one of the training hierarchy and proceed with massed learning trials until he achieves 90% mastery on three consecutive days in the training setting, which will trigger a move to level two." Evidence of the latter was the comfort with which people used words like *diagnosis, prognosis, treatment, treatment room, positive identification of disorders using test batteries*, and *patient* in medical settings. With some effort, we have come to adopt a flexible combination of the consultant, master craftsperson, and coach metaphors as a more generally helpful guide in our work with people with TBI, at least beyond the earliest stages of cognitive recovery.

Our point is not that any of these metaphors or models is good and useful in all clinical circumstances, or that any of them is bad and incapable of driving good clinical activity under some conditions. Rather, we wish to sensitize rehabilitation professionals to the power of unconsciously held metaphors and to invite all workers in brain injury rehabilitation to raise their implicit driving metaphors to a level of consciousness, so that deliberate and wise decisions about the nature of the relationship between professionals and the people they serve (individuals with disability as well as the significant people in their environment) can be made in individual cases.

As long as professionals retain a perception of their role that singularly emphasizes their discipline-specific expertise and their use of that expertise to diagnose and treat patients, it will seem foreign and uncomfortable at best to enter into collaborative relationships with people with disability, their families, and others who lack the special expertise of that discipline. However, for reasons that have been elaborated throughout this book, many aspects of brain injury rehabilitation have been moved to a new level, requiring professionals to embrace a vision of themselves as experts who have a profoundly important contri-

bution to make, but as experts who work in collaboration, who learn through collaboration, and who empower others through collaboration.

Access to Everyday People

A more concrete, but often equally difficult, obstacle to collaboration is the logistic difficulty of bringing potential collaborators together. If, during inpatient rehabilitation, family members only visit in the evening and on weekends, there will be few occasions for collaborative activities with therapists unless the therapists schedule occasional evening and weekend hours, as we recommended earlier. Furthermore, flexible scheduling of this sort helps to create collaborative relationships between rehabilitation therapists and evening and weekend nursing staff, the cornerstone of inpatient brain injury rehabilitation.

An alternative solution is to make active use of videotape communication. Therapists can tape models of important procedures or techniques, which can then be viewed as frequently as necessary by other staff and family members who are in a position to use the helpful procedures. Similarly, family members can videotape interactions with their family member or present other information on video and send it to the therapists with the goal of giving information or requesting feedback. Later in this chapter we describe the use of transitional videos, which can be flexibly used at any time to enhance communication between people who have difficulty scheduling time together, but need to talk about realities that have to be viewed. Logistically easier solutions include frequent telephone conversations, possibly using teleconference capabilities with families who have difficulty meeting with staff, and problem-solving e-mail conversations.

Potential Barriers to Learning

Collaborative relationships between rehabilitation specialists and everyday people may be difficult to establish because specialists take insufficient note of the difficulty of the learning tasks that they present to people at an exceedingly stressful time in their lives.

Quantity and Complexity of Information and Skills

It is useful for specialists to remind themselves of the months or years of academic study and coached clinical practice that they needed in order to master the knowledge and skills that they may otherwise be tempted to present at a Friday afternoon family conference or in a 1-hour inservice session for staff who lack expertise in the professional's area of specialization. Such a presentation is, of course, a prescription for frustration and failure, doubly so if other specialists have the same ill-conceived attempt in mind for the same audience at the same time. Strategies for overcoming this obstacle include appropriately limited teaching objectives, more appropriate teaching approaches (such as those discussed later), less formal venues in which interaction, practice, and feedback are possible, and ongoing educational supports, such as demonstration videos.

Language Barriers

People with no previous education or training in rehabilitation, whether family members or new support staff, understandably have great difficulty grasping important concepts when they are expressed in professional language or without adequate demonstration or other support. When teaching or otherwise communicating with people who lack a technical vocabulary, it is always useful to ask oneself: "Would my grandmother understand this?" If not, the explanations and demonstrations must be improved.

A Potential Threat to Hope

A third potential obstacle to learning in family members is their powerful hope that their loved one will soon recover, making new learning about disability and management procedures unnecessary. That is, for family members to work hard at mastering new information and rehabilitation competencies, they must at some level acknowledge that their loved one's disability will persist, which is not an easy acknowledgment for family members to make within the first few weeks after a catastrophic injury. Staff must be sensitive to this potential reality and remind family members that the discussion is about present and near-term future needs, with no implied judgments about the long term.

Severely Competing Priorities: Exhaustion and Stress

In some cases, collaborative relationships fail to evolve because the potential collaborators do not share the priorities of the specialists seeking collaboration. For example, overworked nurses and support staff may avoid contact with therapists, not because they do not value the collaboration or recognize the importance of their role in relation to the therapist's professional domain; rather, the nurses are simply so busy and exhausted that they cannot squeeze one more activity into their demanding shift. Family members may similarly be consumed by their life of work, travel to the hospital, ongoing financial crises, care for other family members, and more. They may be doing as much as they can do and learning as much as they can possibly learn at that time. Therapists must be sensitive to these limits on time and other resources, and not pressure families and others to do more than they are capable of doing.

In other cases, the breakdown in collaboration may be related less to time constraints and more to conflicts in priorities. Therapists may disagree among themselves about priorities; disagreements may also exist between staff and family, between staff and the individual with TBI, and between the individual and his or her family. When the disagreement is about how best to pursue a goal that is not in dispute, we recommend the hypothesis-testing procedures described in Chapter 3. In contrast, when the conflict is about goals or values, resolution may be more difficult. For example, therapists may wish to engage family members in a more active collaborative role. The family members may resist this role because they see it as inconsistent with family or cultural values that they embrace. In many cases, therapists are well advised to simply respect family wishes and restrict collaborative efforts to those that are consistent with the family's commitments. In other cases, there might be value in soliciting the assistance of other families or other respected advisors (e.g., a priest) in bringing an understandably reluctant family into a collaborative relationship.

Often conflicts between rehabilitation specialists and individuals with TBI are a consequence of two diametrically opposed visions of the individual's needs. People with TBI naturally react to events and make decisions from the perspective of their life, their goals, and what they need to do to pursue their goals. The center of the universe is their ongoing life quite unrelated to the rehabilitation program. In contrast, therapists often define realities from their own perspective, namely the individual's rehabilitation needs within that discipline and the clinical context in which those needs will be met. The center of the universe is the therapy session. Therapists typically increase their effectiveness and strengthen their collaborative relationship when they shift to the person's perspective and wrap their clinical activity around that vision.

Crisis Orientation

If interaction between rehabilitation specialists and everyday people is largely restricted to occasions motivated by crises, there is scant likelihood of solid collaborative relationships evolving. For example, if a behavioral specialist generally meets with direct care staff during or in the immediate

aftermath of a serious behavioral crisis, the implicit agenda may include assignment of blame (a notorious obstacle to collaboration) and the explicit agenda is generally restricted to emergency procedures to restore equilibrium. For everyday people to collaborate in a positive, proactive approach to challenging behavior (or a positive approach to any rehabilitation goal), collaborative conversations must occur at a time of tranquil reflection, which we sometimes refer to as community meetings to emphasize the shared goals and agendas and the equal standing of all collaborators in rehabilitation. Community meetings are an opportunity for staff, possibly the individuals served, and possibly family members, to step back, identify successes as well as challenges, and collaboratively and proactively create plans to address the outstanding challenges.

Overdependence on One Person to Provide Supports

In inpatient rehabilitation, we frequently observe a bonding of family members to one staff person, who could be any member of the team, including an assistant level staff person. Family members then seek that person out for support, present their concerns to that person, and perhaps learn most effectively from that person. There may be no real dangers in this relationship; indeed, it may be useful in some cases to capitalize on the phenomenon by using that bonded staff person as a general conduit for important communications between other staff members and families. Dangers arise, however, when conflicts are thereby created among staff and when family members grow dependent on that person for their well being. The latter is particularly common following discharge from inpatient rehabilitation when needs remain at a high level and families rely on one person to meet those needs. The predictable consequences of such dependence are (a) increasing dependence as the timeless dynamics of learned helplessness unfold, (b) ongoing crises when the support person is unavailable, (c) anger directed at the support person for failing the family when problems inevitably arise, and (d) ultimate burnout in the support person. The solution of this problem is prevention, involving a circle of support, as opposed to a one-person support system, and a jointly developed plan for fading supports over time with the goal of increasing self-reliance and decreasing learned helplessness.

COLLABORATING WITH EVERYDAY PEOPLE: PROCEDURES

General Considerations in Collaboration

Specialists in rehabilitation who wish to succeed as collaborators with the people who are most important in the everyday routines of individuals with TBI must act in a way that is sensitive to the basic rules of collaboration: be available, listen actively, be respectful, clarify roles and expectations, and identify as many occasions as possible for collaboration, including collaboration in assessment and intervention.

Be Available

Collaboration with people one rarely sees is not easy. Earlier we emphasized the value in inpatient rehabilitation of flexible scheduling of therapists so they have ample opportunity to work elbow-to-elbow with the critical 3:00 PM to 11:00 PM nursing staff and the weekend nursing staff. The same hours typically create opportunities for interaction with family members who may be able to visit only in the evenings and on weekends. Creative therapists can use those times to establish collegial working relationships and to engage staff and family members in symmetric, mutually respectful problem-solving activities connected with the rehabilitation program of the person with TBI.

Listen Actively and Nonjudgmentally

Successful collaborators also listen to their co-collaborators, actively seeking information, concerns, insights, and suggestions. Inexperienced clinicians often assume that their job is primarily to tell others what the issues are and what to do about them. Experienced clinicians know that they must listen to others, including family members and other staff at all levels, profiting from their insights and respecting their concerns, thereby creating collegial relationships that yield rich rewards for the person with disability.

Be Respectful: "I Am a Guest in Your Home"

When specialists in rehabilitation consult to family members in their homes or to other professionals on their professional turf, those consulting specialists must remember that they are guests in those homes. In our vocabulary, "I am a guest in your home" carries with it the following obligations:

➤ *Respect Diversity:* Helping people with disability and the significant people in their lives create positive everyday routines must be accomplished within the framework imposed by basic values and practices in that setting, if only because recommendations inconsistent with those values and practices simply will not be implemented.

➤ *Seek Capacity:* Successful collaborators do not begin with an assumption of incapacity. Rather they seek capacity in the important people and settings of the individual's life and intervene only as needs arise that cannot be dealt with by the everyday people in those settings without help.

➤ *Respect Expertise:* Experienced clinicians understand the value of collaboration with everyday people and respect the expertise that each everyday person has to share.

➤ *Understand Grieving:* When staff members erroneously expect family members to proceed sequentially through a rigid series of stages of mourning, ultimately achieving acceptance and adjustment within the first few months after an injury to a loved one, those staff are likely to experience serious and frequent conflict with families. Staff must understand the long-term nature of mourning, the possibility for phases of grieving to be recycled over and over, and the distinct and eminently understandable possibility that *acceptance* will never be achieved, despite satisfactory *adjustments* to the changes in life.

➤ *Identify an Effective Communicator:* Earlier we commented that some families bond to one or a small number of staff members, often because of the comfort they feel communicating with those few people. These natural communication bonds can be used for frequent and positive communication. Alternatively, communication can be channelled through a family counselor specifically trained for this role.

➤ *Ensure That Everyday People Are Supported:* Earlier we highlighted the importance of creating a circle of support for staff and families. In the case of families, this circle often includes relatives, friends, church members, and others. We frequently connect families with other families we know who have much to offer because of their own experiences. Effective pairing of families can contribute mightily to the circle of support.

Clarify Roles and Expectations

Most everyday people, including family members and direct care staff, are more than willing to do whatever it takes to facilitate progress in the person with TBI. However, confusion and anxiety are the dominant outcomes when important people do not know what is expected of them and that the expectations are reasonable. We have promoted negotiation and collaborative development of plans, which may not seem consistent with clear role definition and expectations. But they are. However

the plans are developed, they should result in clear roles and expectation, including roles for everyday people.

Collaborate in Assessment

In Chapter 3, we focused our comments on functional assessment, understood as a process of ongoing, collaborative, contextualized hypothesis testing. One of the many advantages of the collaborative aspect of this approach to assessment is that it promotes collegiality and a habit of collaboration from the initial stages of intervention.

Collaborate in Intervention

Throughout the book, we have described intervention through everyday routines, necessitating collaboration with the people who are part of and shape those routines. When intervention plans have their basis in collaborative, contextualized assessment, collaboration in functional intervention naturally follows.

Collaborating With Everyday People: Education and Support Options

Everyday people may or may not possess the technical knowledge and procedural competencies needed to play their role in functional, contextualized intervention. Several options are available to assist those who have needs in this area.

Informational Inservices and Family Conferences

In rehabilitation and special education settings, support staff generally receive their orientation and education from inservice training sessions, if indeed they receive it at all. We add this qualification because we frequently hear teaching assistants in schools complain that they received no orientation and education to prepare them for their important role with complex students. Family members often receive their orientation in family conferences with a characteristically full agenda. The shortcomings of these training venues are well known and were mentioned earlier.

Decontextualized Competency-Based Training

We use the term *competency-based training* to refer to inservice training sessions that involve practice of competencies or procedures, with appropriate modeling and feedback as needed. Educational opportunities of this sort have the distinct advantage over informational inservices in that those receiving the training have the opportunity to apply the information and receive some coaching, however limited, in their application. However, there remain two serious shortcomings with this method. First, people who lack the skill or competency in question typically need more than 2 or 3 hours of exposure and practice to master the skill. Second, the practice is out of context, which carries with it all of the threats to transfer of training that we have highlighted throughout the book. Just as academic and clinical preparation programs for rehabilitation professionals do not expect clinicians-in-training to transfer skills learned in a classroom directly to independent clinical practice without the coached, contextualized practice available in their practicum or internship experiences, so also rehabilitation programs should not expect healthcare support staff or family members to transfer skills learned in a decontextualized inservice session without additional support. Therefore, this type of training is best understood as a first stage, making possible the inclusion of the skill on the staff person's job description and preparing the way for meaningful contextualized teaching, described next.

Apprenticeship

Under *apprenticeship*, we include a set of teaching procedures that are collaborative in the sense that the teacher and learner work together to enhance the "product," that teaching occurs as much as possible in the context of the activity in question (as it does in a true apprenticeship), and that the teacher works with the apprentice to ensure that the product is of high quality, pulling back levels of support as the apprentice acquires competence. We have recently acquired considerable experience with an apprenticeship model of education and training in connection with a New York State Health Department Program, designed in part to create supports for adults with TBI in community settings. Among the most challenging members of this population are those with behavioral disorders after the injury. These are the individuals we have been serving through the program for 3 years.

Knowing that many of the individuals returning to their communities from nursing homes, psychiatric hospitals, or other restrictive settings will be served by staff with a history of working in geriatric centers or working with people with developmental disabilities, mental health needs, or spinal cord injury, we began the program by developing a TBI Manual and conducting approximately 40 two-day workshops around the state. The workshop phase was followed by the development of an apprenticeship training program. The apprentices, who may be direct care staff or certified rehabilitation professionals from any disciplinary background, with formal educations ranging from high school equivalency diplomas to Ph.D.s, volunteer for the program with the goal of improving their skills with this population. As they work with adults with behavior and other problems, we provide them with support and teaching from the set of options described in the next sections.

Our work with these apprentices has strengthened our evaluation of apprenticeship procedures and confirmed our skepticism about decontextualized training. Some of our best apprentices attended the 2-day workshop and received the manual, commented positively about what they received from the 2 days, then returned to their work site and made few changes in their everyday practices, including practices that clearly were not consistent with the principles described and illustrated in the workshop about which they had so positively commented! As we have observed several times, this failure of transfer should come as no surprise in light of what is known about the difficulty of transfer of training in humans, regardless of their level of intelligence and education. Many of the apprentices reported to us that they knew in the abstract what they should be doing, but had great difficulty with concrete implementation of the ideas in their setting.

Coaching in Vivo. By adding coaching procedures to the general concept of apprenticeship, we have mixed a metaphor in a way that we think is potentially useful, despite the literary sensitivities that may be offended. Situational coaching is well illustrated by an interaction that we had recently with one of our apprentices. He was working with an adult, Bob, with severe memory problems and inhibition impairment, including frequent socially inappropriate, sexually oriented comments. Bob had been asked to type his schedule on a computer, but instead was composing a sexually explicit letter to a female staff person. The apprentice, who was at that time overseeing activities in the TBI group room, reminded Bob of his assignment. Bob perceived this as nagging, became angry, cursed, and continued with his letter. The apprentice then calmly reminded Bob that letters of this sort are offensive and inappropriate. Bob continued with the letter.

The apprentice then approached us (we were observing at the time) and asked for help. We engaged the apprentice and Bob in a brief discussion about the letter, which Bob insisted on completing. We then proposed an experiment: Bob would finish the letter, show it to the woman, and ask her for her reaction. He would then compose an alternative letter judged to be friendly and complimentary, without the offensiveness of the sexually explicit material, show that to various women in the center, and record their reactions. He agreed—and his agreement was recorded and signed by all of us—that he would use this experiment to make decisions about how best to achieve his goal, which was to interact positively and more frequently with women. The completed experiment clearly revealed that he met his goal with the inoffensive letters and blocked his goal with the offensive letters. Results of the experiment were summarized and posted at his workstation. From that point on, staff simply used the word *experiment* to remind Bob, without nagging, of the interactive style that he had come to understand was successful for him.

After we completed the initial negotiation about the experiment with Bob, we videotaped Bob and the apprentice replicating the intervention. For Bob, the video could potentially serve as a reminder that he had made a commitment. For the staff person (i.e., the apprentice), the video was used as a "game film." He reviewed the tape much as athletes review their performance in games with the goal of evaluating and improving that performance.

In this case, the apprentice had heard us discuss the process of engaging clients in experiments as a respectful way to resolve conflicts and avoid potentially inflammatory confrontation (see Chapter 3), had watched model videotapes, and had read discussions of the process, but was struggling with its functional implementation in his everyday routine interactions with potentially volatile individuals with TBI. He later reported that the 15 minutes of situational coaching that he received that day was the beginning of his effective implementation of a collaborative, experimental approach to intervention with all of the people with whom he worked.

Guided Self-Observation on Video. In Chapter 3 we discussed self-observation as a component of assessment and presented a protocol for guided self-observation. The same protocol can be used during the apprenticeship phase of staff training. The experiences of the apprentices in our New York TBI Apprenticeship Program indicate that guided self-observation on video is among the most useful apprenticeship procedures and in some cases is a necessary component of training. Our experience with this procedure is so positive that we now include, as a precondition for participation in the Apprenticeship Program, that potential apprentices agree to video themselves interacting with individuals with TBI and to create time for guided observation of the videotaped interaction. In many cases, apprentices need no guidance; as they watch their routines of interaction, they identify for themselves the respects in which the interaction can be improved.

Community Meetings. As we use the term, community meetings can be a time for staff, or staff and family members, to engage in collaborative problem solving, sharing information about what is working, and ensuring that all staff have the script that, for the present, is working. Community meetings are quite different from staffings in that there are no formal reports and the focus is not on the latest crisis, but rather on the overall story, what is positive about that story, and how to make the story better. In these meetings, we encourage staff to share their visions and brainstorm about how best to realize those visions. Understood in these terms, community meetings are a time to support, encourage, and learn from one another. For this reason, we include them in this list of effective teaching and support procedures. Elsewhere, we discussed community meetings specifically for the *clients* in a program who may benefit from a periodic meeting in which they reflect as a group on their experiences in rehabilitation and work at supporting one another.

Peer-Peer Training and Support. In busy work settings and in busy families, scheduling time for all potential everyday coaching partners to receive instruction and practice in relevant competencies is difficult and often impossible. One solution to this chronic scheduling problem is to create training chains. Competencies are passed from one person to another much as one communicates by means of a chain letter. For example, evening staff can receive coaching from a therapist and pass the competency on to the night staff; parents can receive coaching from a therapist and pass the competency on to siblings and other relatives. Similarly, family members can help one staff person understand an important feature of interaction with the person with TBI and that staff member can then pass the insight on to other staff.

For this system to work in an institutional setting, managers must ensure that there is a culture in place that supports peer support and teaching. We occasionally encounter organizations in which staff members who offer suggestions to peers are thought to be stepping out of line and are punished by their peers for doing so. In our opinion, this is a symptom of an unhealthy work environment, requiring managers to help staff understand that peer support and peer discussions of what works and what does not work are not only permitted, they are a job expectation.

Training Videos

Rehabilitation specialists typically have years of academic education and clinical training before they are certified to work as independent practitioners with individuals with disability. It is obviously unrealistic to suppose that people without this education and training, whether they are support staff, family members, or other specialists trained in a different speciality area of rehabilitation, can acquire comparable competence in the skills of that speciality even given the best and most practical training opportunities among those described in the previous sections.

Under these circumstances, a very useful support is a videotaped illustration of how best to implement a specific procedure, teach, manage a difficult behavior, or interact most positively. Commercially available videotapes may be useful in some cases, but generally present illustrations too distant from the specific realities of the individual in question to communicate effectively. Therefore, many rehabilitation hospitals routinely create videotapes showing staff modeling types of interaction or intervention procedures that are useful for the individual. These videotapes are then given to all of the nursing shifts, family members, or professional and support staff who will be serving the individual after discharge so that they can watch, repeatedly if necessary, a good model of the interaction or intervention that has been recommended. In our experience, these videos serve an important purpose, particularly with the dramatic reduction in average length of stay in rehabilitation hospitals in the 1980s and 1990s. Even more useful, in our experience, are the transitional or self-advocacy videotapes described in the next section.

Collaboratively Produced Transitional/ Self-Advocacy Videos: Ylvisaker, Szekeres, and Feeney (1998) presented a protocol for collaborating with a person with a disability in producing a self-advocacy videotape that, in most cases, is used to facilitate a transition that requires that a new set of people learn to know the person and gain competence in serving that person. The transition could be from hospital to home and a day or outpatient program, from hospital to school, from one level of schooling or day program to another, or from one residential setting to another. Alternatively, the tape could be produced as communication from one setting to another during the same period of time, for example, from the day program to the group home or vice versa, from school to family home or vice versa, or from outpatient therapists to school staff or vice versa.

The collaborators in the production of the video include the person with a disabil-

ity, who takes as much of a leadership role as possible with whatever support is necessary, family members, staff, and possibly others. The primary goal of the video is to introduce the individual, including his or her strengths, positive attributes, interests, and needs, and demonstrate the types of support or intervention that are most useful at that time. An equally important goal for many people with disability is to enable them to assume control over orienting new professional or support staff, which necessitates organized reflection on strengths, needs, and strategies to achieve goals. When understood as a routine practice in supporting people with disability, this collaborative activity meets several of the conditions outlined by Wehmeyer and Schwartz (1997) in their discussion of self-determination. Many people with whom we have worked in producing such a video have stated that the process gave them a sense of power and control that they had generally lacked since their injury and that they achieved greater clarity about their needs when required to explain those needs in an effective way to people who needed to understand.

In our experience, the collaboration involved in the production is also useful for and appreciated by families. We include family members in decisions about what is most important to show in the video and often include them in the presentation of their family member. If possible, we use family members to demonstrate important intervention or support procedures. Their preparation for this role may be productive for them. The role also communicates a sense of empowerment that may have been lacking if they had previously played a largely passive role in relation to rehabilitation professional.

Finally, when staff from diverse professional backgrounds are required to collaborate with each other, with family members, and with the individual with TBI in deciding what is most critical to illustrate and how best to illustrate it, their commitment to collaboration may be increased along with their appreciation for the perspective of the individual and family.

SUMMARY

In this chapter we highlighted the value of collaboration—multiple levels of collaboration—in TBI rehabilitation. We also described procedures that can be used to create collaborative relationships among staff, between staff and individuals with TBI, and between both of these parties and the everyday people in the life of the person with TBI.

The epilogue that follows, written by Jason Lewin, illustrates and summarizes the themes of this book. We have worked collaboratively with Jason for 4 years. We have also collaborated with his family, friends, and other supports. The point of our collaboration with them was in part to facilitate the development of their collaborative relationship with Jason.

Jason now collaborates with us in a number of ways. He is our copresenter at TBI workshops; he designs graphic illustrations for us, including the one on the cover of this book; he works as a peer counselor in an intervention setting where we consult. Jason's story and his evaluation of a collaborative, everyday approach to rehabilitation are a fitting summary of the themes of this book.

Epilogue

My name is Jason S. Lewin and I've had a severe traumatic brain injury since 21 June, 1991. My goal in this epilogue is to tell you a bit about my life before my injury, paint a bleak picture of my life over the first few years after the injury, and describe some of the efforts that have enabled me to resume control of my life and put it back on a satisfying path. Recreating success and a sense of meaning for myself has been hard. But I've received the assistance of people who deliver their rehabilitation services according to the principles presented in this book—people who helped me take control rather than trying to take control of me. I've read the book and I know Mark and Tim very well. I hope that you will read my story as support for the approach to brain injury rehabilitation that they have described.

I was on my way home from work, on my motorcycle, when an oncoming car made a left turn directly in front of me. We collided. I was in a coma officially for 5 weeks, although I do not remember anything from 5 minutes preaccident until 6 weeks post. I was left with injuries to the frontal, temporal, parietal, and occipital lobes of my brain. I also had a hypoxic injury to the brain, as well as many, many internal and orthopedic injuries. It is truly a miracle that I survived the accident—even more a miracle that I am able to speak to you in this way.

THE DOWNWARD SPIRAL: LIFE WITH NO CONTROL

Following my regaining consciousness, most of my problems were behavioral. The first major episode was an altercation with my wife, which led to a suicide attempt and my divorce. I had been released from my first rehabilitation facility 3 months prior, with no aftercare.

At the time of my accident I was engaged to be married. I was working three jobs and helping to plan my wedding for late August, 1991. While I was in the hospital and comatose, my fiancé was seldom around. Her greatest interest seemed to be getting a good lawyer and a sizable lawsuit settlement. As I emerged from the coma, she rarely visited until I started to remember things; then she started coming by. When I was released from rehab, she and I married—as I had spent our original wedding date in the rehabilitation hospital.

As soon as our vows were exchanged, she tried to become my lord and master. She told me, "If you ever ride a motorcycle again, I'll leave you." Her father told me that if I rode again, he would shoot me—and he showed me the weapon. My greatest passion, motorcycling, was forbidden. My wife took over all the household chores that I had done before the accident, and enjoyed doing. She convinced me to break contact with my family. She also divided me from all of my friends. My wife took control over who I socialized with and what we did. She was consumed with getting me back to work and bringing money into the house. I was excessively depressed and could not "just snap out of it," as she repeatedly commanded. With no aftercare from the rehab, I had nothing to check reality with.

After 3 months of that stress, I could not handle any more. I got excessively drunk at a Christmas party. Once home, I started destroying our apartment and took a massive overdose of digoxin. The police came and I was hauled off to a hospital, then to a psychiatric hospital. I spent the next 2 months in psych wards. I blamed my actions on unlivable conditions with my wife. On Christmas day, 1991, while I was on a psych ward, my wife told me that she was going to divorce me. Three and a half months later we were legally divorced. My marriage lasted 3 months together, and 3 months separated, for a total of 6 months.

I thought I had gone crazy. The psych hospitals did nothing but intensify that opinion. I was put on Prozac, an antidepressant. That helped—for 5 months. I took the news of my impending divorce in stride; I reinstated my old friendships and created new ones; I even got back together with my family. I was released from the hospital with minimal aftercare—aftercare that did not understand brain injury, but treated me as just another psych patient. Finally living independently for the first time in all of my 25 years, I continued psychological counseling and taking Prozac. About 3 months after my release, overwhelming feelings of anger and paranoia firmly set in. They began while I was still in the hospital, but over time they just became worse and worse. After a billing dispute, I ceased therapy and Prozac.

Initially, I crashed. Prozac had controlled levels of serotonin in my brain for 5 months. Without it, my body did not know what to do. I became more and more angry at the woman who had hit my motorcycle—for causing me to have to endure an intolerable life.

In June, 1992 I was found ineligible for SSD/SSI. The Social Security Administration (SSA) determined that I was not severely disabled by my brain injury and orthopedic injuries. I was livid. I wrote a nastygram to the SSA, both locally and to their Baltimore office, appealing the deci-

sion and demanding reconsideration. I also sent a copy of the letter to my attorney and turned the matter over to his care. In response, the SSA repeatedly lost my paperwork and delayed their decision for 3 years. They lost everything except the nastygram I had written. It was only through the diligence and persistence of my attorney that a decision was finally reached—in my favor! But at the time of the rejection, I was livid, not only at the SSA, but also at the woman who had hit me. In my view, she had crippled me both physically and mentally. I was not able to work, and without any support from the government, there was no financial way for me to survive, much less thrive as I had done before the injury. Everything looked black, and all the result of one woman's negligence on the day of 21 June, 1991. I wanted blood—retribution. I continued to look for employment, without success. My anger and desire heightened. By the time a month had gone by, I was planning to get retribution; July, 1992.

On the advice of my attorney, I took a vacation. I spent 2 days in Colorado Springs, 2 weeks in Santa Cruz, and a week on the road. I found peace and an "at home" feeling in Colorado. My time in California was spent with a friend of the family. After 3 weeks, I returned home.

I continued to look for employment. After another month I got a job working for a retail clothing store as an assistant manager. I could handle the floor work and dealing with customers, but I could not make sense of the paperwork or the computer/cash register. After 1 month there, I received a partial settlement from my lawsuit. I quit work and went back to college to complete my bachelor's degree in industrial design. I had already completed 3 out of 5 years for the degree at the time of the accident, but had stopped college for two reasons. The first was to wait for the head of my department to retire the next year. He and I had worked together previously and I had done some personal work for him. We had professional differences, to say the least. I was not going to graduate with him as the head of the department. The second reason was that, as long as I was out of college and getting married, I had to work. At the time of the accident, I was working three jobs and bringing home about $40,000 per year after taxes. With a new head of my department and the money from the partial settlement, I decided the best investment I could make was completing my education. So, back to college I went.

I found the work extremely taxing. It was challenging before my injury, but not to the same extent. Before the injury I had attended college, worked two jobs, had a full social life, and maintained a 3.4 grade point average. After my injury, I was not working, taking only two classes, and receiving Cs—with no social life. I blamed the difference on the brain injury. I should have been getting As, but struggled for Cs. The anger was fueled.

Other behavioral problems surfaced on the road.

I bought a HarleyDavidson, something I had dreamed of since childhood. Riding one day, another woman made a left turn directly in front of me. I had to lock the brakes and almost dump the bike to avoid hitting her. I followed her, passed her, and then had to stop at a traffic lamp—I was in front of her. I got off the motorcycle and started back to her car. I was out for blood. Luckily for her, she pulled around my motorcycle, ran a red light, and got away before I could do anything to her.

One day, an old man pulled out of a driveway in front of my car. Again I had to lock the brakes and steer harshly to avoid impact. At the next traffic lamp, he stopped in front of me. I was blowing my horn. He gave me the finger. I pulled up next to him. I was yelling at him. His door started to open. I lost it. I thought, "O.K., you want to go down? Fine, I'll take you down." I got out of my car and went after him. He was out of his car. I walked around to the front of his car shouting, "You stupid motherfucker . . ." when he hit me with a wooden

cane on the neck. The cane hit me so hard that it broke. I tackled him to the ground making sure that my knee went into his chest. On top of him, I started choking him and pounding his head on the pavement. One of my passengers pulled me off of him. I kicked him in the head with a steel-toed work boot and left. That was summer, 1992.

Over the next year and a half, things were calm. I continued college—and continued frustration and anger about the accident. I got involved with marijuana. I had tried it a number of times before my injury and it had no effect on me. After my injury, some was going around at a Halloween party. I tried it again—it worked and I liked it. So during this time I continued to smoke a lot of pot. I also got involved with a woman over the summer of 1993 and she moved in with me.

Home life with this woman, Jenifer, was not bliss. We did not fight much, but we were not compatible. With her knowledge and approval, I started seeking other women. Jenifer continued to live with me in my two bedroom apartment, but we were distant. I started seeing another woman, Julie, in another city. We would write, call, and see each other on weekends as work permitted.

One morning Jenifer showed me a letter that she had written to Julie the day before. That letter told Julie harm would befall her if she continued to date me. Again, I lost it. I threw Jenifer out of the apartment. She came back with her mother. We all started yelling at each other. Jenifer's mother hit me in the face. I threw both of them out and called the police. The police came and said that Jenifer could stay in my apartment and that they would take me to jail. I got the apartment manager, who explained that Jenifer could not stay in the apartment and we moved all of her belongings into the hallway. On a 1 to 10 scale, my anger level was 9.99. I was all primed and ready to go off.

I went to my class at the university. After 15 minutes there, I realized that I was too agitated to take in any useful information. I left and headed home. Along the way, I was driving very aggressively. I weaved in and out of traffic, passing everyone on the freeway. In the extreme right lane a white car was trying to stay with me. I thought he was trying to race me. That fueled my anger; now it had become a contest. We continued up the freeway going between 90 and 100 miles per hour. I was in the extreme left lane. Ahead of me was a Cadillac moving slowly; there was no one to her right. I could tell it was a "her" from her big hairdo. When I was about a quarter mile behind her, I flashed my lights, telling her to move over. She responded by flipping me both middle fingers over her shoulders. Because of my high speed, I caught up to her very quickly. I flashed my lights again. She responded by slamming on her brakes. I had to steer harshly to avoid hitting her Cadillac with my small Nissan. I pulled in front of her and slammed on my brakes. Further up, I saw my exit. I slowed down and started moving right to exit. She pulled up alongside me. She was giving me the middle finger and shouting "Fuck you!" That was it! I'd had enough. I pulled out my pellet pistol and started shooting at her. She pulled away quickly; I exited the freeway.

I could not get into the correct lane of my exit, so I continued up a service road to the next exit. At the traffic light, there she was in front of me—the woman in the Cadillac. I had already reached my breaking point. I was going to kill her. I followed her into a convenience mart, got out of my car with the pistol, and marched up to her car. She was getting out; I started yelling at her. She pulled a little girl out of the car whom I'd not seen previously. I assumed the little girl was hers; I could not kill this woman in front of her daughter. We yelled at each other for 5 minutes; the rest of the market was frozen. I left without even striking the woman.

When I got home, my apartment was surrounded by police. On 27 January, 1994, I was arrested and taken to jail. In a few hours, I was taken to the arraignment and

bail was set. Luckily, I had enough money in my wallet to cover the bail, so I bailed myself out. I had been charged with only misdemeanor offenses—much to the disappointment of the judge.

Two weeks later, my attorney called and told me to report to the courthouse. I was arraigned on a felony charge. My life had just taken a turn I did not want. I could live with the misdemeanors, but a felony conviction would block me from achieving my ultimate goal, being a college professor. Suicide had been a recurrent thought since I emerged from my coma. At this point, it seemed more justifiable than at any other time. The gears in my head started turning. Leaving the arraignment, my lawyer asked if I was going to be all right. I replied, "Yeah Steve, I'll be just fine."

I had not made up my mind to commit suicide, but I wanted the means available if I did decide to. I went to a sporting goods store and bought a 12-gauge shotgun plus ammunition. While at home contemplating the issue, my youngest brother barged into my apartment. While I was talking with him, two friends I had been in the Marine Corps with arrived. The discussion got heated and we were all yelling at each other. My brother grabbed the weapon and we wrestled for it. We went half over my armchair; the two Marine friends jumped on my back. My brother fired the weapon. At that point the friends got off my back and my brother squirmed out from under me, went through my screen door, and jumped off my balcony with the weapon.

My choice was made for me. I knew that the police would come and I would go straight to jail. I slashed my wrists with an X-Acto knife, got in my car, and just started driving. My eyeglasses had been knocked off during the struggle, so I could not see where I was going. Obviously, cutting my wrists did not work—the incisions were too clean and the blood clotted.

After driving for 2 hours, I recognized the city as the one my girlfriend, Julie, lived in. I fumbled my way to her house. I spent the night there. The next morning I returned to my home city to face what was going to happen. I went to my attorney's office. Seeing the cuts on my arms, he had me check into a hospital psych ward. I got to the ward on Friday evening. Nothing happened then, or over the weekend. Part of my state's Patient's Bill of Rights is that the patient will take part in all decision making about his treatment, and that he will be given a written statement as to when he will be discharged and how to appeal the discharge plan. Unfortunately, the hospital did not follow that Bill of Rights. On Monday morning my doctor, seeing me for the first time, told me that I was discharged and that the two men in the room were U.S. Marshals. I was arrested and taken to jail without any treatment from the hospital. Today the hospital is suing me for $3,000.00 +, for the "care" they gave me.

Anyway, I was in jail. The District Attorney made a deal that if I attended and completed a program for head injury rehabilitation, I would be convicted of only a misdemeanor and serve probation. I went to a rehabilitation facility in New England. Upon arriving there, I saw that it was in the middle of nowhere. Even if I did want to run away, there was no place to go.

The rehab was pure hell. It was worse than jail; it was run as a medium-security prison. The staff were all local rednecks. It is my opinion that the staff relieved the boredom there by using physical force on their "clients." I was stuffed into a small log cabin with 16 other clients. There was no space to be alone. There was also a lot of fighting between clients, because of the cramped quarters. The rehab controlled what I did, where I did it, and who I did it with—they controlled every second of my life there. For me there is little worse than a total lack of control.

Before I signed in at the rehab, they told me and my attorney that they would do everything to keep the police uninvolved in what happened there. This was not to be. As I said, I think the staff would relieve boredom by using physical force on clients. I learned quickly to see when this was

about to happen, especially because it happened to me a great deal. Staff called it Behavior Modification Training, or BMT. They would sit around and pick who their target was, then set that client off as an excuse to use BMT on him. Their brand of BMT involved physically taking the client down and forcing him to act as the staff commanded. The client was always outnumbered, so he always lost. As I said, I learned to see when the BMT was going to start, which is the reason I left the rehab. After having words with a staff member, I saw he was coming for me. I got up and hit him first. I was immediately isolated from the rest of the population there. The next day a state trooper arrested me and took me to a local jail.

At that arraignment, the rehab director told the judge that my actions were not due to my brain injury, but that I was psychopathic—a menace to myself and to society. Facility staff also said the same in reports about me. They said I chose to lose my temper. Those reports would come back to haunt me right up through the final trial about my motorcycle accident. Anyway, I was bailed out of that New England jail a couple of days later and returned to my home city's jail in New York State, where I was held without bail—from the shotgun incident. I had spent 3 months in New England, but I had also learned that attempting to control me in the name of rehabilitation was a big mistake. Many other people with traumatic brain injuries have told me the same thing.

I was back in central New York, in jail without bail. The District Attorney was still demanding therapy for my brain injury. I had weekly meetings with the Office of Mental Health (OMH). I could not get out of jail to get therapy, and I could not get anyone to come into the jail to give me therapy. I kept telling my plight to the OMH people and after 3 months, they told me that if I was committed to a justice system psychiatric hospital, I would get therapy. I went for it.

Upon arriving at the hospital, I was asked what my problem was. I replied,

"My temper." The nurse then asked what things caused me to loose my temper. I went down the whole list of things, as I knew them. When I met my doctor, she told me that I was not going to receive any therapy, but simply be evaluated for 30 days and sent back to jail. Again, my temper was aroused. I was mad at the doctor for not even caring about what I needed and mad at the OMH officials for lying to me. The hospital was much more restrictive than jail, which did nothing but upset me more. After a week there, the same nurse who had done my intake went right down the list of things I had told her would set me off. We had words; as punishment I was being taken to the "Time Out Room." I had reached my breaking point. Holding the door to the room open was the nurse who had set me off—I punched her on the head. I was immediately put in restraints.

The month at the hospital passed. During that month my girlfriend left me and moved to an unknown place. My pride and temper were both upset. At the end of a month there, I was taken to court in that city and arraigned on assault for the incident with the nurse. Once back at the hospital, I sat down to a meeting with my doctor and attorney. After a few minutes, someone else came into the room and whispered something into the doctor's ear. That person left, the doctor stood up and announced, "The sheriffs are here; they will take you back to jail." I had not expected this. No one had told me that it was going to happen, much less when. I lost it again. I was wrestled to the floor by staff and the sheriffs, who put handcuffs on me tightly. They then drove me back to my home city.

Back at my home jail, I was placed on the psych floor for a week, then moved into the general population. My attorney had arranged that I could be released into my mother's care in order to receive therapy for my brain injury. So, at 28 years old, I was released to live with mommy and my two brothers—the brother who had pulled the trigger on the shotgun, getting me thrown in jail without bail, and the other brother who maintained that I was a menace to society and should be kept in jail until I died of old age. In order to get therapy, I moved into a very, very tense situation. And to make things even worse, the sheriffs put numerous restrictions on me; I was basically under house arrest. Life was splendid! I now lived in a place where I wasn't wanted and didn't want to be, and from which I had no way out. I lasted 6 weeks there—all so that I would not have a felony conviction.

One morning over coffee, my mother and I were having words. I got up and walked around the block to cool off. When I got back, the second brother was up. My mother and I started up again. I was losing my temper again. In frustration I said, "Fuck it" and threw my coffee cup against the wall.

My brother jumped up, "That's it, Jason. You're going back to jail." I started for the door. My mother grabbed me and held me back; we were yelling at each other. My brother came over, picked up a sizable houseplant from the ledge and threw it at me, hitting me in the stomach.

I said, "Oh, you want to throw shit at me; here you go." I picked up pieces of the coffee cup and threw them at him for at least 1 minute. My sister-in-law got involved. I headed out the door, got in my car, and started to back out of the drive. My mother was standing behind my car, holding it so I would not leave. I could not back over my mother, but I put the car in first gear and drove into the garage, hoping that the car would explode. My mother moved from behind my car. I backed into the street and peeled out of our housing project. I still do not know why I did this, but I turned around and went back to the house when I reached the main road. As I pulled up, my mother was coming out of the house. She put me in her car and we drove off.

We went to a friend's house in still another city, then to the local psychiatric clearing house. I was put involuntarily in a local hospital psych ward. As a result of the melee at my mother's house, still more felony and misdemeanor charges were piled on me and my chances for a plea bargain were gone. I was going to be a convicted felon. While on the psych ward, I maintained that all I needed was a place to live and to be left alone. After 3 or 4 months on the ward, I met with Patricia Greene, from the New York State Department of Health, and Tim Feeney, a behavioral psychologist. They were the first people to agree with me. The hospital wanted to put me in a group home for psychiatric patients. My parents wanted me out of the hospital, but with 24-hour supervision.

Anyway, after 5 months and numerous discharge meetings, I was released to my own house, on the outskirts of the city. I went through the court proceedings and for the last 4 years have been trying to build my life again.

REBUILDING A LIFE OF SELF-CONTROL

Following discharge from the psychiatric hospital, I was placed on the New York State Home and Community Based Services for Traumatic Brain Injury Waiver through the Department of Health (NYS-DOH HCBS/TBI Waiver). As part of that program, my Independent Living Center had stipulated that I was to have someone with me to help reintegrate me into the community. I waited and waited for this person to appear. I kept asking the center when they would have someone for me. That went on for many weeks. All the while I was becoming—the hard way—more integrated into the community. There was one person, R, whom I had worked with in my first rehab and who I knew was available. I thought he would make a good community reentry support person, but the center would not hire him because he lacked a college degree.

I was becoming frustrated and angry at the center, so I decided to help them out. Working with Tim Feeney, I made a short videotape introducing myself, explaining what I expected out of a staff person and what some of my issues were. Tim and Mark refer to these videos as transitional, self-advocacy videotapes and use them to serve a variety of purposes for the people they work with. The tape I made was intentionally intimidating—my head was shaved bald, punk rock played in the background, and I smoked on screen. I was trying to scare off people I call "do-gooders," those who come into the human services profession trying to lighten up everyone's day, but who have nothing upstairs. In my experience, they don't know how to handle a crisis. They often misperceive that there is a crisis when there is none. They patronize the people they work with, collect their paycheck, and go home, telling themselves what a good job they've done. I didn't want someone like that. I wanted someone who was dedicated to his work and could communicate effectively with me. So I made the video by putting my worst foot forward. My caseworker at the center was moved. She watched the video, looked at me and said, "That's scary." She didn't understand that was the way I wanted it. But she did show it to a number of prospective workers. They were all scared off. The tape worked wonderfully. As I watched the tape over and over, it also gave me greater insight into myself, even though I had written the script.

More time went by. I was upset with the center regarding the community reintegration person. Finally, in early 1996 I wrote a letter concerning the matter and asking why R could not be hired. I sent copies of the letter to my caseworker, her boss, the head of the center, and many people in the Department of Health (DOH). Within 1 week, R was scheduled to work with me. With the support of Tim Feeney, he worked with me for 6 months. By the time he was hired, I was already fairly well integrated into the community by my friends, family, and the necessities of life.

MY REVIEW OF WHAT WORKS AND WHAT DOESN'T WORK

I want to talk to you about brain injury rehabilitation, using a What Works? and What Doesn't Work? exercise that Tim and Mark constantly urge people to apply to their own lives and decision making. In my experience, some things work, others don't. I have seen two types of rehabilitation, traditional medical model intervention and collaborative, person-centered intervention as Tim and Mark describe it in this book. In my case and in almost every single case I have seen since, the latter of these two types supports the most positive outcome and the highest degree of self-control over the long run.

What Doesn't Work?

I have already described a number of interventions that didn't work for me. For example, jail didn't work. When I was released from jail, I was not only suicidal, but homicidal as well. Biofeedback didn't work. When agitated, my mind raced too fast to employ the relaxation techniques. Psych hospitals and wards didn't work. I have a brain injury; I'm not mentally ill. Furthermore, most psychiatrists I've worked with don't know much about brain injury or brain injury rehabilitation.

In general, medical model rehabilitation was ineffective for me because it focused too much on test data and training that had little to do with me and my life. It also took responsibility away from me and placed it in the hands of the caregiver. It did the same with freedom of choice. When I was in New England, I was homicidal and their attempts at rehab simply did not work. I had no choice. I had to follow their routine. Medical model rehab was too rigid to work with my real-life behavioral issues, which was the area that I needed help with. Staff simply tried to control my behavior with consequences. This has never worked with me and will never work with me. In some cases, there was little attempt at actual rehab for me. I was not an active part of the rehabilitation, more a target of it.

What Works?

What has worked for me in the rehab process? Choice and control, a network of support, prevention, reality checks, talking to me (not at me), giving me responsibility, and enabling me to be in charge of my program.

Choice and Control: Within the collaborative rehabilitation process, I was and continue to be the central focus and primary decision maker. I was given choices when getting out of the hospital. I chose to live in my home community (May 1995), with supports. I chose the supports I would have, initially working with Tim Feeney and an Independent Living Center. Other, more natural supports were my family and friends. One of my friends actually moved to my new city from an hour away. I spent most of my time with her. But, in concert with Tim, I chose my supports and created plans to use those supports. Tim's constant focus was on my goals and what was working and not working to help me achieve those goals. I always felt in control, but I needed guidance creating and following plans that worked for me.

Because agitation is a real problem for me, Tim asked me to keep track of my agitation levels at the beginning and end of each day. I thought that was a good idea, but it would not tell me anything about what set me off. So I started keeping track of my agitation levels throughout the day. I created an internal "barometer"—a 100-point scale that I used to measure my level of agitation. With Tim's help, I created a set of rules to follow based on my barometric readings. I have learned a lot about myself through doing this. Also I have been better able to manage my life. I set up a plan for each day. On the same sheet, I keep track of what I actually do and my level of agitation. If I see my levels start to climb too high, I may have to alter my schedule for later in the day. There is a point where I should no longer drive. There is another, higher point where I cannot be around people, so I isolate myself until I am calm enough to rejoin the group. Tim and Mark refer to this in the book as self-control of antecedents. I call it my control and I need it.

A Network of Support: My supports include my family and friends. I recently became engaged, so my first support is my fiancé. But there are others as well. My mother and father are there for me. Tim Feeney has been a great support in my life. There are also friends and professionals—most of whom I consider friends more than professionals, such as my attorney.

How do I use this support network? When I have a problem, I first identify what type of problem it is. Sometimes I need help doing this. If I do, I turn to my fiancé, my mother, Tim, or one of my other support team. Sometimes, many of my support team members will meet and discuss problem areas. When this happens, I am always present, and the conversation is directed toward me. Realizing that I need help identifying the nature of the problem —and that I need to deliberately create and follow concrete plans, especially when times are tough—is probably the biggest difference between me and "normal" people and between my life now and my life as it would have been without the injury.

Prevention and Scripting: Prevention, including writing a script to follow during difficult situations, is the best tool for avoiding and, if necessary, dealing with a crisis. One of my biggest helps in prevention is the scale I use with my agitation. There is also writing scripts for life events. In writing a script, I sit down—usually with one of my support team—and look at an upcoming event. We will play that event out to every possible outcome, and in doing so come up with how I should respond to those possible outcomes.

For example, I recently decided to move to Albany, New York to pursue an education in brain injury and rehabilitation. Right now I live 1 hour east of my mother, who has been a great support to me. For all her good traits, when it comes to me and

how I will get by in this world, my mother is sort of kooky. Moving to Albany will put me at least 3 hours away from her. Also, Albany is a fast paced city compared to where I now live. Once the decision to move was made, my mother had to be told. Because of the magnitude of the news, and knowing how my mother worries about me, I foresaw the potential for much weeping, wailing, and gnashing of teeth—a crisis. I predicted her concerns: "What supports will Jason have? What about the traffic in Albany? You know how Jason gets in traffic. Albany is so far away, how will I get there if Jason needs me?. . . ." So I sat down with Tim Feeney, and we came up with scripts for all of my mother's potential concerns. We also came up with ways for me to behave during the delivery of the news, and ways for me to behave if my mother started going batty on me.

As it worked out, we were right about her concerns, but I never had to resort to the backup strategy. Tim and I knew that I would have to redirect the conversation with my mother from time to time, so we planned how I would do that. That redirection was all that was needed. This is one fairly benign example, but the concept of developing scripts for tough situations works. I have used it a number of times. It may also be used for more complex situations. I have also seen this scripting process work for people with far greater disability than mine. This is one way for people with brain injury to take control of their lives even if they have difficulty making good judgments in the thick of battle.

Reality Checks: A reality check is just that. I know that my perceptions are somewhat warped by my brain injury. I may perceive problems or threats that are simply not real. When I start to question something, I go to someone I trust and ask if he or she sees the same thing happening that I do. This person is usually someone in my support team, but it does not have to be. Based on the feedback I get, I can adjust my behavior appropriately. In the book, Tim and Mark illustrate the usefulness of this "check it out" strategy with people who have pretty severe disability after brain injury. It works.

In most traditional, medical model rehab programs, professionals talk among themselves. The "client" is not talked to, much less consulted about treatment plans—or if he is, he is the last to know something. In the collaborative process, the "client" talks to everybody and is included in all important decision making. That is how my program works. I talk with everybody who will have an impact on my life. And the amazing thing is, by talking to me it is surprising how many reality checks are possible and how much prevention occurs.

Responsibility and Personally Meaningful Activities: Enabling me to assume responsible roles as a contributor (not just a receiver of services) has been as great a help to me as anything—which also relates to me being in charge of my own program. Since my last psychiatric hospital discharge almost 4 years ago, little by little I have been given more and more responsibility. Now I am a peer counselor to a group of people (not "clients") who are dealing with issues both of brain injury and substance abuse. For me, knowing that someone is depending on me both fills me with a great sense of responsibility and makes me feel better about myself.

In the fall of 1995, Tim asked me to speak at a seminar in Albany, sponsored by the New York State Department of Health. I was enthused by the idea because I knew that a lot of brain injury service providers were going to be there. I felt it was important for them to see a survivor's point of view. I talked about how brain injury can be a downward spiral. I no longer see brain injury as only a downward spiral, because I have been given more responsibility and because the collaborative approach has worked so well for me.

Later in 1995 Tim and Mark asked me to design the cover of a manual to be used in their brain injury seminars, called "Creating a Satisfying Life After Brain Injury." I was schooled as an industrial designer, and although this was only a graphic exercise, it was a chance to use my skills. It was also a chance to show many people across the state a picture of what brain injury feels like. The same graphic is on the cover of the book you are reading. After the image was done, Mark and Tim asked me to be a part of their Satisfying Life seminars, talking about staff training. I took the task very seriously. This was my opportunity to tell staff how to work with people who have had traumatic brain injuries. Mark, Tim, and I toured New York State over the next 3 years giving the seminars. The feedback we got made me feel wonderful, like I was really giving something to these people. That began in 1996.

During that time, Tim asked me to start the role I play now as a peer counselor. At first I was uncomfortable and skeptical; but now it is one of the most fulfilling things I do. I have seen, with my own eyes, the impact I have made on some of the people in the TBI-substance abuse program. That is very satisfying and gives me a sense of worth. Along with the counseling, the Department of Health asked me to create an image for their Best Practices conference. I did, and it has become a logo for the DOH brain injury program. The same type of feeling followed—worth and satisfaction. Finally, I was asked to write this Epilogue. The feelings of responsibility and satisfaction are equally great. Creating a satisfying life after brain injury does not simply mean recovering functions. It must include becoming successfully engaged in activities that are meaningful to the person.

Although it has been 4 years in the making, little by little I have been given more and more responsibility. With each step, I have a greater sense of self-worth. The more I get into it, the more I like it. That is why I decided to move to Albany and pursue an education in brain injury rehabilitation. This is going to be a part of my life, and a very satisfying part I expect.

Being in Charge: The last thing that has worked for me is being in charge of my own program. I have been given choices, as everyone should be in life. My life has been the result of my choices. I do not have someone over me deciding what I will do. It has been my choice. This also relates to acceptance of responsibility—if I choose badly, I have no one to blame but myself. I spent 3 years after my injury making a series of bad choices. I needed help to create habits of thoughtful planning and decision making. I finally got that help and am now generally making good decisions.

This is my life. I can do with it as I see fit. It is the God-given right of everybody to do precisely that. Just because I have a brain injury, it does not mean that I cannot choose for myself.

Tim Feeney and I have been working together for 4 years, using the collaborative approach to brain injury rehabilitation. In the process, I have learned what I must do to achieve the goals that I set for myself. I have also worked with Mark Ylvisaker in the area of communication. All told, it has been a huge success. This is not to say that my life is a bed of roses. It's not. I have had to see things about myself that I did not want to see. There have been times when I have felt my life was spinning out of control. There have been some really black times during these 4 years.

What I have had to see is that my life is not so bad, certainly not as bad as it could have been right now. It's easy to wallow in self-pity; I have done and sometimes continue to do more than my share of that. But through working with Mark and Tim, I have seen that there is a contribution I can make to the world. Right now I could still be in that New England rehab, with no choice in my life, and paying nearly $1,000.00 per day to be there. I could still be in a psychiatric hospital as a result of my bad decisions, again with no choice in my life. I could be in prison as a result of my crimes, still without choice. In all of these places, I would be removed from family and friends. I also would be removed from any chance of brain injury rehab that worked.

Instead of being someplace I do not want to be, I am leading a life of my own choosing. Still there have been some black times in my life, even after I had seen these things. For example, the litigation process associated with the original motorcycle accident was very stressful. But with great effort I kept my composure and decided in the end to settle for less than I thought was fair. The first major fight with my current fiancé left me feeling suicidal. But I followed the plans that are tied to my agitation barometer, and survived that difficult time. This is another example of anticipation and prevention—keystones of my current life. I know that there will be more tough times. But now I know how to control my destiny —how to collaborate with my support team to create a plan for tough times. This sense of control helps more than anything to fight my depression.

What have I learned? I have learned a great deal about myself and how my mind —my logic—works. I have learned that having a choice in life, being given responsibility, and making genuine contributions are life savers. Had it not been for these components of my life, I am certain that I would have committed suicide by now. What stops me from killing myself is the effect it would have on those that I care about, the responsibilities I have, and the contributions I can make.

The collaborative approach that Tim and Mark describe in this book and live in their lives as rehabilitation professionals means working with people who have had an injury and with the everyday people in their lives to help them achieve what they want to achieve in life. It requires having them all work together, but the person they are working for is always in charge of where his life is going. That is what I have. And this is the only approach that has worked for me. The collaborative approach is humane and successful. Try it; it's your life.

Sincerely,

Jason S. Lewin

References

Abelson, R.P. (1981). Psychological status of the script concept. *American Psychologist, 36,* 715–729.

Ackerly, S.S. (1964). A case of paranatal frontal lobe defect observed for thirty years. In J.M. Warren & K. Ackert (Eds.), *The frontal granular cortex and behavior* (pp. 192–218). New York: McGraw-Hill.

Adams, J.H., Graham, D.I., Scott, G., Parker, L.S., & Doyle, D. (1980). Brain damage in fatal non-missile head injury. *Journal of Clinical Pathology, 33,* 1132–1145.

Adolphs, R., Tranel, D., Damasio, H., & Damasio, A.R. (1994). Impaired recognition of emotion in facial expressions following bilateral damage to the human amygdala. *Nature, 372,* 669–672.

Adolphs, R., Tranel, D., Damasio, H., & Damasio, A.R. (1995). Fear and the human amygdala. *Journal of Neuroscience, 15,* 5879–5891.

Aggleton, J.P. (1992). *The amygdala: Neurobiological aspects of emotion, memory, and mental dysfunction.* New York: Wiley-Liss.

Alberts, M.S., & Binder, L.M. (1991). Premorbid psychosocial factors that influence cognitive rehabilitation following traumatic brain injury. In J.S. Kreutzer & P.H. Wehman (Eds.), *Cognitive rehabilitation of persons with traumatic brian injury: A functional approach* (pp. 95–103). Baltimore, MD: Paul H. Brookes Publishing Co.

Alderman, N. (1983). Central executive deficit and response to operant conditioning methods. *Neuropsychological Rehabilitation, 6,* 161–186.

Alexander, M.P., Benson, D.F., & Stuss, D.T. (1989). Frontal lobes and language. *Brain and Language, 37,* 656–691.

Allman, J., & Brothers, L. (1994). Faces, fear, and the amygdala. *Nature, 372,* 613–614.

Aman, M.G., & Singh, N.N. (1988). *Aberrant behavior checklist.* East Aurora, NY: Slosson Educator Publications.

Anderson, S.W., Damasio, H., Tranel, D., & Damasio, A.R. (1988). Neuropsychological correlates of bilateral frontal lobe lesions in humans. *Society for Neuroscience, 14,* 1288.

Anderson, S.W., & Tranel, D. (1989). Awareness of disease states following cerebral infarction, dementia, and head trauma: Standardized assessment. *The Clinical Neuropsychologist, 3,* 327–339.

Annegars, J.F. (1983). The epidemiology of head trauma in children. In K. Shapiro (Ed.), *Pediatric head trauma* (pp. 1–10). Mt. Kisco, NY: Futura Publishing.

Annegars, J.F., Grabow, J.O., Kurland, L.T., & Laws, E.R. (1980). The incidence, causes, and secular trends of head trauma in Olmstead County, Minnesota, 1953–1974. *Neurology, 30,* 912.

Asarnow, R.F., Satz, P., Light, R., & Neumann, E. (1991). Behavior problems and adaptive functioning in children with mild and severe closed head injury. *Journal of Pediatric Psychology, 16,* 534–555.

Ashman, A.F., & Conway, R.N.F. (1989). *Cognitive strategies for special education.* London: Routledge.

Auerbach, S.H. (1986). Neuroanatomical correlates of attention and memory disorders in traumatic brain injury: An application of neurobehavioral sybtypes. *Journal of Head Trauma Rehabilitation, 1,* 3–4.

Awh, E., Smith, E., & Jonides, J. (1995). Human rehearsal processes and the frontal lobes: PET evidence. In J. Grafman, K.J. Holyoak, & F. Boller (Eds.), *Structure and functions of the human prefrontal cortex* (pp. 97–117). New York: The New York Academy of Sciences.

Bachman, D.L. (1992). The diagnosis and management of common neurologic sequelae of closed head injury. *Journal of Head Trauma Rehabilitation, 7,* 50–59.

Baddeley, A. (1986). *Working memory*. Oxford, UK: Clarendon Press.

Baddeley, A.D. (1992). Working memory. *Science, 255*, 556–559.

Baddeley, A.D. (1995). The psychology of memory. In A.D. Baddeley, B.A. Wilson, & F.N. Watts (Eds.), *Handbook of memory disorders* (pp. 3–25). New York: Wiley.

Baddeley, A.D., & Wilson, B.A. (1994). When implicit memory fails: Amnesia and the problem of error elimination. *Neuropsychologia, 32*, 53–68.

Baer, D. (1981). *How to plan for generalization*. Manhattan, KS: H&H Enterprises.

Baer, D.M., Wolf, M.M., & Risley, T.R. (1987). Some still current dimensions of applied behavior analysis. *Journal of Applied Behavior Analysis, 20*, 313–327.

Bailey, D.B. (1987). Collaborative goal-setting with families: Resolving differences in values and priorities for services. *Topics in Early Childhood Special Education, 7*, 59–71.

Bailey, J.S., & Pyles, D.A. (1989). Behavioral diagnostics. *Monographs of the American Association on Mental Retardation, 12*, 85–106.

Bambara, L.M., Koger, F., Katzer, T., & Davenport, T.A. (1995). Embedding choice in the context of daily routines. *Journal of the Association of Persons with Severe Handicaps, 20*, 185–195.

Bandura, A. (1977). *Social learning theory*. Englewood Cliffs, NJ: Prentice-Hall.

Bannerman, D.J., Sheldon, J.B., Sherman, J.A., & Harchik, A.E. (1990). Balancing the right to habilitation with the right to personal liberties: The rights of people with developmental disabilities to eat too many doughnuts and take a nap. *Journal of Applied Behavior Analysis, 23*, 79–89.

Barkley, R.A. (1997). Behavioral inhibition, sustained attention, and executive functions: Constructing a unified theory of ADHD. *Psychological Bulletin, 121*, 65–94.

Beardshaw, V., & Towell, D. (1990). *Assessment and case management: Implications for the implementation of "caring people."* London: King's Fund Institute.

Bechara, A., Damasio, A.R., Damasio, H., & Anderson, S.W. (1994). Insensitivity to future consequences following damage to the human prefrontal cortex. *Cognition, 50*, 7–12.

Bechara, A., Tranel, D., Damasio, H., Adolphs, R., Rockland, C., & Damasio, A.R. (1995). Double dissociation of conditioning and declarative knowledge relative to the amygdala and the hippocampus in humans. *Science, 269*, 1115–1118.

Becker, M.E., & Vakil, E. (1993). Behavioral psychotherapy of the frontal-lobe injured patient in an outpatient setting. *Brain Injury, 7*, 515–523.

Bellamy, G.T., Newton, J.S., LeBaron, N.M., & Horner, R.H. (1990). Quality of life and lifestyle outcomes: A challenge for residential programs. In R.L. Schalock (Ed.), *Quality of life: Perspectives and issues* (pp. 127–137). Washington, DC: American Association of Mental Retardation.

Benton, A. (1991). Prefrontal injury and behavior in children. *Developmental Neuropsychology, 7*, 275–281.

Ben-Yishay, Y., Piasetsky, E.B., & Rattok, J. (1987). A systematic model for ameliorating disorders in basic attention. In M.J. Meir, L. Diller, & A.L. Benton (Eds.), *Neuropsychological rehabilitation* (pp. 165–181). London: Churchill Livingstone.

Berk, L.E., & Winsler, A. (1995). Scaffolding children's learning: Vygotsky and early childhood education. *NAEYC Research and Practice Series, 7*. Washington, DC: National Association for the Education of Young Children.

Berkman, K.A., & Meyer, L.H. (1988). Alternative strategies and multiple outcomes in the remediation of severe self injury: Going "all-out" nonaversively. *Journal of the Association of Persons with Severe Handicaps, 13*, 76–86.

Bernstein, G.S. (1982). Training behavior change agents: A conceptual review. *Behavior Therapy, 13*, 1–23.

Biddle, K.R., McCabe, A., & Bliss, L.S. (1996). Narrative skills following traumatic brain injury in children and adults. *Journal of Communication Disorders, 29*, 447–470.

Bigler, E.D. (1988). Frontal lobe damage and neuropsychological assessment. *Archives of Clinical Neuropsychology, 3*, 279–297.

Bigler, E. (1990). *Traumatic brain injury: Mechanisms of damage*. Austin, TX: Pro-Ed.

Bijou, S.W., & Baer, D. (1978). *Behavior analysis and child development*. Englewood Cliffs, NJ: Prentice-Hall.

Bijou, S.W., Peterson, R.F., & Ault, M.H. (1968). A method to integrate descriptive and experimental field studies at the level of data and empirical concepts. *Journal of Applied Behavior Analysis, 1,* 175–191.

Bijur, P.E., Haslum, M., & Golding, J. (1990). Cognitive and behavioral sequelae of mild head injury in children. *Pediatrics, 86,* 337–344.

Bjorklund, D.F. (Ed.). (1990). *Children's strategies: Contemporary views of cognitive development.* Hillsdale, NJ: Lawrence Erlbaum and Associates.

Blackman, P., & LeJeune, H. (Eds.). (1990). *Behavior analysis in theory and practice: Contributions and controversies.* Hillsdale, NJ: Lawrence Erlbaum and Associates.

Bodrova, E., & Leong, D.J. (1996). *Tools of the mind: The vygotskyan approach to early childhood education.* Englewood Cliffs, NJ: Prentice-Hall.

Bond, M. (1990). Standardized methods of assessing and predicting outcome. In M. Rosenthal, E.R. Griffin, M.R. Bond, & J. Miller (Eds.), *Rehabilitation of the adult and child with traumatic brain injury* (pp. 59–74). Philadelphia, PA: F.A. Davis.

Booth, S.R., & Fairbank, D.W. (1984). Videotape feedback as a behavior management technique. *Behavioral Disorders, 9,* 55–59.

Braunling-McMorrow, D., Lloyd, K., & Fralish, K. (1986). Teaching social skills to head injured adults. *Journal of Rehabilitation, 52,* 39–44.

Brazzeli, M., Colombo, N. DellaSala, S., & Spinnler, H. (1994). Spared and impaired cognitive abilities after bilateral frontal lobe damage. *Cortex, 30,* 27–51.

Brismar, B., Engstrom, A., & Rydberg, U. (1983). Head injury and intoxication: A diagnostic and therapeutic dilemma. *Acta Chirurgica Scandinavica, 149,* 11–14.

Brooks, D.N. (1983). Disorders of memory. In M. Rosenthal, E. Griffith, M. Bond, & J.D. Miller (Eds.), *Rehabilitation of the head injured adult* (pp. 185–196). Philadelphia: F.A. Davis.

Brooks, D.N., Campsie, L., Symington, C., Beattie, A., Bryden, J., & McKinlay, W. (1987). The effects of severe head injury upon patient and relative within seven years of injury. *Journal of Head Trauma Rehabilitation, 2,* 1–13.

Brooks, D.N., Campsie, L., Symington, C., Beattie, C., & McKinlay, W. (1986). The five year outcome of severe blunt head injury. A relative's view. *Journal of Neurology, Neurosurgery, and Psychiatry, 49,* 764–770.

Brooks, D.N., & McKinlay, W. (1983). Personality and behavioral change after severe blunt head injury—a relative's view. *Journal of Neurology, Neurosurgery, and Psychiatry, 46,* 336–344.

Brotherton, F.A., Thomas, L.L., Wisotzek, I.E., & Milan, M.A. (1988). Social skills training in the rehabilitation of patients with traumatic closed head injury. *Archives of Physical Medicine and Rehabilitation, 69,* 827–832.

Browder, D.M. (1991). *Assessment of individuals with severe disabilities: An applied behavior approach to life skills assessment* (2nd Ed.). Baltimore: Paul H. Brookes Publishing Co.

Brown, A.L. (1975). The development of memory: Knowing, knowing about knowing, and knowing how to know. In H.W. Reese (Ed.), *Advances in child development and behavior* (Vol. 10, pp. 103–152). New York: Academic Press.

Brown, A.L. (1979). Theories of memory and problems of development, activity, growth, and knowledge. In F.I.M. Craik & L. Cermak (Eds.), *Levels of processing and memory* (pp. 225–258). Hillsdale, NJ: Lawrence Erlbaum and Associates.

Brown, A.L., Campione, J.C., Weber, L.S., & McGilly, K. (1992). *Interactive learning environments: A new look at assessment and instruction.* Berkeley: University of California, Commission on Testing and Public Policy.

Brown, F. (1991). Creative daily scheduling: A nonintrusive approach to challenging behaviors in community residences. *Journal of the Association for Persons with Severe Handicaps, 16,* 75–84.

Brown, F., Belz, P., Corsi, L., & Wenig, B. (1993). Choice diversity for people with severe disabilities. *Education and Training in Mental Retardation, 28,* 318-326.

Brown, F., & Snell, M. (1993). Meaningful assessment. In M.E. Snell (Ed.), *Instruction of students with severe disabilities* (4th ed., pp. 61–98). New York: Merrill.

Brown, G., Chadwick, O., Shaffer, D., Rutter, M., & Traub, M. (1981). A prospective study of children with head injuries. III. Psychiatric sequelae. *Psychological Medicine, 11,* 63–78.

Bruner, J. (1975). The ontogenesis of speech acts. *Journal of Child Language, 2,* 1–20.

Bruner, J. (1978). How to do things with words. In J. Bruner & A. Garton (Eds.), *Human growth and development*. Oxford, UK: Oxford University Press.

Bruner, J. (1985). Vygotsky: A historical and conceptual perspective. In J.V. Wertsch (Ed.), *Culture, communication and cognition: Vygotskyan perspectives* (pp. 21–34). Cambridge, UK: Cambridge University Press.

Buckner, R.L., Peterson, S., Ojemann, J., Miezin, F., Squire, L., & Raichle, M. (1995). Functional anatomical studies of explicit and implicit memory. *Journal of Neuroscience, 15,* 12–29.

Burke, G.M., (1990). Unconventional behavior: A communicative interpretation in individuals with severe disabilities. *Topics in Language Disorders, 10,* 75–85.

Buschke, H., & Fuld, P.A. (1974). Evaluating storage, retention, and retrieval in disordered memory and learning. *Neurology,* 1019–1025.

Butler, R.W., & Namerow, N.S. (1988). Cognitive retraining in brain injury rehabilitation: A critical review. *Journal of Neurological Rehabilitation, 2,* 97–101.

Campbell T.F., & Dollaghan, C.A. (1990). Expressive language recovery in severely brain-injured children and adolescents. *Journal of Speech and Hearing Disorders, 55,* 567–581.

Campione, J.C., & Brown, A.L. (1984). Learning ability and transfer propensity as sources of individual differences in intelligence. In P.H. Brooks, R. Sperber, & C. McCauley (Eds.), *Learning and cognition in the mentally retarded* (pp. 137–150). Baltimore, MD: University Park Press.

Campione, J.C., & Brown, A. L. (1990). Guided learning and transfer. In N. Fredrickson, R. Glaser, A. Lesgold, & M. Shafto (Eds.), *Diagnostic monitoring of skill and knowledge acquisition* (pp. 141–172). Hillsdale, NJ: Lawrence Erlbaum and Associates.

Carnevale, G.J. (1996). Natural-setting behavior management for individuals with traumatic brain injury: Results of a three-year caregiver training program. *Journal of Head Trauma Rehabilitation, 11,* 27–38.

Carr, E.G., & Carlson, J.I. (1993). Reduction of severe behavior problems in the community using a multicomponent treatment approach. *Journal of Applied Behavior Analysis, 26,* 157–172.

Carr, E.G., & Durand, V.M. (1985a). Reducing behavior problems through functional communication training. *Journal of Applied Behavior Analysis, 18,* 75–85.

Carr, E.G., & Durand, V.M. (1985b). The social-communicative basis of severe behavior problems in children. In S. Reiss & R. Bootzin (Eds.), *Theoretical issues in behavior therapy.* New York: Academic Press.

Carr, E.G., Levin, L., McConnachie, G., Carlson, J.I, Kemp, D.C., & Smith, C.E. (1994). *Communication-based intervention for problem behavior: A user's guide for producing positive change.* Baltimore, MD: Paul H. Brookes Publishing Co.

Carr, E.G., McConnachie, G., Levin, L., & Kemp, D. (1993). Communication-based treatment of severe behavior problems. In R. VanHouten & S. Axelrod (Eds.), *Behavior analysis and treatment* (pp. 231–267). New York: Plenum Press.

Carr, E.G., Reeve, C.E., & Magito-McLaughlin, D. (1997). Contextual influences on problem behavior in people with developmental disabilities. In L.K. Koegel, R.L. Koegel, & G. Dunlap (Eds.), *Positive behavioral support: Including people with difficult behavior in the community* (pp. 403–423). Baltimore, MD: Paul H. Brookes Publishing Co.

Case, R. (1992). The role of the frontal lobes in the regulation of cognitive development. *Brain and Cognition, 20,* 51–73.

Chandler, L.K., Fowler, S.A., & Lubek, R.C. (1992). An analysis of the effects of multiple setting events on the social behavior of preschool children with special needs. *Journal of Applied Behavior Analysis, 25,* 249–264.

Chapman, P.F., Kairiss, E.W., Keenan, C.L., & Brown, T.H. (1990). Long-term synaptic potentiation in the amygdala. *Synapse, 6,* 271–278.

Chapman, S., Culhane, K., Levin, H., Harward, H., Mendelsohn, D., Ewing-Cobbs, L., Fletcher, J., & Bruce, D. (1992). Narrative discourse after closed head injury in children and adolescents. *Brain and Language, 43,* 42–65.

Chapman, S.B. (1997). Cognitive-communication abilities in children with closed head injury. *American Journal of Speech-Language Pathology, 6,* 50–58.

Chapman, S.B., Levin, H.S., Matejka, J., Harward, H.N., & Kufera, J. (1995). Discourse ability in head injured children: Consideration of linguistic, psychosocial, and cognitive factors. *Journal of Head Trauma Rehabilitation, 10*, 36–54.

Chapman, S.B., Watkins, R., Gustafson, C., Moore, S., Levin, H.S., & Kufera, J.A. (1997). Narrative discourse in children with closed head injury, children with language impairment, and typically developing children. *American Journal of Speech-Language Pathology, 6*, 66–76.

Chester, C.C., Henry, K., & Tarquinio, T. (1998). Assistive technology for children with traumatic brain injury. In M. Ylvisaker (Ed.), *Traumatic brain injury rehabilitation: Children and adolescents* (pp. 107–124). Boston, MA: Butterworth-Heinemann.

Christopher, J.J., Hansen, D.J., & MacMillan, V.M. (1991). Effectiveness of a peer-helper intervention to increase children's social interaction: Generalization, maintenance, and social validity. *Behavior Modification, 15*, 22–50.

Cicerone, K.D., & Wood, J.C. (1987). Planning disorder after closed head injury: A case study. *Archives of Physical Medicine and Rehabilitation, 68*, 111–115.

Cockrell, J.L. (1991). Pharmacologic treatment in pediatric rehabilitation: Potential adverse effects. *NeuroRehabilitation, 1*, 7–11.

Cohen, N.J., & Eichenbaum, H. (1993). *Memory, amnesia, and the hippocampal system.* Cambridge, MA: MIT Press.

Cohen, S.B., Joyce, C.M., Rhoades, K.W., & Welks, D.M. (1995). Educational programming for head injured students. In M. Ylvisaker (Ed.), *Head injury rehabilitation: Children and adolescents* (pp. 383–409). San Diego, CA: College-Hill Press.

Colvin, G., & Sugai, G. (1989). *Managing escalating behavior.* Eugene, OR: Behavior Associates.

Condeluci, A. (1991). *Interdependence: The route to community.* Orlando, FL: Deutsch.

Condeluci, A. (1992). Brain injury rehabilitation: The need to bridge paradigms. *Brain Injury, 6*, 543–551.

Conroy, M.A., & Fox, J.J. (1994). Setting factors and challenging behaviors in the classroom: Incorporating contextual factors into effective intervention plans for children with aggressive behaviors. *Journal of Prevention of School Failure, 38*, 29–34.

Cooper, C.J., Walker, D.P., Sasso, G.M., Reimers, T.M., & Donn, L.K. (1990). Using parents as therapists to evaluate the appropriate behavior of their children: Applica-

tions to a tertiary diagnostic clinic. *Journal of Applied Behavior Analysis, 23*, 285–296.

Cooper, L.J., Wacker, D.P., Thursby, D., Plagmann, L.A., Harding, J., Millard, T., & Derby, M. (1992). Analysis of the effects of task preferences, task demands, and adult attention on child behaviors in outpatient and classroom settings. *Journal of Applied Behavior Analysis, 19*, 823–840.

Corrigan, J.D., Rust, E., Lamb-Hart, G.L. (1995). The nature and extent of substance abuse problems in persons with traumatic brain injury. *Journal of Head Trauma Rehabilitation, 10*, 29–46.

Craine, S.F. (1982). The retraining of frontal lobe dysfunction. In L.E. Trexler (Ed.), *Cognitive rehabilitation: Conceptualization and intervention.* New York: Plenum Press.

Crépeau, F., Scherzer, B.P., Belleville, S., & Desmarais, G. (1997). A qualitative analysis of central executive disorders in a real-life work situation. *Neuropsychological Rehabilitation, 7*, 147–165.

Cummings, J.L. (1993). Frontal-subcortical circuits and human behavior. *Archives of Neurology, 50*, 873–880.

Curl, R.M., Fraser, R.T., Cook, R.G., & Clemmons, D. (1996). Traumatic brain injury vocational rehabilitation: Preliminary findings for the coworker as trainer project. *Journal of Head Trauma Rehabilitation, 11*, 75–85.

Daigneault, S., Braun, C.M.J., & Montes, J.L. (1997). Pseudodepressive personality and mental inertia in a child with a focal left-frontal lesion. *Developmental Neuropsychology, 13*, 1–22.

Dalby, P.R., & Obrzut, J.E. (1991). Epidemiologic characteristics and sequelae of closed head-injured children and adolescents: A review. *Developmental Neuropsychology, 7*, 35–68.

Damasio, A.R. (1989). Time-locked multiregional retroactivation: A systems-level proposal for the neural substrates of recall and recognition. *Cognition, 33*, 25–62.

Damasio, A.R. (1990). Category-related defects as a clue to the neural substrates of knowledge. *Trends in Neuroscience, 13*, 95–98.

Damasio, A.R. (1994). *Descartes' error.* New York: Avon Books.

Damasio, A.R., Tranel, D., & Damasio, H. (1990). Individuals with sociopathic behavior caused by frontal lobe damage fail to respond automatically to socially charged stimuli. *Behavioral Brain Research, 14*, 81–94.

Damasio, A.R., Tranel, D., & Damasio, H. (1991). Somatic markers and the guidance of behavior: Theory and preliminary testing. In H.S. Levin, H.M. Eisenberg, & A.L. Benton (Eds.), *Frontal lobe function and dysfunction* (pp. 217–229). New York: Oxford University Press.

Daniels, H. (Ed.). (1996). *An introduction to Vygotsky.* New York: Routledge.

Davis, C.A., Brady, M.P., Hamilton, R., McEvoy, M.A., & Williams, R.E. (1994). Effects of high probability requests on the social interactions of young children with severe disabilities. *Journal of Applied Behavior Analysis, 27,* 619–637.

Dehaene, S., & Changeux, J-P. (1995). Neuronal models of prefrontal cortical functions. In J. Grafman, K. Holyoak, & F. Boller (Eds.), *Structure and functions of the human prefrontal cortex* (pp. 305–319). New York: New York Academy of Sciences.

Demb, J.B., Desmond, J.E., Wagner, A.D., Vaidya, C.J., Glover, G.H., & Gabrieli, J.D.E. (1995). Semantic encoding and retrieval in the left inferior prefrontal cortex: A functional MRI study of task difficulty and process specificity. *Journal of Neuroscience, 15,* 4870–4878.

Denckla, M.B. (1996). Research on executive function in a neurodevelopmental context: Application of clinical measures. *Developmental Neuropsychology, 12,* 5–15.

Dennett, D.C., & Kinsbourne, M. (1992). Time and the observer: The where and when of consciousness in the brain. *Behavioral and Brain Sciences, 15,* 183–247.

Dennis, M. (1991). Frontal lobe function in childhood and adolescence: A heuristic for assessing attention regulation, executive control, and the intentional states important for social discourse. *Developmental Neuropsychology, 7,* 327–358.

Dennis, M. (1992). Word-finding in children and adolescents with a history of brain injury. *Topics in Language Disorders, 13,* 66–82.

Dennis, M., & Barnes, M. (1990). Knowing the meaning, getting the point, bridging the gap, and carrying the message: Aspects of discourse following closed head injury in childhood and adolescence. *Brain and Language, 39,* 428–446.

Dennis, M., Barnes, M.A., Donnelly, R.E., Wilkinson, M., & Humphreys, R.P. (1996). Appraising and managing knowledge: Metacognitive skills after childhood head injury. *Developmental Neuropsychology, 12,* 77–103.

Dennis, M., & Lovett, M. (1990). Discourse ability in children after brain damage. In Y. Joanette & H.H. Brownell (Eds.), *Discourse ability and brain damage: Theoretical and empirical perspectives* (pp. 199–223). New York: Springer-Verlag.

DePaepe, P., Reichle, J., & O'Neill, R. (1993). Applying general-case instructional strategies when teaching communicative alternatives to challenging behaviors. In J. Reichle & D.P. Wacker (Eds.), *Communication alternatives to challenging behaviors* (pp. 237–262). Baltimore, MD: Paul H. Brookes Publishing Co.

Deshler, D.D., & Schumaker, J.B. (1988). An instructional model for teaching students how to learn. In J.L. Graden, J.E. Zins, & M.J. Curtis (Eds.), *Alternative educational delivery systems: Enhancing instructional options for all students* (pp. 391–411). Washington, DC: National Association of School Psychologists.

Devinsky, O., & Luciano, D. (1993). The contributions of cingulate cortex to human behavior. In B.A. Vogt, & M. Gabriel (Eds.), *Neurobiology of the cingulate cortex and limbic thalamus* (pp. 427–556). Boston: Birkhauser.

Diamond, A. (1991). Guidelines for the study of brain-behavior relationships during development. In H.S. Levin, H.M. Eisenberg, & A.L. Benton (Eds.), *Frontal lobe function and dysfunction* (pp. 339–378). New York: Oxford University Press.

Diamond, A., & Goldman-Rakic, P.S. (1989). Comparison of human infants and rhesus monkeys on Piaget's AB task: Evidence for dependence on dorsolateral prefrontal cortex. *Experimental Brain Research, 74,* 24–40.

Diller, L., & Gordon, W.A. (1981). Interventions for cognitive deficits in brain-injured adults. *Journal of Consulting and Clinical Psychology, 49,* 822–834.

Donnellan, A.M., Mirenda, P.L., Mesaros, R.A., & Fassbender, L.L. (1984). Analyzing the communicative functions of aberrant behavior. *Journal of the Association for Persons with Severe Handicaps, 9,* 201–212.

Doss, S., & Reichle, J. (1989). Establishing alternatives to the emission of socially motivated excess behavior: A review. *Journal of the Association of Persons with Severe Handicaps, 14,* 101–112.

Dowrick, P.W. (1979). Single dose medication to create a self-model film. *Child Behavior Therapy, 1*, 193–198.

Dowrick, P.W. (1983). Video training of alternatives to cross-gender identity behaviors in a 4-year-old boy. *Child and Family Behavior Therapy, 5*, 59–65.

Dowrick, P.W., & Raeburn, J.M. (1995). Self-modeling: Rapid skill training for children with physical disabilities. *Journal of Developmental and Physical Disabilities, 7*, 25–37.

Dowrick, P.W., & Biggs, S.J. (1983). *Using video: Psychological and social applications.* New York: John Wiley and Sons.

Duncan, J. (1986). Disorganisation of behavior after frontal lobe damage. *Cognitive Neuropsychology, 3*, 271–290.

Dunlap, G., dePerczel, M., Clarke, S., Wilson, D., Wright, S., White, R., & Gomez, A. (1994). Choice-making to promote adaptive behavior for students with emotional and behavioral challenges. *Journal of Applied Behavior Analysis, 27*, 505–518.

Dunlap, G., Johnson, L.F., & Robbins, F.R. (1990). Preventing serious behavior problems through skill development and early intervention. In A.C. Repp & N.N. Singh (Eds.), *Current perspectives in the use of nonaversive and aversive interventions with developmentally disabled persons* (pp. 273–286). Sycamore, IL: Sycamore Publishing Co.

Dunlap, G., & Kern, L. (1993) Assessment and intervention for children within the instructional curriculum. In J. Reichle & D.P. Wacker (Eds.), *Communicative alternatives to challenging behavior* (pp. 177–204). Baltimore: Paul H. Brookes Publishing Co.

Dunst, C.J., Johanson, X.X., Trivette, C.M., & Hamby, D. (1991). Family oriented early interventions policies and practices: Family centered or not? *Exceptional Children, 58*, 115–126.

Dunst, C., Trivette, C., & Deal, A. (1988). *Enabling and empowering families.* Cambridge, MA: Brookline Books.

Dunst, C.J., Trivette, C.M., Gordon, N.J., & Pletcher, L.L. (1989). Building and mobilizing informal family support networks. In G.H.S. Singer & L.K. Irvin (Eds.), *Support for caregiving families: Enabling positive adaptation to disability* (pp. 121–141). Baltimore: Paul H. Brookes Publishing Co.

Durand, V.M. (1990). *Severe behavior problems: A functional communication training approach.* New York: Guilford Press.

Durand, V.M., Berotti, D., & Weiner, J. (1993). Functional communication training: Factors affecting effectiveness, generalization, and maintenance. In J. Reichle & D.P. Wacker (Eds.), *Communicative alternatives to challenging behavior: Integrating functional assessment and intervention strategies* (pp. 317–340). Baltimore, MD: Paul H. Brookes Publishing Co.

Durand, V.M., & Carr, E.G. (1991). Functional communication training to reduce challenging behavior: Maintenance and application to new settings. *Journal of Applied Behavior Analysis, 24*, 251–264.

Durand, V.M., & Crimmins, D.B. (1992). *The Motivation Assessment Scale.* Topeka, KS: Monaco & Associates.

Dywan, J., & Segalowitz, S.J. (1996). Self- and family-ratings of adaptive behavior after traumatic brain injury: Psychometric scores and frontally generated RRPs. *Journal of Head Trauma Rehabilitation, 11*, 79–75.

Eames, P. (1988). Behavior disorders after severe head injury: Their nature and causes and strategies for management. *Journal of Head Trauma Rehabilitation, 3*, 1–6.

Eames, P. (1990). Organic basis of behavioral disorders after traumatic brain injury. In R.L. Wood (Ed.), *Neurobehavioral sequelae of traumatic brain injury* (pp. 134–150). London: Taylor & Francis.

Ehrlich, J.S. (1988). Selective characteristics of narrative discourse in head-injured and normal adults. *Journal of Communication Disorders, 21*, 1–9.

Eichenbaum, H., & Otto, T. (1992). The hippocampus: What does it do? *Behavioral and Neural Biology, 57*, 2–36.

Eichenbaum, H., Otto, T., & Cohen, N.J. (1994). Two functional components of the hippocampal memory system. *Behavioral and Brain Sciences, 17*, 449–518.

Elkinson, L.L., & Elkinson, N. (1989). Collaborative consulting: Improving parent-teacher communication. *Academic Therapy, January*, 261–269.

Emery, R.E., Binkoff, J.A., Houts, A.C., & Carr, E.G. (1983). Children as independent variables: Some clinical implications of child effects. *Behavior Therapy, 14*, 398–412.

Engelmann, S., & Carnine, D. (1991). *Theory of instruction: Principles and application.* Eugene, OR: ADI Press.

Englemann, S., & Colvin, G.T. (1988). *Generalized compliance training.* Austin, TX: Pro-Ed.

Eslinger, P.J., Biddle, K.R., & Grattan, L.M. (1997). Cognitive and social development in children with prefrontal cortex lesions. In N.A. Krasnegor, G.R. Lyon, & P.S. Goldman-Rakic (Eds.), *Devlopment of the prefrontal cortex: Evolution, neurobiology, and behavior* (pp. 295–335). Baltimore, MD: Paul H. Brookes Publishing Co.

Eslinger, P.J., & Damasio, A.R. (1985). Severe disturbance of higher cognition following bilateral frontal lobe oblation: Patient EVR. *Neurology, 35,* 1731–1741.

Eslinger, P.J., Damasio, A.R., Damasio, H., & Grattan, L.M. (1989). Developmental consequences of early frontal lobe damage. *Journal of Clinical and Experimental Neuropsychology, 11,* 50–62.

Eslinger, P.J., & Grattan, L.M. (1993). Frontal lobe and frontal-striatal substrates for different forms of human cognitive flexibility. *Neuropsychologia, 31,* 17–28.

Eslinger, P.J., Grattan, L.M., Damasio, H., & Damasio, A.R. (1992). Developmental consequences of childhood frontal lobe damage. *Archives of Neurology, 49,* 764–769.

Evans, P. (1993). Some implications of Vygotsky's work for special education. In H. Daniels (Ed.), *Charting the agenda: Education activity after Vygotsky.* London: Routledge.

Ewing-Cobbs, L., Levin, H.S., Eisenberg, H.M., & Fletcher, J.M. (1987). Language functions following closed head injury in children and adolescents. *Journal of Clinical and Experimental Neuropsychology, 9,* 575–592.

Ewing-Cobbs, L., Levin, H.S., Fletcher, J.M., Miner, M.E., & Eisenberg, H.M. (1989). *Posttraumatic amnesia in children: Assessment and outcome.* Paper presented at the International Neuropsychological Society Annual Meeting, Vancouver, BC.

Ewing-Cobbs, L., Miner, M., Fletcher, J.M., & Levin, H.S. (1989). Intellectual, motor, and language sequelae following closed head injury in infants and preschoolers. *Journal of Pediatric Psychology, 14,* 531–544.

Feeney, T.J., & Ylvisaker, M. (1995). Choice and routine: Antecedent behavioral interventions for adolescents with severe traumatic brain injury. *Journal of Head Trauma Rehabilitation, 10,* 67–86.

Feeney, T.J., & Ylvisaker, M. (1997). A positive, communication-based approach to challenging behavior after TBI. In A. Glang, G.H.S. Singer, & B. Todis (Eds.), *Children with acquired brain injury: The school's response* (pp. 229–254). Baltimore: Paul H. Brookes Publishing Co.

Fernandez-Ballesteros, R., & Staats, A.W. (1992). Paradigmatic behavioral assessment, treatment, and evaluation: Answering the crisis in behavioral assessment. *Advances in Behavioral Research and Therapy, 14,* 1–27.

Feuerstein, R. (1979). *The dynamic assessment of retarded performers: The Learning Potential Assessment Device, theory, instruments, and techniques.* Baltimore, MD: University Park Press.

Fey, M. (1986). *Language intervention with young children.* San Diego, CA: College-Hill Press.

Filley, C.M., Cranberg, M.D., Alexander, M.P., & Hart, E.J. (1987). Neurobehavioral outcome after closed head injury in childhood and adolescence. *Archives of Neurology, 44,* 194–198.

Finset, A., & Andresen, S. (1990). The process diary concept: An approach in training orientation, memory, and behavior control. In R.L. Wood & I. Fussey (Eds.), *Cognitive rehabilitation in perspective* (pp. 99–116). London: Taylor & Francis.

Fivush, R. (1991). The social construct of personal narratives. *Merrill-Palmer Quarterly, 37,* 59–81.

Fivush, R., & Fromhoff, F.A. (1988). Style and structure in mother-child conversations about the past. *Discourse Processes, 11,* 337–355.

Fivush, R., & Reese, E. (1992). The social construction of autobiographical memory. In M.A. Conway, D.C. Rubin, H. Spinnler, & W.A. Wagenaar (Eds.), *Theoretical perspectives on autobiographical memory* (pp. 115–132). Amsterdam: Kluwer Academic Publishers.

Flannery, K.B., & Horner, R.H. (1994). The relationship between predictability and problem behaviors for students with severe disabilities. *Journal of Behavioral Education, 4,* 157–176.

Flavell, J.H. (1985). *Cognitive development.* Englewood Cliffs, NJ: Prentice-Hall.

Flavell, J., Miller, P., & Miller, S. (1993). *Cognitive development* (3rd ed.). Englewood Cliffs, NJ: Prentice-Hall.

Fletcher, J.M., Ewing-Cobbs, L., McLaughlin, E.J., & Levin, H.S. (1985). *Cognitive and psychosocial sequelae of head injury in children: Implications for assessment and management.* Austin: University of Texas.

Fletcher, J.M., Ewing-Cobbs, L., Miner, M., & Levin, H.S. (1990). Behavioral changes after closed head injury in children. *Journal of Consulting and Clinical Psychology, 58*, 93–98.

Fletcher, J.M., Levin, H.S., & Butler, I.J. (1995). Neurobehavioral effects of brain injury on children: Hydrocephalus, traumatic brain injury, and cerebral palsy. In M.C. Roberts (Ed.), *Handbook of pediatric psychology* (2nd ed., pp. 362–383). New York: Guilford Press.

Fletcher, J.M., Miner, M.E., & Ewing-Cobbs, L. (1987). Age and recovery from head injury in children. In H. Levin, J. Grafman, & H. Eisenberg (Eds.), *Neurobehavioral recovery from head injury* (pp. 279–291). New York: Oxford University Press.

Fowler, R. (1996). Supporting students with challenging behaviors in general education settings: A review of behavioral momentum techniques and guidelines for use. *The Oregon Conference Monograph, 8*, 137–155.

Fox, J., & Conroy, M. (1995). Setting events and behavioral disorders of children and youth: An interbehavioral field analysis for research and practice. *Journal of Emotional and Behavioral Disorders, 3*, 130–140.

Franzen, M.D. (1991). Behavioral assessment and treatment of brain-impaired individuals. In M. Hersen, R.M. Eisler, & P.M. Miller (Eds.), *Progress in behavior modification* (Vol. 27, pp. 56–85). Newbury Park, CA: Sage Publications.

Furman, L.N., & Walden, T.A. (1990). Effect of script knowledge on preschool children's communicative interaction. *Developmental Psychology, 26*, 227–233.

Fuster, J.M. (1989). *The prefrontal cortex: Anatomy, physiology, and neuropsychology of the frontal lobe* (2nd ed.). New York: Raven Press.

Fuster, J.M. (1990). Prefrontal cortex and the bridging of temporal gaps in the perception–action cycle. *Annals of the New York Academy of Science, 608*, 318–329.

Fuster, J.M. (1991). The prefrontal cortex and its relation to behavior. *Progress in Brain Research, 87*, 201–211.

Gans, J.S. (1987). Facilitating staff/patient interaction in rehabilitation. In B. Caplan (Ed.), *Rehabilitation psychology desk reference* (pp. 185–218). Gaithersburg, MD: Aspen.

Gaultieri, T., & Cox, D.R. (1991). The delayed neurobehavioral sequelae of traumatic brain injury. *Brain Injury, 5*, 219–232.

Giangreco, M.F., Cloninger, C.J., & Iverson, V.S. (1993). *Choosing options and accommodations for children (COACH): A guide to planning inclusive education*. Baltimore, MD: Paul H. Brookes Publishing Co.

Giangreco, M.F., Edelman, S.W., Luiselli, T.E., & MacFarland, S.Z.C. (1997). Helping or hovering? Effects of instructional assistant proximity on students with disabilities. *Exceptional Children, 64*, 7–18.

Glang, A.E., Singer, G.H.S., Cooley, E.A., & Tish, N. (1992). Tailoring direct instruction techniques for use with students with brain injury. *Journal of Head Trauma Rehabilitation, 7*, 93–108.

Glang, A., Singer, G.H.S., & Todis, B. (Eds.). (1997). *Students with acquired brain injury: The school's response*. Baltimore: Paul H. Brookes Publishing Co.

Glisky, E.L., & Schacter, D.L. (1987). Acquisition of domain-specific knowledge in organic amnesia: Training for computer-related work. *Neuropsychologia, 25*, 893–906.

Glisky, E.L., & Schacter, D.L. (1989). Models and methods of memory rehabilitation. In F. Boller & J. Grafman (Eds.), *Handbook of neuropsychology. Vol. 3: Sec. 5. Memory and its disorders* (pp. 233–246). Amsterdam: Elsevier Science Publishers.

Gluck, M.A., & Myers, C.E. (1995). Representation and association in memory: A neurocomputational view of hippocampal function. *Current Directions in Psychological Science, 4*, 23–29.

Goldman, P.S. (1971). Functional development of the prefrontal cortex in early life and the problem of neuronal plasticity. *Experimental Neurology, 32*, 366–387.

Goldman, P.S. (1972). Developmental determinants of cortical plasticity. *Acta Neurobiology Experiments, 32*, 495–511.

Goldman-Rakic, P. (1987). Development of cortical circuitry and cognitive function. *Child Development, 58*, 601–622.

Goldman-Rakic, P. (1993). Specification of higher cortical functions. *Journal of Head Trauma Rehabilitation, 8*, 13–23.

Goldstein, A.P., Sprafkin, R.P., Gershaw, N.J., & Klein, P. (1980). *Skillstreaming the adolescent: A structured learning approach to teaching prosocial skills*. Champaign, IL: Research Press.

Goldstein, F.C., & Levin, H.S. (1989). Manifestations of personality change after closed head injury. In E. Perecman (Ed.), *Integrating theory and practice in clinical neuropsychology* (pp. 217–243). Hillsdale, NJ: Lawrence Erlbaum and Associates.

Grafman, J. (1989). Plans, actions, and mental sets: Managerial knowledge units in the frontal lobes. In E. Perecman (Ed.), *Integrating theory and practice in clinical neuropsychology* (pp. 93–138). Hillsdale, NJ: Lawrence Earlbaum Associates.

Grafman, J. (1995). Similarities and distinctions among current models of prefrontal cortical functions. In J. Grafman, K. Holyoak, & F. Boller (Eds.), *Structure and functions of the human prefrontal cortex* (pp. 337–368). New York: New York Academy of Sciences.

Grafman, J., Holyoak, K.J., & Boller, F. (Eds.). (1995). *Structure and functions of the human prefrontal cortex.* New York: New York Academy of Sciences.

Grafman, J., Sirigu, A., Spector, L., & Hendler, J. (1993). Damage to the prefrontal cortex leads to decomposition of structured event complexes. *Journal of Head Trauma Rehabilitation, 8,* 73–87.

Graham, D.I., Adams, J.H., & Doyle, D. (1978). Ischemic brain damage in fatal nonmissle head injuries. *Journal of Neurological Sciences, 39,* 213–234.

Graham, S., & Harris, K.R. (1996). Addressing problems in attention, memory, and executive functioning: An example from self-regulated strategy development. In G.R. Lyon & N.A. Krasnegor (Eds.), *Attention, memory, and executive function* (pp. 349–365). Paul H. Brookes Publishing Co.

Grattan, L.M., & Eslinger, P.J. (1990). Influence of cerebral lesion site upon the onset and progression of interpersonal deficits following brain injury. *Journal of Clinical and Experimental Neuropsychology, 12,* 33–39.

Grattan, L.M., & Eslinger, P.J. (1991). Frontal lobe damage in children and adults: A comparative review. *Developmental Neuropsychology, 7,* 283–326.

Grattan, L.M., & Eslinger, P.J. (1992). Long-term psychological consequences of childhood frontal lobe lesion in patient DT. *Brain and Cognition, 20,* 185–195.

Greenspan, A.I., & MacKenzie, E.J. (1994). Functional outcome after pediatric head injury. *Pediatrics, 94,* 425–432.

Gresham, F.M. (1988). Social skills: Conceptual and applied aspects of assessment, training, and social validation. In J.C. Witt, S.N. Elliot, & F.M. Gresham (Eds.), *Handbook of behavior therapy in education.* New York: Plenum Press.

Groher, M.E., & Ochipa, C. (1992). The standardized communication assessment of individuals with traumatic brain injury. *Seminars in Speech and Language, 13,* 252–262.

Haas, J., Cope, D.N., & Hall, K. (1987). Premorbid prevalence of poor academic performance in severe head injury. *Journal of Neurology, Neurosurgery, and Psychiatry, 50,* 52–56.

Hagen, C. (1981). Language disorders secondary to closed head injury. *Topics in Language Disorders, 1,* 73–87.

Hall, K.M., Karzmark, P., Stevens, M., Englander, J., O'Hare, P., & Wright, J. (1994). Family stressors in traumatic brain injury: A two-year follow-up. *Archives of Physical Medicine and Rehabilitation, 75,* 876–884.

Halle, J.W. (1989). Identifying stimuli in natural settings: An analysis of stimuli that acquire control during training. *Journal of Applied Behavior Analysis, 24,* 579–589.

Halle, J.W., & Spradlin, J.E. (1993). Identifying stimulus control of challenging behavior: Extending the analysis. In J. Reichle & D.P. Wacker (Eds.) *Communicative alternative to challenging behavior:* (pp. 83–109). Baltimore, MD: Paul H. Brookes Publishing Co.

Hallowell, E.M., & Ratey, J.J. (1994). *Driven to distraction.* New York: Touchstone.

Harchik, A.E., & Putzier, V.S., (1990). The use of high probability requests to increase compliance with instructions to take medication. *Journal of the Association for Persons with Severe Handicaps, 15,* 40–43.

Harchik, A.E., Sherman, J.A., & Bannerman, D.J. (1993). Choice and control: New opportunities for people with developmental disabilities. *Annals of Clinical Psychiatry, 5,* 151–162.

Haring, T.G., & Kennedy, C.H. (1990). Contextual control of problem behavior in students with severe disabilities. *Journal of Applied Behavior Analysis, 23,* 235–243.

Harlow, J. (1868). Recovery from passage of an iron bar through the head. *Massachusetts Medical Society Publications, 2,* 329–347.

Harrell, M., Parenté, F., Bellingrath, E.G., & Lisicia, K.A. (1992). *Cognitive rehabilitation of memory*. Gaithersburg, MD: Aspen Publishers.

Hart, T., & Jacobs, H. (1993). Rehabilitation and management of behavior disturbances following frontal lobe injury. *Journal of Head Trauma Rehabilitation, 8*, 1–12.

Hartley, L.L. (1995). *Cognitive-communicative abilities following brain injury: A functional approach*. San Diego, CA: Singular Publishing Group.

Hartley, L.L., & Jensen, P.J. (1991). Narrative and procedural discourse after closed head injury. *Brain Injury, 5*, 267–285.

Haynes, W., Pindzoal, R., & Emerick, L. (1992). *Diagnosis and evaluation in speech pathology* (4th ed.). Englewood Cliffs, NJ: Prentice-Hall.

Hebb, D.O. (1945). Man's frontal lobes: A critical review. *Archives of Neurology and Psychiatry, 54*, 10–24.

Hecimovic, A., Fox, J.J., Shores, R.E., & Strain, P.S. (1985). An analysis of integrated and segregated free play settings and the generalization of newly acquired social behaviors of socially withdrawn preschoolers. *Behavioral Assessment, 7*, 367–388.

Heilman, K.M. (1991). Anosagnosia: Possible neuropsychological mechanisms. In G.P. Prigatano & D.L. Schacter (Eds.), *Awareness of deficit after brain injury* (pp. 53–61). New York: Oxford University Press.

Heilman, K.M., Watson, R.T., & Valenstein, E. (1993). Neglect and related disorders. In K.M. Heilman & E. Valenstein (Eds.), *Clinical neuropsychology* (3rd ed., pp. 279–336). New York: Oxford University Press.

Herrnstein, R.J. (1961). Relative and absolute strength of responses as a function of frequency of reinforcement. *Journal of the Experimental Analysis of Behavior, 4*, 267–272.

Herrnstein, R.J. (1970). On the law of effect. *Journal of the Experimental Analysis of Behavior, 21*, 159–164.

Hersh, N., & Treadgold, L. (1994). NeuroPage: The rehabilitation of memory dysfunction by prosthetic memory and cueing. *NeuroRehabilitation, 4*, 187–197.

Hilton, A., & Henderson, C.J. (1993). Parent involvement: A best practice or forgotten practice? *Education and Training in Mental Retardation, 28*, 199–211.

Hinkeldey, N.S., & Corrigan, J.D. (1990). The structure of head–injured patients' neurobehavioral complaints: A preliminary study. *Brain Injury, 4*, 115–133.

Holst, P., & Vikki, J. (1988). Effect of frontomedial lesions on performance on the Stroop Test and word fluency tasks. *Journal of Clinical and Experimental Neuropsychology, 10*, 79.

Holyoak, K.J., & Kroger, J.K. (1995). Forms of reasoning: Insight into prefrontal functions. In J. Grafman, K.J. Holyoak, & F. Boller (Eds.), *Structure and functions of the human perifrontal cortex* (pp. 253–263). New York: The New York Academy of Sciences.

Horner, R.H. (1994). Functional assessment: Contributions and future directions. *Journal of Applied Behavior Analysis, 27*, 401–404.

Horner, R.H., & Budd, C.M. (1985). Acquisition of manual sign use: Collateral reduction of maladaptive behavior, and factors limiting generalization. *Education and Training of the Mentally Retarded, 20*, 39–47.

Horner, R.H., & Day, H.M. (1991). The effects of response efficiency on functionally equivalent competing behaviors. *Journal of Applied Behavior Analysis, 24*, 719–732.

Horner, R.H., Dunlap, G., & Koegel, R.L. (Eds.). (1988). *Generalization and maintenance: Lifestyle changes in applied settings*. Baltimore, MD: Paul H. Brookes Publishing Co.

Horner, R.H., Dunlap, G., Koegel, R., Carr, E., Sailor, W., Anderson, Albin, R., & O'Neill, R. (1990). Toward a technology of "nonaversive" behavioral support. *Journal of the Association of Persons with Severe Handicaps, 15*, 125–132.

Horner, R.H., McDonnell, J.J., & Bellamy, G.T. (1986). Teaching generalized skills: General case instruction in simulation and community settings. In R.H. Horner, L.H. Meyer, & H.D.B. Fredericks (Eds.), *Education of learners with severe handicaps: Exemplary service strategies* (pp. 289–314). Baltimore, MD: Paul H. Brookes Publishing Co.

Horner, R.H., O'Neill, R.E., & Flannery, K.B. (1993). Effective behavior support plans. In M. Snell (Ed.), *Instruction of students with severe disabilities* (pp. 184–214). New York: Merrill.

Horner, R.H., Vaughn, B.J., Day, H.M., & Ard, Jr., W.R. (1997). The relationship between setting events and problem behavior. In L.K. Koegel, R.L. Koegel, & G. Dunlap (Eds.), *Positive behavioral support: Including people with difficult behavior in the community* (pp. 381–402). Baltimore, MD: Paul H. Brookes Publishing Co.

Hudson, J.A. (1990a). Constructive processes in children's event memory. *Developmental Psychology, 26,* 180–187.

Hudson, J.A. (1990b). The emergence of autobiographical memory in mother-child conversations. In R. Fivush & J.A. Hudson (Eds.), *Knowing and remembering in young children* (pp. 166–196). New York: Cambridge University Press.

Hudson, J.A., & Nelson, K. (1983). Effects of script structure on children's story recall. *Developmental Psychology, 19,* 625–635.

Hudson, J.A., & Nelson, K. (1986). Repeated encounters of a familiar link: Effects of familiarity on children's autobiographical memory. *Cognitive Development, 1,* 253–271.

Hudson, J.E. (1993). Understanding events: The development of script knowledge. In M. Bennett (Ed.), *The development of social cognition* (pp. 142–167). New York: Guilford Press.

Hudson, J.E., & Fivush, R, (1993). Planning in the preschool years: The emergence of plans from general event knowledge. *Cognitive Development, 6,* 253–271.

Hunkin, N.A., Parkin, A.J., Bradley, V.A., Burrows, E.H., Aldrich, F.K., Jansari, A., & Burdon-Cooper, C. (1995). Focal retrograde amnesia following closed head injury: A case study and theoretical account. *Neuropsychologia, 33,* 509–523.

Iwata, B.A., Vollmer, T.R., & Zarcone, J.R. (1990). The experimental (functional) analysis of behavior disorders: Methodology, applications, and limitations. In A.C. Repp & N.N. Singh (Eds.), *Perspectives on the use of nonaversive and aversive interventions for persons with developmental disabilities* (pp. 301–330). Sycamore, IL: Sycamore Publishing Co.

Izard, C.E. (1992) Four systems for emotion activation: Cognitive and noncognitive. *Psychological Review, 100,* 68–90.

Jacobs, H.E. (1990). Identifying post-traumatic behavior problems: Data from psychosocial follow-up studies. In R.L. Wood (Ed.), *Neurobehavioral sequelae of traumatic brain injury* (pp. 37–51). London: Taylor & Francis.

Jacobs, H.E. (1993). *Behavior analysis guidelines and brain injury rehabilitation: People, principles, and programs.* Gaithersburg, MD: Aspen Publishing.

Jacobs, H.E. (1997). The clubhouse: Addressing work-related behavioral challenges through a supportive social community. *Journal of Head Trauma Rehabilitation, 12,* 14–27.

Jaffe, K.M., Fay, G.C., Lincoln, N.L., Martin, K.M., Shurtleff, H.A., Rivara, J.B., & Winn, H.R. (1993). Severity of pediatric traumatic brain injury and neurobehavioral recovery at one year—a cohort study. *Archives of Physical Medicine and Rehabilitation, 74,* 587–595.

Johnson, D.W., & Johnson, R. (1991a). *Joining together: Group theory and group skills* (4th ed.). Englewood Cliffs, NJ: Prentice-Hall.

Johnson, D.W., & Johnson, R. (1991b). *Learning together and alone: Cooperation, competition, and individualization* (3rd ed.). Englewood Cliffs,NJ: Prentice-Hall.

Kaiser, A.P., & McWhorter, C.M. (Eds.). (1990). *Preparing personnel to work with persons with severe disabilities.* Baltimore, MD: Paul H. Brookes Publishing Co.

Kantor, J.R. (1959). *Interbehavioral psychology.* Granville, OH: Principia.

Kaplan, E. (1988). A process approach to neuropsychological assessment. In T. Boll & B.K. Bryant (Eds.), *Clinical neuropsychology and brain function: Research, measurement, and practice* (pp. 129–167). Washington, DC: American Psychological Association.

Kaplan, S.P. (1990). Social support, emotional distress and vocational outcome among persons with brain injuries. *Rehabilitation Counseling Bulletin, 34,* 16–23.

Kaplan, S.P. (1991). Psychological adjustment three years after traumatic brain injury. *The Clinical Neuropsychologist, 5,* 360–369.

Kapur, N. (1995). Memory aids in the rehabilitation of memory disordered patients. In A.D. Baddeley, B.A. Wilson, & F.N. Watts (Eds.), *Handbook of memory disorders* (pp. 533–556). London: John Wiley & Sons.

Katz, D.I. (1992). Neuropathology and neurobehavioral recovery from closed head injury. *Journal of Head Trauma Rehabilitation, 7,* 1–15.

Kavale, K., & Mattson, P. (1983). "One jumped off the balance beam": Meta-analysis of perceptual-motor training. *Journal of Learning Disabilities, 16,* 165–173.

Kendall, E., & Terry, D.J. (1996). Psychosocial adjustment following closed head injury: A model for understanding individual differences and predicting outcome. *Neuropsychological Rehabilitation, 6,* 101–132.

Kennedy, C.H. (1994). Manipulating antecedent conditions to alter the stimulus control of problem behavior. *Journal of Applied Behavior Analysis, 27,* 161–170.

Kennedy, C.H., & Itkonen, T. (1993). Effects of setting events on the problem behavior of students with severe disabilities. *Journal of Applied Behavior Analysis, 26*, 321–327.

Kennedy, C.H., Itkonen, T., & Lindquist, K. (1995). Comparing interspersed requests and social comments for increasing student compliance. *Journal of Applied Behavior Analysis, 28*, 97–98.

Kent, R. (1997). *The speech sciences.* San Diego, CA: Singular Publishing Group.

Kern, L., Childs, K.E., Dunlap, G., Clarke, S., & Falk, G.D. (1994). Using assessment based curricular intervention to improve the classroom behavior of a student with emotional and behavioral challenges. *Journal of Applied Behavior Analysis, 27*, 7–19.

Kern-Dunlap, L., Dunlap, G., Clarke, S., Childs, K.E., White, R.L., & Stewart, M.P. (1992). Effects of a videotape feedback package on the peer interactions of children with serious behavioral and emotional challenges. *Journal of Applied Behavior Analysis, 25*, 355–364.

Kertesz, A. (1994). Frontal lesions and function. In A. Kertesz (Ed.), *Localization and neuroimaging in neuropsychology* (pp. 567–598). New York: Academic Press.

Klonoff, P.S., & Lage, G.A. (1991). Narcissistic injury in patients with traumatic brain injury. *Brain Injury, 6*, 11–21.

Klonoff, P.S., & Lage, G.A. (1995). Suicide in patients with traumatic brain injury: Risk and prevention. *Journal of Head Trauma Rehabilitation, 10*, 16–24.

Klonoff, P.S., Costa, L.D., & Snow, W.G. (1986). Predictors and indicators of quality of life in patients with closed-head injury. *Journal of Clinical and Experimental Neuropsychology, 8*, 469–485.

Knights, R.M., Ivan, L.P., Venturey, E.C.G., Bentivoglio, C., Stoddart, C., Winogren, W., & Bawden, H.N. (1991). The effects of head injury in children on neuropsychological and behavioral functioning. *Brain Injury, 5*, 339–351.

Koegel, R., & Koegel, L.K. (1995). *Teaching children with autism: Strategies for initiating positive interactions and improving learning opportunities.* Baltimore, MD: Paul H. Brookes.

Kolb, B. (1995). *Brain plasticity and behavior.* Mahwah, NJ: Lawrence Erlbaum and Associates.

Kraus, J.F. (1995). Epidemiological features of brain injury in children: Occurrence, children at risk, causes and manner of injury, severity, and outcome. In S.H. Broman & M.E. Michel (Eds.), *Traumatic head injury in children* (pp. 22–39). New York: Oxford University Press.

Kreutzer, J.S., & Wehman, P.S. (Eds.). (1991). *Cognitive rehabilitation for persons with traumatic brain injury.* Baltimore: Paul H. Brookes Publishing Co.

Lalli, J.S., Browder, D.M., Mace, F.C., & Brown, K. (1995). Teacher use of descriptive analysis data to implement interventions to decrease students' maladaptive behavior. *Journal of Applied Behavior Analysis, 28*, 135–163.

Landis, S., & Peeler, J. (1990). *What have we noticed as we've tried to assist people one person at a time?* Chillicothe, OH: Ohio Safeguards.

Lawson, M.J., & Rice, D.N. (1989). Effects of training in use of executive strategies on a verbal memory problem resulting from closed head injury. *Journal of Clinical and Experimental Neuropsychology, 11*, 842–854.

LeDoux, J.E. (1991). Emotion and the limbic system concept. *Concepts in Neuroscience, 2*, 169–199.

LeDoux, J.E. (1993). Emotional memory systems in the brain. *Behavioral Brain Research, 58*, 69–79.

LeDoux, J.E. (1995). Emotion: Clues from the brain. *Annual Review of Psychology, 46*, 209–235.

LeDoux, J.E. (1996). *The emotional brain.* New York: Simon & Schuster.

Lehr, E. (1990). *Psychological management of traumatic brain injuries in children and adolescents.* Gaithersburg, MD: Aspen Publishing.

Leigland, S. (1984). On "setting events" and related concepts. *The Behavior Analyst, 7*, 41–45.

Leont'ev, A. (1978). *Activity, consciousness, and personality.* Englewood Cliffs, NJ: Prentice-Hall.

Levin, H., Benton, A., & Grossman, R. (1982). *Neurobehavioral consequences of closed head injury.* New York: Oxford University Press.

Levin, H.S., Eisenberg, H.M., & Benton, A.L. (Eds.). (1991). *Frontal lobe function and dysfunction.* New York: Oxford University Press.

Levin, H.S., Fletcher, J.M., Kufera, J.A., Harward, H., Lilly, M.A., Mendelsohn, D., Bruce, D., & Eisenberg, H.M. (1996). Dimensions of cognition measured by the Tower of London and other cognitive tasks in head-injured children and adolescents. *Developmental Neuropsychology, 12*, 17–34.

Levin, H.S., & Goldstein, F.C. (1986). Organization of verbal memory after severe head in-

Page 282 header

jury. *Journal of Clinical and Experimental Neuropsychology, 8,* 643–656.

Levin, H.S., Goldstein, F.C., Williams, D.H., & Eisenberg, H.M. (1991). The contribution of frontal lobe lesions to the neurobehavioral outcome of closed head injury. In H.S. Levin, H.M. Eisenberg, & A.L. Benton (Eds.), *Frontal lobe function and dysfunction* (pp. 318–338). New York: Oxford University Press.

Levin, W. (1991). Computer applications in cognitive rehabilitation. In J.S. Kreutzer & P.H. Wehman (Eds.), *Cognitive rehabilitation for persons with traumatic brain injury* (pp. 163–179). Baltimore, MD: Paul H. Brookes Publishing Co.

Lezak, M. (1982). The problem of assessing executive functions. *International Journal of Psychology, 17,* 281–297.

Lezak, M. (1986). Psychological implications of traumatic brain damage for the patient's family. *Rehabilitation Psychology, 31,* 241–250.

Lezak, M. (1987). Relationships between personality disorders, social disturbances, and physical disability following traumatic brain injury. *Journal of Head Trauma Rehabilitation, 2,* 57–69.

Lezak, M. (1988). Brain damage is a family affair. *Journal of Clinical and Experimental Neuropsychology, 10,* 111–123.

Lezak, M. (1993). Newer contributions to the neuropsychological assessment of executive functions. *Journal of Head Trauma Rehabilitation, 8,* 24–31.

Lezak, M.D. (1995). *Neuropsychological assessment* (3rd ed.). New York: Oxford University Press.

Lezak, M., & O'Brien, K. (1988). Longitudinal study of emotional, social, and physical changes after traumatic brain injury. *Journal of Learning Disabilities, 21,* 456–463.

Lhermitte, F. (1983). "Utilization behavior" and its relation to lesions in the frontal lobes. *Brain, 106,* 237–255.

Lhermitte, F. (1986). Human anatomy and the frontal lobes. Part II: Patient behavior in complex and social situations: The "environmental dependency" syndrome. *Annals of Neurology, 19,* 326–334.

Lhermitte, F., Pillon, B., & Serdaru, M. (1986). Human anatomy and the frontal lobes. Part I. Imitation and utilization behavior: A neuropsychological study of 75 patients. *Annals of Neurology, 19,* 205–213.

Liles, B.J., Coelho, C.A., Duffy, R.J., & Zalagens, M.R. (1989). Effects of elicitation procedures on the narratives of normal and closed head-injured adults. *Journal of Speech and Hearing Disorders, 54,* 356–366.

Livingston, M.G., & Brooks, D.N. (1988). The burden on families of the brain injured: A review. *Journal of Head Trauma Rehabilitation, 3,* 6–15.

Lombardi, W.J., & Weingartner, H. (1995). Pharmacological treatment of impaired memory. In A.D. Baddeley, B.A. Wilson, & F.N. Watts (Eds.), *Handbook of memory disorders* (pp. 578–601). New York: John Wiley & Sons.

Lovaas, I. (1977). *The autistic child: Language development through behavior modification.* New York: Irvington.

Lucyshyn, J.M., & Albin, R.W. (1993). Comprehensive support to families of children with disabilities and behavior problems: Keeping it "friendly." In G.H.S. Singer & L.E. Powers (Eds.), *Families, disability, and empowerment: Active coping skills and strategies for family interventions* (pp. 365–407). Baltimore, MD: Paul H. Brookes Publishing Co.

Lucyshyn, J.M., Nixon, C., Glang, A., & Cooley, E. (1996). Comprehensive family support for behavior change in children with ABI. In G.H.S. Singer, A. Glang, & J. Williams (Eds.), *Children with acquired brain injury: Educating and supporting families* (pp. 99–136). Baltimore, MD: Paul H. Brookes Publishing Co.

Luria, A.R., (1965). Two kinds of motor perseveration in massive injuries to the frontal lobes. *Brain, 88,* 1–10.

Luria, A.R. (1966). *Higher cortical functions in man* (2nd ed.). (B. Haigh, Trans.). New York: Basic Books. (Original work published 1962.)

Luria, A.R. (1970). *Traumatic aphasia: Its syndromes, psychology, and treatment.* The Hague: Mouton.

Luria, A.R. (1973a). The frontal lobes and the regulation of behaviour. In K.H. Pribram & A.R. Luria (Eds.), *Psychophysiology of the frontal lobes* (pp. 3–26). New York: Academic Press.

Luria, A.R. (1973b). *The working brain: An introduction to neuropsychology.* New York: Basic Books.

Luria, A.R. (1979). *The making of mind: A personal account of soviet psychology.* Cambridge, MA: Harvard University Press.

MacDonald, J. (1989). *Becoming partners with children: From play to conversation.* Chicago: Riverside Publishing Co.

Mace, F.C., Hock, M.L., Lalli, J.S., West, B.J., Belfore, P., Pinter, E., & Brown, K. (1988). Behavioral momentum in the treatment of noncompliance. *Journal of Applied Behavior Analysis, 21,* 123–132.

Mace, F.C., Lalli, J.S., Shea, M.C., Lalli, E., West, R., Roberts, M.L., & Nevin, J.A. (1990). The momentum of human behavior in a natural setting. *Journal of the Experimental Analysis of Behavior, 54,* 163–172.

Mace, F.C., Mauro, B.C., Boyajian, A.E., & Eckert, T.L. (1997). Effects of reinforcer quality on behavioral momentum: Coordinated applied and basic research. *Journal of Applied Behavior Analysis, 30,* 1–20.

Mace, F.C., Page, T.J., Ivanck, M.T., & O'Brien, S. (1986). Analysis of environmental determinants of aggression and disruption in mentally retarded children. *Applied Research in Mental Retardation, 7,* 203–221.

Mace, F.C., & Roberts, M.L. (1993). Factors affecting selection of behavioral interventions. In J. Reichle & D.P. Wacker (Eds.), *Communicative alternatives to challenging behavior* (pp. 113–133). Baltimore, MD: Paul H. Brookes.

Madigan, K.A., Hall, T.E., & Glang, A. (1997). Effective assessment and instructional practices for students with ABI. In A. Glang, G.H.S. Singer, & B. Todis (Eds.), *Students with acquired brain injury* (pp. 123–183). Baltimore, MD: Paul H. Brookes.

Malloy, P., Bihrle, A., Duffy, J., & Cimino, C. (1993). The orbitomedial frontal syndrome. *Archives of Clinical Neuropsychology, 8,* 185–201.

Mandler, G. (1967). Organization in memory. In K.W. Spence & J.T. Spence (Eds.), *The psychology of learning and motivation* (Vol. 1, pp. 327–372). New York: Academic Press.

Mann, L. (1979). *On the trail of process: A historical perspective on cognitive processes and their training.* New York: Grune & Stratton.

Marlowe, W. (1989). Consequences of frontal lobe injury in the developing child. *Journal of Clinical and Experimental Neuropsychology, 12,* 105–112.

Marlowe, W.B. (1992). The impact of a right prefrontal lesion on the developing brain. *Brain and Cognition, 20,* 205–213.

Marsh, N.V., & Knight, R.G. (1991). Behavioral assessment of social competence following severe head injury. *Journal of Clinical and Experimental Neuropsychology, 13,* 729–740.

Martin, G., & Pear, J. (1996). *Behavior modification: What it is and how to do it* (5th ed.). Upper Saddle River, NJ: Prentice-Hall.

Martzke, J.S., Swan, C.S., & Varney, N.R. (1991). Posttraumatic anosmia and orbital frontal damage: Neuropsychological and neuropsychiatric correlates. *Neuropsychology, 5,* 213–225.

Mateer, C.A., & Mapou, R.L. (1996). Understanding, evaluating, and managing attention disorders following traumatic brain injury. *Journal of Head Trauma Rehabilitation, 11,* 1–16.

Mateer, C., & Sohlberg, M.M. (1992). Process-oriented approaches to treatment of attention and memory disorders following traumatic brain injury. *Seminars in Speech and Language, 13,* 280–292.

Mateer, C.A., & Williams, D. (1991). Effects of frontal lobe injury in childhood. *Developmental Neuropsychology, 7,* 359–376.

Mateer, C.A., & Williams, D. (1992). Developmental impact of frontal lobe injury in middle childhood. *Brain and Cognition, 20,* 196–204.

Mattson, A.S., & Levin, H.S. (1990). Frontal lobe dysfunction following closed head injury: A review of the literature. *Journal of Nervous and Mental Disorders, 178,* 282–291.

Mayer, N.H., Keating, D.J., & Rapp, D. (1986). Skills, routines, and activity patterns of daily living: A functional nested approach. In B.P. Uzzell & Y. Gross (Eds.), *Clinical neuropsychology of intervention* (pp. 205–222). Boston: Martinus Nijhoff.

McCabe, A., & Peterson, C. (Eds.). (1991). *New directions in developing narrative structure.* Hillsdale, NJ: Lawrence Erlbaum and Associates.

McClelland, J.L., McNaughton, B.L., & O'Reilly, R.C. (1995). Why there are complementary learning systems in the hippocampus and neocortex: Insights from the successes and failures of connectionist models of learning and memory. *Psychological Review, 102,* 419–457.

McDonald, S. (1992a). Communication disorders following closed head injury: New approaches to assessment and rehabilitation. *Brain Injury, 6,* 283–292.

McDonald, S. (1992b). Differential pragmatic language loss following severe closed head injury: Inability to comprehend conversational implicature. *Applied Psycholinguistics, 13,* 295–312.

McDonald, S. (1993). Pragmatic language skills after closed head injury: Ability to meet the informational needs of the listener. *Brain and Language, 44,* 28–46.

McIntosh, S., Vaughn, S., & Zaragoza, N. (1991). A review of social interventions for students with learning disabilities. *Journal of Learning Disabilities, 24,* 451–458.

McKinlay, W.W., & Brooks, D.N. (1984). Methodological problems in assessing psychological recovery following severe head injury. *Journal of Clinical Neuropsychology, 6,* 87–99.

McKinlay, W.W., Brooks, D.N., Bond, M.R., Martinage, D.P., & Marshall, M.M. (1981). The short-term outcome of severe blunt head injury as reported by relatives of the injured persons. *Journal of Neurology, Neurosurgery, and Psychiatry, 44,* 529.

McKinlay, W.W., & Hickox, A. (1988). How can families help in the rehabilitation of the head injured? *Journal of Head Trauma Rehabilitation, 3,* 64–72.

Meichenbaum, D. (1993). The "potential" contributions of cognitive behavior modification to the rehabilitation of individuals with traumatic brain injury. *Seminars in Speech and Language, 14,* 18–30.

Mendelsohn, D., Levin, H.S., Bruce, D., Lilly, M.A., Harward, H., Culhane, K., & Eisenberg, H.M. (1992). Late MRI after head injury in children: Relationship to clinical features and outcome. *Child's Nervous System, 8,* 445–452.

Mentis, M., & Prutting, C. (1987). Cohesion in the discourse of head injured and normal adults. *Journal of Speech and Hearing Research, 30,* 88–98.

Mentis, M., & Prutting, C.A. (1991). Analysis of topic as illustrated in a head-injured and a normal adult. *Journal of Speech and Hearing Research, 34,* 583–595.

Meyer, L.H., & Evans, I.A. (1989). *Nonaversive intervention for behavior problems: A manual for home and community.* Baltimore, MD: Paul H. Brookes Publishing Co.

Meyer, L.H., & Evans, I.M. (1994). Meaningful outcomes in behavioral intervention: Evaluating positive approaches to the remediation of challenging behaviors. In J. Reichle & D.P. Wacker (Eds.), *Communicative alternatives to challenging behavior* (pp. 407–428). Baltimore, MD: Paul H. Brookes Publishing Co.

Michael, J. (1982). Distinguishing between discriminative and motivational functions of stimuli. *Journal of the Experimental Analysis of Behavior, 37,* 149–155.

Michael, J. (1989). Motivative relations and establishing operations. In J. Michael (Ed.), *Verbal and non-verbal behavior: Concepts and principles* (pp. 40–53). Kalamazoo: Western Michigan University.

Michael, J. (1993). Establishing operations. *The Behavior Analyst, 16,* 191–206.

Miller, G.A., Galanter, E.H., & Pribram, K.H. (1960). *Plans and the structure of behavior.* New York: Holt, Rinehart, & Winston.

Miller, J.D., & Jones, P.A. (1990). Minor head injury. In M. Rosenthal, E.R. Griffith, M.R. Bond, & J.D. Miller (Eds.), *Rehabilitation of the adult and child with traumatic brain injury* (2nd ed.) (pp. 236–247). Philadelphia, PA: F.A. Davis.

Miller, J.D., Pentland, B., & Berrol, S. (1990). Early evaluation and management. In M. Rosenthal, E.R. Griffith, M.R. Bond, & J.D. Miller (Eds.), *Rehabilitation of the adult and child with traumatic brain injury* (2nd ed., pp. 21–51). Philadelphia, PA: F.A. Davis.

Mira, M., Tyler, J., & Tucker, B. (1988). *Traumatic head injury in children and adolescents: A sourcebook for teachers and other school personnel.* Austin, TX: Pro-Ed.

Moore, A.D., & Stambrook, M. (1992). Coping strategies and locus of control following traumatic brain injury: Relationship to long-term outcome. *Brain Injury, 6,* 89–94.

Moore, A.D., Stambrook, M., Peters, L.C., Cardoso, E.R., & Kassum, D.A. (1990). Long-term multidimensional outcome following traumatic brain injuries and traumatic brain injuries with multiple trauma. *Brain Injury, 4,* 379–389.

Morgan, M., & LeDoux, J.E. (1995). Differential contribution of dorsal and ventral medial prefrontal cortex to the acquisition and extinction of conditioned fear. *Behavioral Neuroscience, 109,* 681–688.

Morris, E.K. (1988). Contexualism: The worldview of behavior analysis. *Journal of Experimental Child Psychology, 46,* 289–323.

Morris, E.K. (1992). The aim, progress, and evolution of behavior analysis. *The Behavior Analyst, 15,* 3–29.

Morton, M.V., & Wehman, P. (1995). Psychosocial and emotional sequelae of individuals with traumatic brain injury: A literature review and recommendations. *Brain Injury, 9,* 81–92.

Mount, B., & Zwernik, K. (1986). *It's never too early, it's never too late.* St. Paul, MN: Metropolitan Council, Publication No. 421-88-109.

Neef, N.A., & Iwata, B.A. (1994). Current research on functional analysis methodologies: An introduction. *Journal of Applied Behavior Analysis, 27,* 211–214.

Nelson, K. (1973). Structure and strategy in learning to talk. *Monograph of the Society for Research in Child Development, 38,* Serial No. 149.

Nelson, K. (1981). Social cognition in a script framework. In J. Flavell & L. Ross (Eds.). *Social cognitive development.* Cambridge, UK: Cambridge University Press.

Nelson, K. (1986). *Event knowledge: Structure and function in development.* Hillsdale, NJ: Lawrence Erlbaum and Associates.

Nelson, K. (1992). Emergence of autobiographical memory at age 4. *Human Development, 35,* 172–177.

Nelson, K.E., Camarata, S.M., Welsh, J., Butkovsky., & Camarata, M. (1996). Effects of imitating and conversational recasting treatment on the acquisition of grammar in children with specific language impairment and younger language-normal children. *Journal of Speech, Language, and Hearing, 39,* 839–859.

Nelson, N.W. (1994). Curriculum-based language assessment and intervention across the grades. In G.P. Wallach & K.G. Butler (Eds.), *Language-learning disabilities in school-age children and adolescents* (pp. 104–131). New York: Macmillan.

Nevin, J.A. (1988). Behavioral momentum and the partial reinforcement effect. *Psychological Bulletin, 103,* 44–56.

Nevin, J.A. (1992). An integrative model for the study of behavioral momentum. *Journal of the Experimental Analysis of Behavior, 57,* 301–316.

Newman, J., & Baars, B.J. (1993). A neural attentional model for access to consciousness: A global workspace perspective. *Concepts in Neuroscience, 4,* 255–290.

O'Brien, J., & Lyle, C. (1987). *Design for accomplishment.* Decatur, GA: Responsive Systems Associates.

O'Keefe, J. (1989). Is consciousness the gateway to the hippocampal cognitive map? A speculative essay on the neural basis of mind. *Brain and Mind, 10,* 59–98.

O'Neill, R.E., Horner, R.H., Albin, R.W., Storey, K., & Sprague, J.R. (1990). *Functional analysis of problem behavior: A practical assessment guide.* Sycamore, IL: Sycamore Publishing Co.

O'Neill, R., & Reichle, J. (1993). Addressing socially motivated challenging behaviors by establishing communicative alternatives. In J. Reichle & D.P. Wacker (Eds.), *Communicative alternatives to challenging behavior* (pp. 205–236). Baltimore, MD: Paul H. Brookes Publishing Co.

O'Shanick, G.J. (1990). Neuropsychopharmacological approaches to traumatic brain injury. In J.S. Kreutzer, & P. Wehman (Eds.), *Communty integration following traumatic brain injury* (pp. 15–27). Baltimore, MD: Paul H. Brookes Publishing Co.

O'Shanick, G.J. (1998). Pharmacologic intervention in children and adolescents with TBI. In M. Ylvisaker (Ed.), *Traumatic brain injury rehabilitation: Children and adolescents* (pp. 53–59). Newton, MA: Butterworth-Heinemann.

Oddy, M. (1984). Head injury and social adjustment. In N. Brooks (Ed.), *Closed head injury: Psychological, social, and family consequences* (pp. 108–192). New York: Oxford University Press.

Oder, W., Goldenberg, G., Spatt, J., Poreka, I., Bibder, H., & Deeke, L. (1992). Behavioural and psychosocial sequelae of severe closed head injury and cerebral blood: A SPECT study. *Journal of Neurology, Neurosurgery, and Psychiatry, 55,* 475–480.

Palinscar, A.S., & Brown, A.L. (1989). Classroom dialogues to promote self-regulated comprehension. In J. Brophy (Ed.), *Teaching for understanding and self-regulated learning* (Vol. 1). Greenwich, CT: JAI Press.

Palinscar, A.S., Brown, A.L., & Campione, J.C. (1994). Models and practices of dynamic assessment. In G.P. Wallach & K.G. Butler (Eds.), *Language-learning disabilities in school-age children and adolescents* (pp. 132–134). New York: Macmillan.

Pang, D. (1985). Pathophysiologic correlates of neurobehavioral syndromes following closed head injury. In M. Ylvisaker (Ed.), *Head injury rehabilitation: Children and adolescents* (pp. 3–70). Newton, MA: Butterworth-Heinemann.

Parenté, R. (1994). Effects of monetary incentives on performance after brain injury. *NeuroRehabilitation, 4,* 198–203.

Parenté, R., & Anderson-Parenté, J.K. (1989). Retraining memory: Theory and application. *Journal of Head Trauma Rehabilitation, 4,* 55–65.

Pascual-Leone, A., Grafman, J., & Hallett, M. (1995). Procedural learning and prefrontal cortex. In J. Grafman, K.J. Holyoak, & F.

Boller (Eds.), *Structure and functions of the human prefrontal cortex* (pp. 61–70). New York: The New York Academy of Sciences.

Patterson, K., & Hodges, J.R. (1995). Disorders of semantic memory. In A.D. Baddeley, B.A. Wilson, & F.N. Watts (Eds.), *Handbook of memory disorders* (pp. 167–186). New York: John Wiley.

Pelco, L., Sawyer, M., Duffield, G., Prior, M., & Kinsella, G. (1992). Premorbid emotional and behavioural adjustment in children with mild head injuries. *Brain Injury, 6*, 29–37.

Perrott, S.B., Taylor, H.G., & Montes, J.L. (1991). Neuropsychological sequelae, family stress, and environmental adaptation following pediatric head injury. *Developmental Neuropsychology, 7*, 69–86.

Peters, M.D., Gluck, M., & McCormick, M. (1992). Behaviour rehabilitation of the challenging client in less restrictive settings. *Brain Injury, 6*, 299–314.

Peterson, C., & Seligman, M.E.P. (1985). The learned helplessness model of depression: Current status of theory and research. In E.E. Beckham & W.R. Leber (Eds.), *Handbook of depression: Treatment, assessment, and research* (pp. 914–939). Homewood, IL: The Dorsey Press.

Petrides, M. (1995). Functional organization of the human frontal cortex for mnemonic processing. In J. Grafman, K.J. Holyoak, & F. Boller (Eds.), *Structure and functions of the human prefrontal cortex* (pp. 85–96). New York: The New York Academy of Sciences.

Petterson, L. (1991). Sensitivity to emotional cues and social behavior in children and adolescents after head injury. *Perceptual and Motor Skills, 73*, 1139–1150.

Pierce, K.L., & Schreibman, L. (1994). Teaching daily living skills to children with autism in unsupervised settings through pictorial self-management. *Journal of Applied Behavior Analysis, 27*, 471–481.

Pierce, W.D., & Epling, W.F. (1995). *Behavior analysis and learning.* Englewood Cliffs, NJ: Prentice-Hall.

Pollock, I.W. (1994a). Individual psychotherapy. In J.M. Silver, S.C. Yudofsky, & R.E. Hales (Eds.), *Neuropsychiatry of traumatic brain injury* (pp. 671–702). Washington, DC: American Psychiatric Press.

Pollock, I.W. (1994b). Reestablishing an acceptable sense of self. In R.C. Savage & G.F. Wolcott (Eds.), *Educational dimensions of aquired*

brain injury (pp. 303–317). Austin, TX: Pro-Ed.

Ponsford, J. (1990). The use of computers in the rehabilitation of attention disorders. In R.L. Wood & I. Fussey (Eds.), *Cognitive rehabilitation in perspective* (pp. 48–67). London: Taylor & Francis.

Ponsford, J.L., Olver, J.H., Curren, C., & Ng, K. (1995). Prediction of employment status two years after traumatic brain injury. *Brain Injury, 9*, 11–20.

Posner, M. (1992). Attention as a cognitive and neural system. *Current Directions in Psychological Science, 1*, 11–14.

Posner, M., & Peterson, S. (1990). The attention system of the human brain. *Annual Review of Neuroscience, 13*, 25–42.

Posner, M.I., & Dehaene, S. (1994). Attentional networks. *Trends in Neuroscience, 17*, 75–79.

Postman, L., & Kruesi, E. (1977). The influence of orienting tasks on the encoding and recall of words. *Journal of Verbal Learning and Verbal Behavior, 2*, 353–369.

Powers, L.E., Singer, G.H.S., Stevens, T., & Sowers, J. (1992). Behavioral parent training in home and community generalization settings. *Education and Training in Mental Retardation, 27*, 13–27.

Premack, D. (1959). Toward empirical behavioral laws: 1. Positive reinforcement. *Psychological Review, 66*, 229–233.

Pressley, M., & Associates (1990). *Cognitive strategy instruction that really improves children's academic performance.* Cambridge, MA: Brookline Books.

Pressley, M., & El-Dinary, P.B. (1992). Memory strategy instruction that promotes good information processing. In D.J. Herrmann, H. Weingartner, A. Searleman, & C. McEvoy (Eds.), *Memory improvement: Implications for memory theory* (pp. 79–100). New York: Springer-Verlag.

Pressley, M. (1993). Teaching cognitive strategies to brain-injured clients: The good information processing perspective. *Seminars in Speech and Language, 14*, 1–16.

Pressley, M. (1995). More about the development of self-regulation: Complex, long-term, and thoroughly social. *Educational Psychology, 30*, 207–212.

Pribram, K.H. (1986). The hippocampal system and recombinant processing. In R. Isaacson & K.H. Pribram (Eds.), *The hippocampus* (pp. 329–370.) New York: Plenum.

Pribram, K.H. (1987). The subdivisions of the frontal cortex revisted. In E. Perecman (Ed.), *The frontal lobes revisited* (pp. 11–39). New York: IRBN Press.

Pribram, K.H. (1997). The work in working memory: Implications for development. In N.A. Krasnegor, G.R. Lyon, & P.S. Goldman-Rakic (Eds.), *Development of the prefrontal cortex: Evolution, neurobiology, and behavior* (pp. 359–378). Baltimore, MD: Paul H. Brookes Publishing Co.

Price, B., Doffnre, K., Stowe, R., & Mesulum, M. (1990). The comportmental learning disabilities of early frontal lobe damage. *Brain, 113*, 1383–1393.

Prigatano, G.P. (1986). *Neuropsychological rehabilitation after brain injury.* Baltimore, MD: Johns Hopkins University Press.

Prigatano, G.P., & Fordyce, D.J. (1986). Cognitive dysfunction and psychosocial adjustment after brain injury. In G.P. Prigatano (Ed.), *Neuropsychological rehabilitation after brain injury.* Baltimore, MD: Paul H. Brookes.

Prigatano, G.P. (1987). Neuropsychological deficits, personality variables, and outcome. In M. Ylvisaker & E.M.R. Gobble (Eds.), *Community re-entry for head injured adults* (pp. 1–23). Boston: College-Hill Press.

Prigatano, G.P. (1991). Disordered mind, wounded soul: The emerging role of psychotherapy in rehabilitation after brain injury. *Journal of Head Trauma Rehabilitation, 6*, 1–10.

Prigatano, G.P., Altman, I.M., & O'Brien, T. (1990). Behavioral limitations that traumatic brain-injured patients tend to underestimate. *Clinical Neuropsychologist, 4*, 163–176.

Prigatano, G.P., Roueche, J.R., & Fordyce, D.J. (1985). Nonaphasic language disturbances after closed head injury. *Language Sciences, 1*, 217–229.

Provencal, G. (1987). Culturing commitment. In S. Taylor, D. Biklen, & J. Kroll (Eds.), *Community integration for people with severe disabilities* (pp. 67–84). New York: Teachers College Press.

Ratner, N., & Bruner, J. (1978). Games, social exchange, and the acquisition of language. *Journal of Child Language, 5*, 391–402.

Reese, E., Haden, C.A., & Fivush, R. (1993). Mother-child conversations about the past: Relationships of style and memory over time. *Cognitive Development, 8*, 403–430.

Reichle, J., & Johnston, S.S. (1993). Replacing challenging behavior: The role of communication intervention. *Topics in Language Disorders, 13*, 61–76.

Reichle, J., & Wacker, D.P. (Eds.). (1993). *Communicative alternatives to challenging behavior.* Baltimore, MD: Paul H. Brookes Publishing Co.

Rogoff, B. (1990). *Apprenticeship in thinking: Cognitive development in social context.* New York: Oxford University Press.

Rogoff, B., & Misty, J. (1990). The social and function context of children's remembering. In R. Fivush & J.D. Hudson (Eds.), *Knowing and remembering in young children.* New York: Cambridge University Press.

Rosen, C.D., & Gerring, J.P. (1986). *Head trauma: Strategies for educational reintegration.* San Diego, CA: College-Hill Press.

Rosenthal, M., & Bond, M.R. (1990). Behavioral and psychiatric sequelae. In M. Rosenthal, E. Griffith, M.R. Bond, & J.D. Miller (Eds.), *Rehabilitation of the adult and child with traumatic brain injury* (pp. 179–192). Philadelphia: F.A. Davis.

Ruff, R.M., Baser, C.A., Johnston, J.W., Marshall, L.F., Klauber, S.K., Klauber, M.R., & Minteer, M. (1989). Neuropsychological rehabilitation: An experimental study with head-injured patients. *Journal of Head Trauma Rehabilitation, 4*, 20–36.

Rutherford, W.H. (1977). Diagnosis of alcohol ingestion in mild head injuries. *The Lancet, 1*, 1021–1023.

Rutter, M., Chadwick, O., & Shaffer, D. (1983). Head injury. In M. Rutter (Ed.), *Developmental neuropsychiatry.* New York: Guilford Press.

Sanchez-Fort, M.R., Brady, M.P., & Davis, C.A. (1995). Using high probability requests to increase low probability communication behavior in young children with severe disabilities. *Education and Training in Mental Retardation and Developmental Disabilities, 30*, 151–165.

Santayana, G. (1905). *The life of reason.* New York: C. Scribner's Sons.

Sarno, M.T. (1980). The nature of verbal impairment after closed head injury. *Journal of Nervous and Mental Disease, 168*, 685–692.

Sarno, M.T. (1984). Verbal impairment after closed head injury: Report of a replication study. *Journal of Nervous and Mental Disease, 172*, 475–479.

Sarno, M.T., Buonaguro, A., & Levita, E. (1986). Characteristics of verbal impairment in closed head injured patients. *Archives of Physical Medicine and Rehabilitation, 67,* 400–405.

Sasso, G.M., Reimers, T.M., Cooper, L.J., Wacker, D. Berg, W., Steege, M., Kelly, L., & Allaire, A. (1992). Use of descriptive and experimental analyses to identify the functional properties of abberant behavior in school settings. *Journal of Applied Behavior Analysis, 25,* 809–821.

Sattler, J.M. (1993). *Assessment of children* (4th ed.). San Diego, CA: Sattler Publishing.

Savage, R.C., & Wolcott, G.F. (Eds.). (1994). *Educational dimensions of acquired brain injury.* Austin, TX: Pro-Ed.

Saver, J.L., & Damaiso, A.R. (1991). Preserved access and processing of social knowledge in a patient with acquired sociopathy due to ventromedial frontal damage, *Neuropsychologia, 29,* 1241–1249.

Schacter, D. (1987). Memory, amnesia, and frontal lobe dysfunction. *Psychobiology, 15,* 21–36.

Schacter, D., & Church, B. (1992). Auditory priming: Implicit and explicit memory for words and voices. *Journal of Experimental Psychology, 18,* 915–930.

Schacter, D.L., & Glisky, E.L. (1986). Memory remediation: Restoration, alleviation, and the acquisition of domain-specific knowledge. In B. Uzzell & Y. Gross (Eds.), *Clinical neuropsychology of intervention* (pp. 257–282). Boston: Martinus Nijhoff.

Schank, R., & Abelson, A. (1977). *Scripts, plans, goals, and understanding.* Hillsdale, NJ: Lawrence Erlbaum.

Schneider, P., & Watkins, R.V. (1996). Applying Vygotskyan developmental theory to language intervention. *Language, Speech, and Hearing Services in the Schools, 27,* 157–170.

Schmidt, N.D. (1997). Outcome-oriented rehabilitation: A response to managed care. *Journal of Head Trauma Rehabilitation, 12,* 44–50.

Schneider, W., & Pressley, M. (1989). *Memory development between 2 and 20.* New York: Springer-Verlag.

Scholnick, E.K., & Friedman, S.L. (1993). Planning in context: Developmental and situational characteristics. *International Journal of Behavioral Development, 16,* 145–167.

Schwartz, M.F. (1995). Re-examining the role of excecutive functions in routine action production. In J. Grafman, K.J. Holyoak, & F. Boller (Eds.), *Structure and functions of the human prefrontal cortex* (pp. 321–335). New York: The New York Academy of Sciences.

Schwartz, M.F., Mayer, N.H., Fitzpatrick DeSalme, E.J., & Montgomery, M.W. (1993). Cognitive theory and the study of everyday action disorders after brain damage. *Journal of Head Trauma Rehabilitation, 8,* 59–72.

Schweinhart, L.J. & Weikart, D.P. (1986). Consequences of three preschool curriculum models through age 15. *Early Childhood Research Quarterly, 1,* 15.

Schweinhart, L.J., & Weikart, D.P. (1993). Success by empowerment: The High/Scope Perry preschool study through age 27. *Young Children, 49,* 54–58.

Seligman, M.E.P. (1974). Depression and learned helplessness. In R.J. Freidman & M.M. Katz (Eds.), *The psychology of depression: Contemporary theory and research.* New York: Winston-Wiley.

Self, H., Benning, T., Marston, D., & Magnusson, D. (1991). Cooperative teaching project: A model for students at risk. *Exceptional Children, 58,* 26–34.

Shaffer, H.R. (1996). Joint involvement episodes as context for development. In H. Daniels (Ed.), *An introduction to Vygotsky* (pp. 251–280). New York: Routledge.

Shallice, T. (1982). Specific impairments in planning. *Philosophical Transactions of the Royal Society of London (Biology), 298,* 199–209.

Shallice, T. (1988). *From neuropsychology to mental structure.* Cambridge, UK: Cambridge University Press.

Shallice, T., & Burgess, P.W. (1991a). Higher order cognitive impairments and frontal lobe lesions in man. In H. Levin, H.M. Eisenberg, & A.L. Benton (Eds.), *Frontal lobe function and dysfunction* (pp. 125–138). London: Oxford University Press.

Shallice, T., & Burgess, P.W. (1991b). Deficits in strategy application following frontal lobe damage in man. *Brain, 114,* 727–741.

Sherwin, E.D., & O'Shanick, G.J. (1998). From denial to poster child: Growing past the injury. In M. Ylvisaker (Ed.), *Traumatic brain injury rehabilitation: Children and adolescents* (pp. 331–343). Boston: Butterworth-Heinemann.

Silver, B.V., Boake, C., & Cavazos, D.I. (1994). Improving functional skills using behavioral procedures in a child with anoxic brain injury. *Archives of Physical Medicine and Rehabilitation, 75,* 742–745.

Silver, J.M., & Yudofsky, S.C. (1994). Psychopharmacology. In J.M. Silver, S.C. Yudofsky, & R.E. Hales (Eds.), *Neuropsychiatry of trau-*

matic brain injury (pp. 631–670). Washington, DC: American Psychiatric Press.

Singer, G.H.S., Glang, A., & Williams, J.M. (Eds.). (1996). *Children with acquired brain injury: Educating and supporting families.* Baltimore, MD: Paul H. Brookes.

Singley, M.K., & Anderson, J.R. (1989). *Transfer of cognitive skill.* Cambridge, MA: Harvard University Press.

Sirigu, A., Zalla, T., Pillon, B., Grafman, J., Dubois, B., & Agid, Y. (1995). Planning and script analysis following frontal lobe lesions. In J. Grafman, K. Holyoak, & F. Boller (Eds.), *Structure and functions of the human prefrontal cortex* (pp. 277–288). New York: New York Academy of Sciences.

Skinner, B.F. (1938). *The behavior of organisms: An experimental analysis.* New York: Appleton.

Skinner, B.F. (1953). *Science and human behavior.* New York: Macmillan

Skinner, B.F. (1969). *Contingencies of reinforcement.* New York: Appleton-Century Crofts.

Skinner, B.F. (1974). *About behaviorism.* New York: Alfred Knopf.

Slifer, K.J., Cataldo, M.D., Babbitt, R.L., Kane, A.C., Harrison, K.A., & Cataldo, M.F. (1993). Behavior analysis and intervention during hospitalization for brain trauma rehabilitation. *Archives of Physical Medicine and Rehabilitiation, 74,* 810–817.

Slifer, K.J., Tucker, C.L., Gerson, A.C., Cataldo, M.D., Sevier, R.C., Suter, A.H., & Kane, A.C. (1996). Operant conditioning for behavior management during posttraumatic amnesia in children and adolescents with brain injury. *Journal of Head Trauma Rehabilitation, 11,* 39–50.

Smull, M.W., & Harrison, S. (1992). *Supporting people with severe reputations in the community.* Alexandria, VA: National Association of State Mental Retardation Program Directors.

Sohlberg, M., & Mateer, C. (1989). *Introduction to cognitive rehabilitation: Theory and practice.* New York: Guilford Press.

Sohlberg, M.M., & Raskin, S.A. (1996). Principles of generalization applied to attention and memory interventions. *Journal of Head Trauma Rehabilitation, 11,* 65–78.

Squire, L.R. (1992). Memory and the hippocampus: A synthesis from findings with rats, monkeys, and humans. *Psychological Review, 99,* 195–231.

Squire, L.R., Knowlton, B., & Musen, G. (1993). The structure and organization of memory. *Annual Review in Psychology, 44,* 453–495.

Squire, L.R., Ojemann, J.G., Miezin, F.M., Petersen, S.E., Videen, T.O., & Raichle, M.E. (1992). Activation of the hippocampus in normal humans: A functional anatomical study of memory. *Proceedings of the National Academy of Sciences of the United States of America, 89,* 1837–1841.

Stainback, S., & Stainback, W. (1990). Facilitating support networks. In W. Stainback & S. Stainback (Eds.), *Support networks for inclusive schooling* (pp. 25–36). Baltimore, MD: Paul H. Brookes Publishing Co.

Stelling, M.W., McKay, S.E., Carr, W.A., Walsh, J.W., & Bauman, R.J. (1986). Frontal lobe lesions and cognitive function in craniopharyngioma survivors. *American Journal of Diseases of Childhood, 140,* 710–714.

Ste-Marie, D.M., Jennings, J.M., Finlayson, A.J. (1996). Process dissociation procedure: Memory testing in populations with brain damage. *Clinical Neuropsychologist, 10,* 25–36.

Stokes, T.F., & Baer, D.M. (1977). An implicit technology of generalization. *Journal of Applied Behavior Analysis, 10,* 349–367.

Stokes, T.F., & Osnes, P.G. (1986). Programming the generalization of children's social behavior. In P.S. Strain, M.J. Guralnick, & H.M. Walker (Eds.), *Children's social behavior: Development, assessment, and modification.* New York: Academic Press.

Strange, P.G. (1992). *Brain biochemistry and brain disorders.* New York: Oxford University Press.

Strain, P., Guralnick, M., & Walker, H.M. (1986). *Children's social behavior: Development, assessment, and modification.* New York: Academic Press.

Stuss, D.T. (1992). Biological and psychological development of executive functions. *Brain and Cognition, 20,* 8–23.

Stuss, D.T., & Benson, D.F. (1986). *The frontal lobes.* New York: Raven Press.

Stuss, D.T., & Buckle, L. (1992). Traumatic brain injury: Neuropsychological deficits and evaluation at different stages of recovery and in different pathologic subtypes. *Journal of Head Trauma Rehabilitation, 7,* 40–49.

Stuss, O.T., Delgodo, M., & Guzman, D.A. (1987). Verbal regulation in the control of motor impersistence. A proposed rehabilitation procedure. *Journal of Neurological Rehabilitation, 1,* 19–24.

Stuss, D.T., Shallice, T., Alexander, M.P., & Picton, T.W. (1992). A multidisciplinary approach to anterior attentional functions. In J. Grafman, K.J. Holoyak, & F. Boller (Eds.), *Structure and functions of the human prefrontal cortex* (pp. 191–211). New York: The New York Academy of Sciences.

Szekeres, S. (1992). Organization as an intervention target after traumatic brain injury. *Seminars in Speech and Language, 13,* 293–307.

Szekeres, S., Ylvisaker, M., & Cohen, S. (1987). A framework for cognitive rehabilitation therapy. In M.Ylvisaker & E. Gobble (Eds.), *Community re-entry for head injured adults* (pp. 87–136). Boston, MA: College-Hill Press.

Taylor, H.G., Drotar, D., Wade, S., Yeates, K., Stancin, T., & Klein, S. (1995). Recovery from traumatic brain injury in children: The importance of the family. In S.H. Broman & M.E. Michel (Eds.), *Traumatic head injury in children* (pp. 188–216). New York: Oxford University Press.

Taylor, H.G., Schatschneider, C., Petrill, S., Barry, C.T., & Owens, C. (1996). Executive dysfunction in children with early brain disease: Outcomes post *Haemophilus Influenzae* meningitis. *Developmental Neuropsychology, 12,* 35–51.

Taylor, J.C., & Carr, E.C. (1992a). Severe problem behaviors related to social interaction. I: Attention seeking and social avoidance. *Behavior Modification, 16,* 305–335.

Taylor, J.C., & Carr, E.C. (1992b). Severe problem behaviors related to social interaction. II: A systems analysis. *Behavior Modification, 16,* 336–371.

Terrace, H.S. (1963). Discrimination learning with and without "errors." *Journal of Experimental Analysis of Behavior, 6,* 1–27.

Teuber, H.L. (1964). The riddle of frontal lobe function in man. In J.M. Warren & K. Akert (Eds.), *The frontal granular cortex and behavior.* New York: McGraw-Hill.

Thatcher, R.W. (1991). Maturation of the human frontal lobes: Physiological evidence of staging. *Developmental Neuropsychology, 7,* 397–419.

Thomsen, I.V. (1974). The patient with severe head injury and his family. *Scandanavian Journal of Rehabilitation and Medicine, 6,* 180–183.

Thomsen, I.V. (1984). Late outcome of very severe blunt head trauma: A 10–15 year second follow-up. *Journal of Neurology, Neurosurgery, and Psychiatry, 47,* 260–268.

Thomsen, I.V. (1987). Late psychosocial outcome in severe blunt head trauma. *Brain Injury, 1,* 131–143.

Thomsen, I.V. (1989). Do young patients have worse outcome after severe blunt head trauma? *Brain Injury, 3,* 157–162.

Thöne, A. (1996). Memory rehabilitation: Recent developments and future directions. *Restorative Neurology and Neuroscience, 9,* 125–140.

Timm, M.A. (1993). The regional intervention program: Family treatment by family members. *Behavioral Disorders, 19,* 34–43.

Toglia, J.P. (1991). Generalization of treatment: A multicontext approach to cognitive perceptual impairment in adults with brain injury. *American Journal of Occupational Therapy, 45,* 505–516.

Tranel, D., & Damasio, A.R. (1995). Neurobiological foundations of human memory. In A. Baddeley, B. Wilson, & F. Watts (Eds.), *Handbook of memory disorders* (pp. 27–50). New York: John Wiley & Sons.

Tranel, D., Anderson, S.W., & Benton, A.I. (1995). Development of the concept of executive function and its relationship to the frontal lobes. In F. Boller & J. Grafman (Eds.), *Handbook of neuropsychology* (pp. 125–148). Amsterdam: Elsevier.

Treadwell, K., & Page, T.J. (1996). Functional analysis: Identifying the environmental determinants of severe behavior disorders. *Journal of Head Trauma Rehabilitation, 11* 62–74.

Turkstra, L.S., & Holland, A.L. (1998). Assessment of syntax after adolescent brain injury: Effects of memory on test performance. *Journal of Speech, Language, and Hearing Research, 41,* 137–149.

van Zomeren, A.H., & van den Burg, W. (1985). Residual complaints of patients two years after severe head injury. *Journal of Neurology, Neurosurgery, and Psychiatry, 48,* 21–28.

Varney, N.R., & Menefee, L. (1993). Psychosocial and executive deficits following closed head injury: Implications for orbital frontal cortex. *Journal of Head Trauma Rehabilitation, 8,* 32–44.

Vaughn, B.J., & Horner, R.H. (1997). Indentifying instructional tasks that occasion problem behaviors and assessing the effects of student versus teacher choice among these tasks. *Journal of Applied Behavior Analysis, 30,* 299–312.

Vaughn, S., McIntosh, R., & Hogan, A. (1990). Why social skills training doesn't work: An alternative model. In T.E. Scruggs & B.Y.L. Wong (Eds.), *Intervention research in learning disabilities* (pp. 279–303). New York: Springer Verlag.

Vilkki, J., Ahola, K., Holst, P., Ohman, J., Servo, A., & Heiskanen, O. (1994). Prediction of psychosocial recovery after head injury with cognitive tests and neurobehavioral ratings. *Journal of Clinical and Experimental Neuropsychology, 16,* 325–338.

Vollmer, T.R., & Iwata, B.A. (1991). Establishing operations and reinforcement effects. *Journal of Applied Behavior Analysis, 23,* 417–429.

von Cramon, D.Y., & Matthes-von Cramon, G. (1994). Back to work with a chronic dysexecutive syndrome? (A case report). *Neuropsychological Rehabilitation, 4,* 399–417.

Vygotsky, L.S. (1978). Interaction between learning and development. In L.S. Vygotsky, *Mind in society: The development of higher psychological processes* (pp. 79–91). (M. Cole, V. John-Steiner, S. Scribner, & E. Souberman, Eds. and Trans.). Cambridge, MA: Harvard University Press. (Original work published 1935).

Vygotsky, L.S. (1978). *Mind in society: The development of higher psychological processes.* (M. Cole, V. John-Steiner, S. Scribner, & E. Souberman, Eds. & Trans.). Cambridge, MA: Harvard University Press.

Vygotsky, L.S. (1981). The genesis of higher mental functions. In J.V. Wertsch (Ed.), *The concept of activity in Soviet psychology* (pp. 144–189). Armonk, NY: M.E. Sharps.

Vygotsky, L.S. (1987). *Thinking and speech.* (N. Minick, ed. and trans.). New York: Plenum.

Waaland, P.K. (1998). Families of children with traumatic brain injury. In M. Ylvisaker (Ed.), *Traumatic brain injury rehabilitation: Children and adolescents* (pp. 345–368). Boston, MA: Butterworth-Heinemann.

Wacker, D.P., Steege, M.W., Northrup, J., Sasso, G., Berg, W., Reimers, T., Cooper, L., Cigrand, K., & Donn, I. (1990). A component analysis of functional communication training across three topographies of severe behavior problems. *Journal of Applied Behavior Analysis, 23,* 417–429.

Wahler, R.G., & Fox, R.M., (1981). Setting events in applied behavior analysis: Towards a conceptual and methodological expansion. *Journal of Applied Behavior Analysis, 14,* 327–338.

Walker, H.M., Schwarz, I.E., Nippold, M.A., Irvin, L.K., & Noell, J.W. (1994). Social skills in school-age children and youth: Issues and best practices in assessment and intervention. *Topics in Language Disorders, 14,* 70–82.

Weddell, R., Oddy, M., & Jenkins, D. (1980). Social adjustment after rehabilitation: A two year follow-up of patients with severe head injury. *Psychological Medicine, 10,* 257–263.

Wehman, P., & Kreutzer, J.S. (1990). *Vocational rehabilitation for persons with acquired brain injury.* Rockville, MD: Aspen Publishing.

Wehman, P., Kregel, J., Sherron, P., Nguyen, S., Kreutzer, J., Fry, R., & Zasler, N. (1993). Critical factors associated with the successful supported employment of patients with severe traumatic brain injury. *Brain Injury, 7,* 31–44.

Wehman, P.H., West, M.D., Kregel, J., Sherron, P., & Kreutzer, J.S. (1995). Return to work for persons with severe traumatic brain injury: A data-based approach to program development. *Journal of Head Trauma Rehabilitation, 10,* 27–39.

Wehmeyer, P., & Kelchner, K. (1995). *The Arc's Self-Determination Scale: Adolescent Version.* Arlington, TX: The Arc of the United States.

Wehmeyer, M., & Schwartz, M. (1997). Self determination and positive adult outcomes: A follow-up study of youth with mental retardation or learning disabilities, *Exceptional Children, 63,* 245–255.

Welsh, M.C., & Pennington, B.F. (1988). Assessing frontal lobe functioning in children: Views from developmental psychology. *Developmental Neuropsychology, 4,* 199–230.

Welsh, M.C., Pennington, B.F., & Groisser, D.B. (1991). A normative-developmental study of executive function: A window on prefrontal function in children. *Developmental Neuropsychology, 7*(2), 131–149.

West, R.L. (1995). Compensatory strategies for age-associated memory impairment. In A.D. Baddeley, B.A. Wilson, & F.N. Watts (Eds.), *Handbook of memory disorders* (pp. 481–500). New York: John Wiley & Sons.

Westby, C.E. (1994). The effects of culture on genre, structure, and style of oral and written texts. In G.P. Wallach & K.G. Butler (Eds.), *Language learning disabilities in school-age children and adolescents* (pp. 180–218). New York: Merrill.

Wetzel, R.J., & Hoschouer, R.L. (1984). *Residential teaching communities: Program development and staff training for developmentally disabled persons.* Dallas, TX: Scott, Foresman and Company.

Wiener, J., & Harris, P.J. (1998). Evaluation of an individualized, context-based social skills training program for children with learning disabilities. *Learning Disabilities Research and Practice, 12*, 40–53.

Willatts, P. (1990). Development of problem-solving strategies in infancy. In D. F. Bjorklund (Ed.), *Children's strategies: Contemporary views of cognitive development* (pp. 23–66). Hillsdale, NJ: Lawrence Erlbaum and Associates.

Williams, D., & Mateer, C.A. (1992). Developmental impact of frontal lobe injury in middle childhood. *Brain and Cognition, 20*, 196–204.

Williams, J.M., & Kay, T. (Eds.). *Head injury: A family matter*. Baltimore, MD: Paul H. Brookes.

Willis, T.M., & LaVigna, G.W. (1989). *Emergency management guidelines*. Los Angeles: Institute for Applied Behavior Analysis.

Wilson, B. (1992). Memory therapy in practice. In B.A. Wilson & N. Moffat (Eds.), *Clinical management of memory problems* (pp. 120–151). London: Chapman & Hall.

Wilson, B.A. (1995). Management and remediation of memory problems in brain-injured adults. In A.D. Baddeley, B.A. Wilson, & F.N. Watts (Eds.), *Handbook of memory disorders* (pp. 452–479). New York: John Wiley & Sons.

Wilson, B.A., Baddeley, A.D., Evans, J., & Shiel, A. (1994). Errorless learning in the rehabilitation of memory-impaired people. *Neuropsychological Rehabilitation, 4*, 307–326.

Wilson, B., & Evans, J. (1996). Error-free learning in the rehabilitation of people with memory impairments. *Journal of Head Trauma Rehabilitation, 11*, 54–64.

Wood, D., Bruner, J. & Ross, G. (1976). The role of tutoring in problem solving. *Journal of Child Psychology and Psychiatry, 17*, 89–100.

Wood, R. L. (1987). *Brain injury rehabilitation: A neurobehavioral approach*. London: Croom-Helm.

Wood, R. L. (1988). Management of behavior disorders in a day treatment setting. *Journal of Head Trauma Rehabilitation, 3*, 53–61.

Wood, R.L. (Ed.). (1990). *Neurobehavioral sequelae of traumatic brain injury*. London: Taylor and Francis.

World Health Organization. (1980). *International classification of impairments, diseases, and handicaps: A manual of classification relating to the consequences of diseases*. Geneva: Author.

Yakovlev, P.I., & Lecours, A.R. (1967). The myelogenetic cycles of regional maturation of the brain. In A. Minkowski (Ed.), *Regional development of the brain in early life*. Oxford, UK: Blackwell.

Ylvisaker, M. (1986). Language and communication disorders following pediatric head injury. *Journal of Head Trauma Rehabilitation, 1*, 48–56.

Ylvisaker, M. (1989). Cognitive and psychosocial outcome following head injury in children. In J.T. Hoff, T.E., Anderson, & T.M. Cole (Eds.), *Mild to moderate head injury* (pp. 203–216). London: Blackwell.

Ylvisaker, M. (1992). Communication outcome following traumatic brain injury. *Seminars in Speech and Language, 13*, 239–251.

Ylvisaker, M. (1993). Communication outcome in children and adolescents with traumatic brain injury. *Neuropsychological Rehabilitation, 3*, 367–387.

Ylvisaker, M. (Ed.). (1998). *Traumatic brain injury rehabilitation: Children and adolescents* (rev. ed.). Newton, MA: Butterworth-Heinemann.

Ylvisaker, M., Chorazy, A., Cohen, S., Nelson, J., Mastrelli, J., Molitor, C., Szekeres, S., & Valko, A (1990). Rehabilitative assessment following head injury in children. In M. Rosenthal, E. Griffith, M. Bond, & J.D. Miller (Eds.), *Rehabilitation of the adult and child with traumatic brain injury* (pp. 558–592). Philadelphia, PA: F.A. Davis.

Ylvisaker, M., & Feeney, T. (1994). Communication and behavior: Collaboration between speech-language pathologists and behavioral psychologists. *Topics in Language Disorders, 15*, 37–52.

Ylvisaker, M., & Feeney, T. (1995). Traumatic brain injury in adolescence: Assessment and reintegration. *Seminars in Speech and Language, 16*, 32–44.

Ylvisaker, M., & Feeney, T. (1996). Executive functions after traumatic brain injury: Supported cognition and self-advocacy. *Seminars in Speech and Language, 17*, 217–232.

Ylvisaker, M., & Feeney, T. (1998). Everyday people as supports: Developing competencies through collaboration. In M. Ylvisaker (Ed.), *Traumatic brain injury rehabilitation: Children and adolescents* (pp. 429–464). Newton, MA: Butterworth-Heinemann

Ylvisaker, M., Feeney, T., & Mullins, K. (1995). School reentry following mild traumatic brain injury: A proposed hospital-to-school protocol. *Journal of Head Trauma Rehabilitation, 10*, 42–49.

Ylvisaker, M., Feeney, T., & Szekeres, S (1998). Social-environmental approaches to communication and behavior. In M. Ylvisaker (Ed.), *Traumatic brain injury rehabilitation: Children and adolescents* (pp. 271–302). Newton, MA: Butterworth-Heinemann.

Ylvisaker, M., Feeney, T., & Urbancyk, B. (1992). Social skills following traumatic brain injury. *Seminars in Speech and Language, 13*(4), 308–321.

Ylvisaker, M., Feeney, T., & Urbanczyk, B. (1993a). A social-environmental approach to communication and behavior after traumatic brain injury. *Seminars in Speech and Language, 14*(1), 74–86.

Ylvisaker, M., Feeney, T., & Urbanczyk, B. (1993b). Developing a positive communication culture for rehabilitation. In C.J. Durgin, N.D. Schmidt, & J. Fryer (Eds.), *Staff development and clinical intervention in brain injury rehabilitation* (pp. 57–85). Gaithersburg, MD: Aspen Publishing.

Ylvisaker, M., & Gioia, G. (1998). Cognitive assessment. In M. Ylvisaker (Ed.), *Traumatic brain injury rehabilitation: Children and adolescents* (pp. 159–179). Newton, MA: Butterworth-Heinemann

Ylvisaker, M., & Gobble, E.M.R. (Eds.). (1987). *Community re-entry for head injured adults.* Newton, MA: Butterworth-Heinemann.

Ylvisaker, M., Hartwick, P., & Stevens, M.B. (1991). School reentry following head injury: Managing the transition from hospital to school. *Journal of Head Trauma Rehabilitation, 6,* 10–22.

Ylvisaker, M., & Szekeres, S. (1989). Metacognitive and executive impairments in head-injured children and adults. *Topics in Language Disorders, 9,* 34–49.

Ylvisaker, M., Szekeres, S., & Feeney, T. (1998). Cognitive rehabilitation: Executive functions. In M. Ylvisaker (Ed.), *Traumatic brain injury rehabilitation: Children and adolescents* (pp. 221–269). Newton, MA: Butterworth-Heinemann.

Ylvisaker, M., Szekeres, S., & Haarbauer-Krupa, J. (1998). Cognitive rehabilitation: Organization and memory. In M. Ylvisaker (Ed.), *Traumatic brain injury rehabilitation: Children and adolescents* (pp. 181–220). Newton, MA: Butterworth-Heinemann.

Zaragoza, N., Vaughn, S., & McIntosh, R. (1991). Social skills interventions and children with behavior problems: A review. *Behavioral Disorders, 16,* 260–275.

Zarcone, J.R., Iwata, B.A., Mazaleski, J.L., & Smith, R.G. (1994). Momentum and extinction effects on self-injurious escape behavior and non-compliance. *Journal of Applied Behavior Analysis, 27,* 649–658.

Zencius, A.H., Wesolowski, M.D., Burke, W.H., & McQuade, D. (1989). Antecedent control in the treatment of brain injured clients. *Brain Injury, 3,* 199–205.

APPENDIX A

New York Brief Behavioral Screening of Persons With Traumatic Brain Injury

PART A. BACKGROUND INFORMATION

1. Name of Individual: _____

2. Name of Reviewer: _____

3. DATE OF REVIEW: _____

4. DOB: _____

5. Date of Injury: _____

6. Date of Placement: _____

7. Current Address:

_____

_____

8. Names & Dates of Previous Placements:

_____

_____

9. Type of Living Arrangement:

   O Individualized Residence

   O Skilled Nursing Facility

   O Specialized Rehabilitation Facility

   O Neurobehavioral Treatment Unit (Locked)

_____

_____

_____

_____

_____

_____

10. Name of Person Providing Information: _____

11. Title/Relationship: _____

12. Length of Time Known the Individual: _____

13. Amount of Time Spent with the Individual (Weekly): _____

14. Brief Report of Preinjury Behaviors (behavioral difficulties; psychiatric diagnoses; legal problems; general social skills, etc.):

15. Current Psychiatric Diagnoses (include DSM-IV Coding):

16. Medications: *Past:*   *Current:*

Name:_____pg. 1

PART B. CURRENT OPPORTUNITIES FOR CHOICE

	Opportunities to Choose:	*Degree of Behavioral Control When Given These Choices:*

1. Access to the Community

0 – 1 – 2 – 3 – 4
Free   None

0 – 1 – 2 – 3 – 4
Indep.   1:1

Frequency:

2. Family visits

0 – 1 – 2 – 3 – 4
Free   None

0 – 1 – 2 – 3 – 4
Indep.   1:1

Frequency:

3. Personal Effects

0 – 1 – 2 – 3 – 4
Free   None

0 – 1 – 2 – 3 – 4
Indep.   1:1

4. Peers

0 – 1 – 2 – 3 – 4
Free   None

0 – 1 – 2 – 3 – 4
Indep.   1:1

5. Daily Routines

0 – 1 – 2 – 3 – 4
Free   None

0 – 1 – 2 – 3 – 4
Indep.   1:1

6. Treatment/Intervention

0 – 1 – 2 – 3 – 4
Free   None

0 – 1 – 2 – 3 – 4
Indep.   1:1

7. Treatment Team

0 – 1 – 2 – 3 – 4
Free   None

0 – 1 – 2 – 3 – 4
Indep.   1:1

Name:_____pg. 2

PART C. BEHAVIORS OF CONCERN

I. Behavioral Excesses

O Physical Assault/Property Destruction (e.g., hitting, punching, kicking, breaking windows, chairs, etc.)

Describe: _____

_____

O Perseverative Behaviors (e.g., repetitively engaging in the same behavior, asking the same question, etc.)

Describe: _____

_____

O Self-Injury (e.g., hitting head against objects, hitting self with fist, etc.)

Describe: _____

_____

O Social Behaviors (e.g., verbal abuse, inappropriate touching, sexual behaviors, etc.)

Describe: _____

_____

Frequency	0	–	1	–	2	–	3	–	4
	Infrequent			Monthly			Weekly		Daily

Typical Intensity of Intervention needed	0	–	1	–	2	–	3	–	4
	Minimal					*Moderate*			*Intensive*
	Verbal Redirection					Removal from Area			Physical Intervention

Supervision needed for safety	0	–	1	–	2	–	3	–	4
	General		Eye Sight			1:1			>1:1

Intensity during most severe incidents	0	–	1	–	2	–	3	–	4
	Minimal					*Moderate*			*Intensive*
	Verbal Redirection					Removal from Area			Physical Intervention

Name:_____pg. 3

2. Mental Health Difficulties:

O Psychotic Behaviors (e.g., hallucinations, delusions, etc.)

Describe: _____

_____

O Mood Disorders (e.g., lability, anxiety, bipolar disorders, depression, etc.)

Describe: _____

_____

O Suicidal Ideation (e.g., speaks of suicide, attempts suicide, etc.)

Describe: _____

_____

O Obsessive/Compulsive Behaviors (e.g., perseveration, ritualistic behaviors, etc.)

Describe: _____

_____

Frequency	0 –	1 –	2 –	3 –	4
	Infrequent	Monthly	Weekly		Daily

Typical Intensity of Intervention needed	0 –	1 –	2 –	3 –	4
	Minimal		*Moderate*		*Intensive*
	Verbal Redirection		Removal from Area		Physical Intervention

Supervision needed for safety	0 –	1 –	2 –	3 –	4
	General	Eye Sight	1:1		>1:1

Intensity during most severe incidents	0 –	1 –	2 –	3 –	4
	Minimal		*Moderate*		*Intensive*
	Verbal Redirection		Removal from Area		Physical Intervention

Name:_____pg. 4

3. Behavioral Deficits:

O Refuses to Participate in Routine Activities

Describe: _____

_____

O Appears Unmotivated to Participate in Activities

Describe: _____

_____

O Requires Frequent Prompts to Maintain Participation in Activities

Describe: _____

_____

O Unable to Maintain Participation in Activities

Describe: _____

_____

Frequency	0	–	I	–	2	–	3	–	4
	Infrequent				Monthly		Weekly		Daily

Typical Intensity of Intervention needed	0	–	I	–	2	–	3	–	4
	Minimal				*Moderate*				*Intensive*
	Verbal Redirection				Removal from Area				Physical Intervention

Supervision needed for safety	0	–	I	–	2	–	3	–	4
	General		Eye Sight			I:I			>I:I

Intensity during most severe incidents	0	–	I	–	2	–	3	–	4
	Minimal				*Moderate*				*Intensive*
	Verbal Redirection				Removal from Area				Physical Intervention

PART D. REVIEW OF PREVIOUS INTERVENTIONS

Specific Behavioral Interventions (check all that apply):

INTERVENTION: *EFFECT ON BEHAVIOR:*

○ Differential Reinforcement Strategies   0   –   I   –   2   –   3   –   4

No   Moderately   Highly
Effect   Effective   Effective

○ Behavioral Contract   0   –   I   –   2   –   3   –   4

No   Moderately   Highly
Effect   Effective   Effective

○ Token System   0   –   I   –   2   –   3   –   4

No   Moderately   Highly
Effect   Effective   Effective

○ Psychotherapy   0   –   I   –   2   –   3   –   4

No   Moderately   Highly
Effect   Effective   Effective

○ Antecedent Control Strategies   0   –   I   –   2   –   3   –   4

No   Moderately   Highly
Effect   Effective   Effective

○ Other   0   –   I   –   2   –   3   –   4
   Describe:_____ No   Moderately   Highly
                                     Effect   Effective   Effective

_____

_____

_____

_____

_____

_____

Name:_____pg. 6

PART E. ANECDOTAL INFORMATION

WHAT WORKS:

From the Perspective of the Individual With Brain Injury:

From the Perspective of Family/Natural Supports:

From the Perspective of Professional Supports:

WHAT DOESN'T WORK:

From the Perspective of the Individual With Brain Injury:

From the Perspective of Family/Natural Supports:

From the Perspective of Professional Supports:

PART F. SUPPORTS

Individual's Description of Supports Needed for Success	Family/Caregiver Description of Supports Needed for Success	Clinical Staff Description of Supports Needed for Success
Medical	**Medical**	**Medical**
Clinical	**Clinical**	**Clinical**
Educational	**Educational**	**Educational**
Vocational	**Vocational**	**Vocational**
Environmental	**Environmental**	**Environmental**
Peer	**Peer**	**Peer**
Other	**Other**	**Other**

PART G. PRIORITIES FOR SERVICES
NEEDED TO LIVE SUCCESSFULLY

Individual's Description of Priorities	Family/Caregiver Description of Priorities	Clinical Staff Description of Priorities
1.	1.	1.
2.	2.	2.
3.	3.	3.
4.	4.	4.
5.	5.	5.

PART H. GENERAL ASSESSMENT THEMES

Describe what about you has changed since your injury:

Describe an ideal day in your life:

List the things that make you angry and the strategies that you use to manage your anger:

Describe some of the qualities that individuals should possess if they want to be successful working with you:

Teaching Positive Communication Alternatives to Challenging Behavior: Proposed Components of an Integrated Communication and Behavior Plan for an Individual With Seriously Challenging Behavior[1]

Teaching Positive Communication Alternatives to Challenging Behavior

The most important focus of John's* communication and behavior plan is a concentrated effort on the part of all staff and family members to teach him positive communication alternatives to his challenging behaviors. This approach to behavior problems is based on the following premises:

*The name was selected arbitrarily to represent any child with TBI.

Premises

1. *All behaviors communicate something.* Initially, the behavior may be unintentional. However, if communication partners consistently reinforce the behavior, it will likely become intentional.

2. *Most behaviors—however unconventional—are adaptive* in that they effectively communicate intended messages.

3. If a challenging behavior (e.g., hitting, screaming, hair pulling) is part of an individual's communication system, it is criti-

[1]Reproduced with permission from M. Ylvisaker, T. Feeney, and S. Szekeres (1998), "Social-Environmental Approaches to Communication and Behavior." In M. Ylvisaker (Ed.), *Traumatic Brain Injury Rehabilitation: Children and Adolescents.* Boston: Butterworth-Heinemann.

cal to *substitute a more acceptable behavior* rather than trying simply to extinguish the challenging behavior. Extinguishing the challenging behavior without teaching a positive communication alternative likely will result in development of a more challenging behavior to communicate the same intention.

4. Ideal teaching of positive communication alternatives occurs *in natural communication contexts with everyday communication partners as the primary agents of change.*

Consistency is one of the keys. Communication partners must develop good communication routines to help the individual acquire good communication routines.

Selection of Communication Intentions to Target

John uses a variety of negative behaviors (e.g., hair pulling, hitting, falling to the floor) to communicate a variety of important messages. Many of the messages that he (at least occasionally) communicates in negative ways fall into two important categories:

1. *Access:* In such cases, John is trying to get something, such as attention, desired activities, desired objects, or stimulation.
2. *Escape:* In such cases, John is trying to escape or avoid something, such as unwanted attention, unwanted activities, unwanted objects, unwanted demands, or unwanted stimulation.

Selection of Positive Communication Alternatives to Teach

Staff and family must work together to select the best communication alternative to promote at any stage in John's intervention. At the outset, it is important that the positive communication alternative have the following characteristics:

1. It is *easy* for John—at least as easy as the negative behavior it will replace.
2. It is *powerful* for John—at least as effective and (it is hoped) more effective in

communicating his message successfully than is the negative behavior it replaces.

3. It is possible for staff and family to *prompt* the positive communication alternative. This characteristic renders gesturing, signing, and pointing to pictures or symbols more useful at the outset than talking. It is possible to prompt the former, but not the latter, physically.

The specific communication behaviors that John uses to communicate important messages will change over time and will become more complex. Staff and family should decide collaboratively when to move from a less to a more complex or conventional means of communicating his messages (e.g., moving from gesture or sign to speech or an augmentative communication device).

Current Plan: Positive Communication Alternatives

1. *Escape:* Sign finished or say no.
2. *Access attention:* Vocalize calmly or tap the other person on the shoulder.
3. *Access activity or object:* Point to activity or object, point to picture or symbol, or say the word.

Teaching Within Routines of Interaction. It is critical for staff and family to ensure that John communicates positively and is rewarded for communicating positively much more frequently than communicating negatively and being rewarded for doing so. Teaching positive communication alternatives must become a *routine* for all staff and family. Ideally, during each day, John will have at least 100 rewarded experiences with positive communication to counterbalance the small number of inevitable, inadvertently rewarded negative communications. The key is to make these teaching interactions *routine.* (See Table 7–1.)

Deciding When Escape and Access Are Acceptable. Staff and family should decide collaboratively when it is acceptable for them to honor John's positive communication of escape or access messages. For example, they may decide that communication is a higher priority now than are physical therapy exercises. Therefore, exercise time would be an acceptable and desirable time at which to prompt and honor John's positive escape communication. At certain times, John is not free to escape undesired activities or to access desired activities. Staff should prepare for those times with the procedures listed later (positive behavioral momentum). In the early stages of training, it is important for staff to recognize the importance of communication-behavior intervention and avoid scheduling a large number of no choice situations that carry the inevitable risk of confrontation and negative behaviors, which may be rewarded unintentionally.

Procedures to Use When Escape or Access Are Not Acceptable. Early in the training, a very large number of times during the course of the day staff should ensure that John has the opportunity to use his positive access or escape communication to access desired activities or to escape undesired activities. However, staff must be prepared with procedures when placing demands on John that are nonnegotiable.

➤ *Cognitive preparation:* Ensure that John is alerted to upcoming events in his schedule so that negative surprise-based responses are avoided.
➤ *Positive behavioral momentum:* Ensure that John has experienced a backlog of success (is "on a roll") before introducing potentially difficult or undesirable tasks.
 1. Identify high-success, high-satisfaction tasks.
 2. Identify low-success, low-satisfaction—but *doable*—tasks.
 3. Engage John in three, four, five, six, or more high success, high-satisfaction tasks (depending on need) before introducing a low-success, low satisfaction task: That is, ensure that John is feeling relaxed and successful before introducing difficult tasks.

➤ *Positive setting events:* Try to ensure that John is in a generally positive state (e.g., not sick, tired, or in pain) before asking him to perform tasks that you know are difficult or stressful for him. In addition, make your interaction with him as pleasant as possible and give him as much control as possible.
➤ *Choice and no-choice:* Teach John the difference between choice and no-choice. For this teaching to be successful, staff and family should use the words *no choice* only for very important times, when it is critical that John comply and when they are willing to persevere in the face of potentially very negative behavior. Make every effort to avoid saying "no choice" and subsequently giving in to him in the face of his fierce resistance. *Choose your battles wisely.* Try to avoid control battles. If you must begin a control battle for some very important reason, ensure that you win it quickly and efficiently; then move on without dwelling on the negative interaction.

Documentation
➤ *Focus on positive communication:* Staff and family should try to chart the number of times per day that John both communicates positively without prompting and with prompting. From the beginning, the total number of positive communications should be very large (perhaps requiring considerable prompting). The percentage of unprompted positive communications should rise over time. This increase is the primary measure of success. With an increase in unprompted positive communications will come an inevitable decrease in negative communications (challenging behaviors). It is important for the documentation system to focus on positive communication alternatives as the primary target behaviors and not just on negative behaviors.
➤ *Progression over time:* Initially, John should be rewarded quite consistently for his positive communication alternatives to challenging behavior. As such alternatives become a more stable part of his

communication repertoire and as the frequency of negative communication behaviors decreases, demands on John's compliance can gradually increase again, and less time can be devoted to teaching communication. As with all aspects of the program, this progression must be coordinated well among staff and between staff and family.

Important Conditions Required for This Intervention to Work

➤ Staff and family must agree to the principles and practices of this intervention. All staff and family members are teachers of positive communication. The most important teachers are those who spend the most time with John (his family members and direct-care staff) and, therefore, interact with him more than others do.

➤ Staff must avoid the temptation to engage John in tests of will. Conflicts should be kept to a minimum. In situations of conflict, John will likely resort to the negative behaviors that he knows have been successful in the past. At least some of these behaviors will likely be rewarded by staff, however good their intentions.

Dealing with Purely Impulsive Behavior

Reportedly, some of John's challenging behavior is purely impulsive, without communicative intent. For example, when unoccupied, on impulse John may touch nearby women inappropriately, with no intent to communicate. The frequency of impulsive negative behaviors must also decrease, because behaviors that begin as purely impulsive can easily become learned components of John's communication system. The two most important procedures in dealing with impulsive behavior are prevention and redirection.

Prevention

To prevent purely impulsive behavior, try to eliminate provocation. For example, women who are not working with John should avoid walking within arm's length of him. Also, try to ensure that John is engaged in meaningful activities as much as possible.

Redirection

When John is beginning to engage in negative impulsive behavior, staff and family members may direct his attention quickly to a neutral activity that breaks the negative behavior pattern. However, redirection must be effected with great caution. If redirection is from a less desired activity to a more desired activity, negative behavior inadvertently may be rewarded, thereby increasing rather than decreasing the negative behavior.

Reacting to Seriously Challenging Behavior

See the behavior specialist's recommended procedures for reacting to negative behaviors and crises on those occasions when preparation, prevention, and redirection have not worked. These procedures must be followed to ensure that everyone remains safe and that John's negative behavior is not reinforced systematically. However, staff and family members must clearly understand that times of crisis are *not* occasions for teaching. Do not try to teach lessons when either John or you are upset. Teaching positive communication alternatives should occur under conditions of low stress.

Interaction Routines for Teaching Positive Communication Alternatives

Guidelines for Interaction

Successful interaction requires guidelines that include careful attention to (1) the general teaching routine, (2) escape and access communication training, and (3) agreement on and indications for situations in which escape and access are acceptable (both in *natural* communication contexts or *contrived* situations).

1. Carefully observe John and interpret his behavior. Identify times at which he is

likely to use challenging behavior to communicate escape or access. Ideally, such times occur when escape- or access-motivated behavior is expected but *hasn't yet begun*. A second-best alternative is to identify the *first sign* of escape- or access-motivated behavior.

2. *Do not wait until John is using challenging behavior.*
3. Prompt the positive communication alternative (e.g., model, shape hands, point hand-over-hand to symbol).
4. Reward the positive communication alternative with escape or access as appropriate.
5. Make it clear that the reward is for the communication alternative. For example, "Thanks for telling me you don't want to do exercises now. We can come back to it later. Let's take a break."
   a. Act before the challenging behavior occurs. *Timing is critical.*
   b. Never reward the challenging behavior.
6. Fade prompts and practice.

Illustrations

Escape: Contrived Communication Situations. Context: In physical therapy sessions, assume that the exercises are not currently a high priority for staff and not a desired activity for John.

Adult (A):	John, how about some exercises?
John (J):	(*Looks unhappy but hasn't acted yet.*)
A:	It looks like you don't want to do this now. Here, show me "finished."
J:	(*Is prompted to use positive communication alternative [PCA].*)
A:	OK! Thanks for telling me! Let's not do it now. We can come back to it later. It's great that you tell me that way that you don't want to do this. Let's do . . . (*or,* Show me what you would like to do for a few minutes . . .*).*

This teaching sequence could be repeated several times during a 20- to 30-minute scheduled exercise session.

Escape: Natural Communication Situations
Context: A staff person wants John to carry his lunchbox as he walks down the hall.

A:	Here, John, carry your lunchbox.
J:	(*Reacts negatively but does not fall to the floor or engage in any other negative communication [NC].*)
A:	I bet you don't want to carry the box, do you? Why don't you tell me "no"?
J:	(*Is prompted to use PCA.*)
A:	Oh!!! Alright! I see you want me to carry it. Thanks for telling me so nicely. Of course I'll carry it when you ask like that.

Access: Contrived Communication Situation
Context: John is with other clients and clearly wants a peer to interact with him. The peer has been alerted to respond when John uses the PCA.

A:	John, I bet you would like to talk with Tim. Why don't you tell him? (*Prompts the PCA.*)
J:	(*Uses the PCA.*)
Peer:	(*Responds to John's PCA.*) Oh, Hi, John. I didn't see you. Thanks for letting me know you want to talk.

Access: Natural Communication Situations
Context: John is at home, and it is time for him to do something he likes to do (e.g., watch television).

A:	John, I wonder what you want to do. I bet you would like to watch TV. Can you let me know? (*Prompts the PCA.*)
J:	(*Uses the PCA.*)
A:	(*Responds to John's PCA.*) Okay, great. Here's the remote. Thanks for telling me that you wanted to watch TV.

Rehabilitation Staff: Communication and Behavioral Competencies[1]

Communication Competencies

Communicating with Patients/Clients

Content   The staff member will:

❏ talk comfortably with patients about topics of interest to them;

❏ use a vocabulary that is meaningful;

❏ use vocabulary that is adequately concrete, yet respectful of the patient's age;

❏ give information needed to keep the patient oriented.

Form   The staff member will:

❏ use gestures, writing, and physical prompts if necessary;

❏ use a natural tone of voice and inflection;

❏ repeat information if necessary;

❏ use short sentences if necessary to ensure understanding;

❏ give adequate processing time between messages;

❏ use simple grammar if necessary;

❏ talk clearly.

Partner Encouragement   The staff member will:

❏ initiate topics of interest to the patient;

❏ use appropriate prompts to encourage communication;

❏ give patients time to respond;

❏ give patients words if they are struggling;

❏ respond to patients' verbal and nonverbal communication;

[1]Adapted with permission from "Developing a Positive Communication Culture for Rehabilitation," by M. Ylvisaker; T. Feeney, and B. Urbanczyk, (1992). In C. Durgin, J. Fryer, & N. Schmidt (Eds.), *Brain Injury Rehabilitation: Clinical Intervention and Staff Development Techniques* (pp. 75–78). Gaithersburg, MD: Aspen Publishers. © 1993 Aspen Publishers, Inc.

- ❑ encourage nonverbal communication;
- ❑ offer choices whenever possible;
- ❑ seek confirmation of patients' understanding;
- ❑ reinforce (e.g., through additional conversation time, praise) successful communication attempts;
- ❑ avoid ridiculing, teasing, or punishing inappropriate or unsuccessful communication.

Communication Environment   The staff member will:

- ❑ minimize distractions;
- ❑ maintain the patient's attention when communicating (e.g., redirect as necessary; use the patient's name; touch the patient to gain attention, if appropriate);
- ❑ interact in a familiar setting;
- ❑ control the number of people present.

Communicating Respect   The staff member will:

- ❑ actively encourage patients' participation in treatment planning at whatever level they are capable of such participation;
- ❑ not talk about patients in their presence;
- ❑ avoid a condescending style (e.g., baby talk) and condescending words (e.g., "sweetie," "honey")
- ❑ communicate respect directly (e.g., "I am sure that it is difficult for an intelligent adult like yourself to accept some of our rules");
- ❑ use polite requests rather than abrupt commands;
- ❑ choose an appropriate time and place to discuss personal issues;
- ❑ pay attention to patients' emotional states and communicate to them that their feelings are understood and are appropriate;
- ❑ never punish, ridicule, or demean patients' atypical behavior;
- ❑ use humor that is appropriate and meaningful to the individual.

Communicating with Family Members

Content   The staff member will:

- ❑ actively invite family members to identify their own concerns and interests, rather than make assumptions about their concerns and interests;
- ❑ actively seek information from family members about the patient that will be useful for the treatment team;
- ❑ provide information to families that will help them to stay informed about their family member's care;
- ❑ clearly explain facility programs, treatment regimens, staff roles, family roles in rehabilitation, and other related matters.

Form   The staff member will:

❑ use meaningful vocabulary and avoid jargon;

❑ speak clearly and use natural inflection;

❑ use illustrations and repetition as needed to ensure comprehension;

❑ communicate openness, warmth, flexibility, and humor (if appropriate);

❑ use techniques of active listening;

❑ use effective and encouraging coaching techniques during family training.

Encouraging Family Participation/Communication   The staff member will:

❑ actively invite family members' participation in assessment, goal setting, and intervention;

❑ actively invite expressions of concern and family problem solving around treatment issues;

❑ act on family recommendations unless harmful to the patient;

❑ be available to family members to discuss their concerns.

Communication Environment   The staff member will:

❑ minimize distractions and interruptions during interaction with family members;

❑ use a private setting to discuss confidential or personal issues.

Communicating Respect   The staff member will:

❑ take family members questions and recommendations seriously and act on them unless contraindicated by the patient's needs;

❑ avoid a condescending or self-righteous manner in communicating with families;

❑ communicate genuine interest in and concern for family members' issues;

❑ respond promptly to family letters or calls;

❑ avoid ridiculing or devaluing a family member's behavior;

❑ respect racial, cultural, ethnic, and religious differences;

❑ respect the family's right to self-determination (freedom of choice).

Communicating With Other Staff

Content   The staff member will:

❑ provide other staff with information that is relevant, useful, reliable, and accurate;

❑ ask relevant questions of other staff (including supervisors) regarding patients, policies, treatment, and other issues;

❑ describe minor concerns to supervisors before they become major concerns.

Form   The staff member will:

❑ speak clearly and concisely, avoiding professional jargon;

❑ use natural inflection and tone of voice;

❑ avoid defensive responses, particularly in connection with professional "turf" issues;

❑ demonstrate initiative in interdisciplinary discussions and at the same time patience, flexibility, and a cooperative attitude;

❑ be supportive of colleagues;

❑ maintain perspective and a sense of humor, particularly during times of stress;

❑ give instructions to subordinates in a respectful manner.

Partner Encouragement   The staff member will:

❑ initiate interaction with other staff;

❑ initiate problem-solving discussions, actively seeking others' opinions;

❑ actively seek out whatever guidance is necessary;

❑ use techniques of "active listening";

❑ make time for communication with other staff;

❑ make expectations of others clear;

❑ maintain active communication during stressful times;

❑ freely admit mistakes.

Communication Environment   The staff member will:

❑ choose the correct time and place to discuss issues, particularly confidential issues;

❑ be respectful of other staff members' needs for work time and quiet in a busy work place.

Communicating Respect   The staff member will:

❑ treat all staff with respect, fairness, and courtesy, regardless of academic degrees, professional training, or level of employment;

❑ assume that all staff members' time with patients is important;

❑ take others' opinions seriously.

Behavioral Competencies

The staff member will:

❑ facilitate positive behavioral routines for the individual with TBI:

    ❑ create a concrete, meaningful daily routine (events, sequences, people, places, activities);

    ❑ create positive setting events (external and internal) before requesting difficult tasks;

    ❑ create positive behavioral momentum before requesting difficult tasks;

    ❑ create as many opportunities for choice as possible; teach choice making if necessary;

    ❑ create positive scripts and roles for the individual;

❏ eliminate chronic behavioral provocations;

❏ ensure that all requested activities are do-able.

❏ Model, prompt, and reward positive communication alternatives to challenging behavior:

  ❏ collaboratively identify the communication intent underlying challenging behavior (e.g., escape task, person, place; access activity, person, place, object);

  ❏ operationally define the communication behavior(s) selected to replace the challenging behaviors;

  ❏ collaboratively decide when it is acceptable to respond affirmatively to the new positive communication acts for escape or access;

  ❏ in appropriate contexts, prompt the positive communication alternative and reward that alternative with escape or access as appropriate. Ensure that there are a large number of successful learning trials daily;

  ❏ fade cues and prompts and/or increase the variety of contexts and tasks in which the child is willing to use positive communication alternatives.

❏ If necessary, teach relevant social knowledge (rules, roles, routines, and scripts), including specific pragmatic communication acts.

❏ If necessary, teach social perception and social decision making.

❏ Prevent behavioral crises:

  ❏ eliminate known provocation for behavioral crises;

  ❏ eliminate known environmental stressors (e.g., noise, activity levels);

  ❏ separate incompatible individuals;

  ❏ avoid threats;

  ❏ avoid power conflicts;

  ❏ avoid demands that cannot be met;

  ❏ distract or redirect individuals to neutral activities in the earliest stages of behavioral outbursts;

  ❏ in the case of a mild behavioral episode, remain focused on the task, thereby directing the individual back to task.

❏ Manage behavioral crises:

  ❏ stay calm;

  ❏ look confident;

  ❏ help the person identify feelings;

  ❏ be a helper not an antagonist;

  ❏ seek help;

  ❏ keep others safe;

❑ avoid:

   ❑ suggesting negative behavior (e.g., "don't hit");

   ❑ threatening with consequences;

   ❑ presenting commands as questions or pleas;

   ❑ having more than one person talk at once;

   ❑ escalating the individual by increasing demands;

   ❑ physical interaction or confrontation;

   ❑ attempting to "teach lessons" during a crisis;

   ❑ rehashing the crisis or re-escalating.

❑ Self-management: If possible, teach the individual to manage his or her own antecedents.

Index